Y0-CBB-506

Performing Advanced Procedures

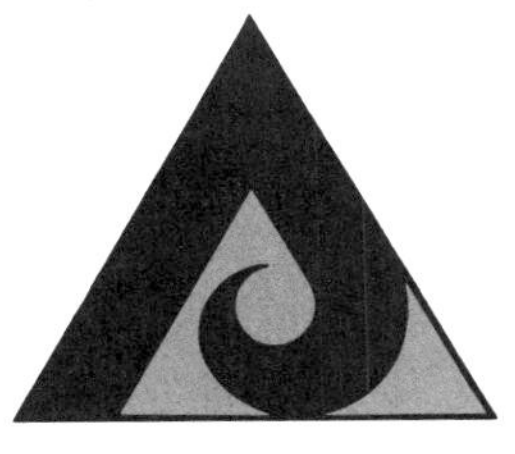

ADVANCED
SKILLS

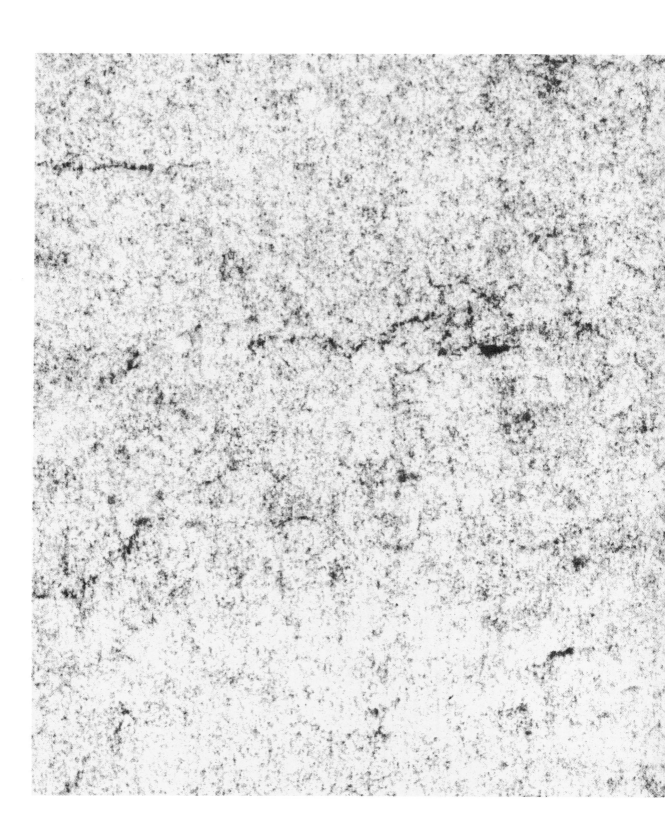

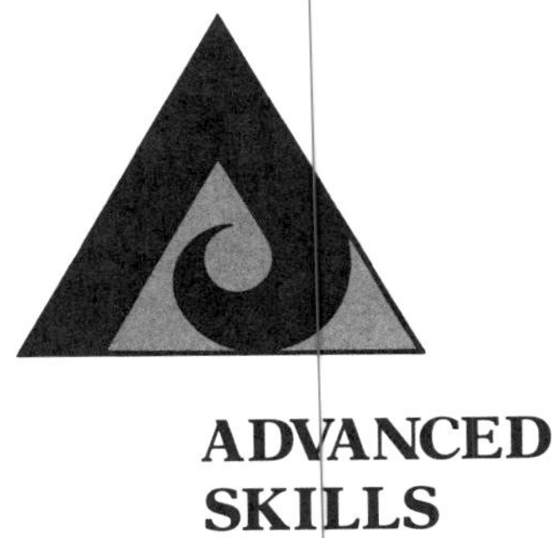

ADVANCED
SKILLS

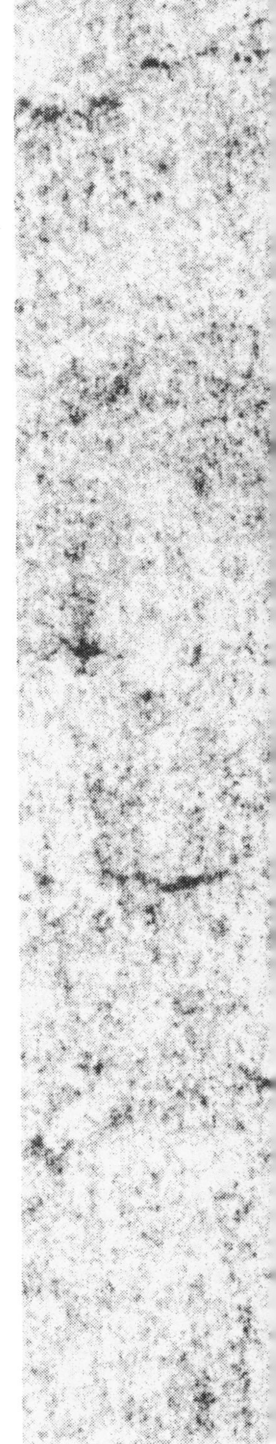

Performing Advanced Procedures

Springhouse Corporation
Springhouse, Pennsylvania

Staff

Executive Director, Editorial
Stanley Loeb

Senior Publisher
Matthew Cahill

Art Director
John Hubbard

Senior Editor
Stephen Daly

Clinical Project Director
Patricia Dwyer Schull, RN, MSN

Editors
Elizabeth Weinstein, Marylou Ambrose, Jody Charnow, Margaret Eckman, Neal Fandek, Kathy Goldberg, Elizabeth Mauro, Gale Sloan

Clinical Editors
Tina R. Dietrich, RN, BSN, CCRN; Mary Jane McDevitt, RN, BS; Sandra M. Nettina, RN,C, MSN, CRNP; Linda F. Roy, RN, MSN, CCRN

Copy Editors
Cynthia C. Breuninger *(supervisor)*, Priscilla DeWitt, Nancy Papsin, Doris Weinstock

Designers
Stephanie Peters *(associate art director)*, Matie Patterson *(senior designer)*, Lynn Foulk, Joseph Laufer

Illustrators
Jackie Facciola, Jean Gardner, Linda Gist, Bob Jackson, Robert Neumann, Judy Newhouse, Mary Stangl

Art Production
Robert Wieder

Typography
David Kosten *(director)*, Diane Paluba *(manager)*, Elizabeth Bergman, Joyce Rossi Biletz, Phyllis Marron, Robin Mayer, Valerie Rosenberger

Manufacturing
Deborah Meiris *(manager)*, Anna Brindisi, T.A. Landis

Production Coordination
Patricia W. McCloskey

Editorial Assistants
Maree DeRosa, Beverly Lane, Mary Madden, Margaret Rastiello

The clinical procedures described and recommended in this publication are based on research and consultation with nursing, medical, and legal authorities. To the best of our knowledge, these procedures reflect currently accepted practice; nevertheless, they can't be considered absolute and universal recommendations. For individual application, all recommendations must be considered in light of the patient's clinical condition and, before administration of new or infrequently used drugs, in light of the latest package-insert information. The authors and the publisher disclaim responsibility for any adverse effects resulting directly or indirectly from the suggested procedures, from any undetected errors, or from the reader's misunderstanding of the text.

Printed in the United States of America.

AS4-010493

Library of Congress Cataloging-in-Publication Data
Performing advanced procedures.
p. cm.—(Advanced skills™)
Includes bibliographical references and index.
1. Nursing—Technique.
I. Springhouse Corporation.
II. Series. [DNLM: 1. Nursing—methods.
WY 100 P438 1993]
RT42.P416 1993
610.73—dc20
DNLM/DLC
93-18366
ISBN 0-87434-554-5 CIP

Contents

Advisory board

At the time of publication, the advisors held the following positions.

Contributors and consultants

At the time of publication, the contributors held the following positions.

Sherry Barnhill, RN, BSN, MAEd
Associate Professor of Nursing
Paducah (Ky.) Community College

Carol A. Basile, RN,C, BSN, CCRN
Research Study Coordinator
Department of Pulmonary and Critical Care
Hospital of the University of Pennsylvania
Philadelphia

Wendy L. Blakely, RN, BSN
Education Instructor
Western Baptist Hospital
Paducah, Ky.

Vicki L. Buchda, RN, MS
Director, Special Care Unit
Maryvale Samaritan Medical Center
Phoenix, Ariz.

Kathleen O. Castiglia, RN, MSN
Critical Care Educator
Desert Samaritan Medical Center
Mesa, Ariz.

Sophia B. Chandler, RN, BSN, CDE
Diabetes Nurse Specialist
Lourdes Hospital
Paducah, Ky.

Bonita Gail Largent Cloyd, RN, BSN, CETN
Enterostomal Therapist
Western Baptist Hospital
Paducah, Ky.

Julia Grove, RN, MSN
Director, Medical-Surgical Services
Community Hospital
Mayfield, Ky.

Susan J. Hart, RN,C, MSN, CCRN
Adjunct Professor, College of Nursing
Seton Hall University
South Orange, N.J.
Staff Nurse, Morristown (N.J.) Memorial Hospital

Connie S. Heflin, RN, MSN
Associate Professor of Nursing
Paducah (Ky.) Community College

Marian J. Hoffman, RN, MSN, CNSN
Clinical Nurse Specialist
Education Nurse Specialist
Lehigh Valley Hospital
Allentown, Pa.

Florence Jones, RN, MSN
Chief Nursing Officer
Community Hospital
Mayfield, Ky.

Marilyn Knoth, RN, MSN
Associate Professor of Nursing
Paducah (Ky.) Community College

Kimberley W. McKinney, RN, BSN
Education Instructor
Western Baptist Hospital
Paducah, Ky.

Faye Overby, RN, CETN
Western Baptist Hospital
Paducah, Ky.

Linda Petrine, RN, MSN, CNN
Renal Nurse Specialist
Lehigh Valley Hospital
Allentown, Pa.

Mary Ruckel Probst, RN, MSN
Adult Acute Care Educator
Desert Samaritan Medical Center
Mesa, Ariz.

Daniele Shollenberger, RN, MSN
Education Nurse Specialist
Lehigh Valley Hospital
Allentown, Pa.

Suzanne D. Skinner, RN, MS
Nursing Education Consultant
Severna, Md.

Julie Tackenberg, RN, MA, CNRN
Department of Neurology
University Medical Center
Tucson, Ariz.

Freda Thompson, RN, MSN
Education Instructor
Western Baptist Hospital
Paducah, Ky.

Sabrina Wilferd, RN, BSN
Director of Quality Management
Community Hospital
Mayfield, Ky.

At the time of publication, the consultants held the following positions.

Charles W. Heckenberger, CRTT, RRT, AS
Staff Respiratory Therapist
Doylestown (Pa.) Hospital

Denise Netz, RN, MSN, CNOR, RNFA
Clinical Instructor
Doylestown (Pa.) Hospital

Linda F. Roy, RN, MSN, CCRN
Clinical Instructor
Critical Care
Doylestown (Pa.) Hospital

FOREWORD

Not long ago, most nurses didn't perform many advanced procedures. But today that's changed. The growing number of acutely ill patients in hospitals — and the growing number of patients who need expert care outside the hospital — has changed the range and complexity of procedures you're expected to perform or assist with.

To keep pace with these changes, you need a reference that covers the most important and the most advanced procedures — from advanced cardiac life support to extracorporeal membrane oxygenation. *Performing Advanced Procedures,* the latest book in the Advanced Skills series, provides you with that and much more. Packed with helpful illustrations and photographs, it takes you step by step through each procedure, explaining in refreshingly clear, instructive language exactly what you're expected to know and do.

The book begins with basic and advanced life support — covering everything from cardiopulmonary resuscitation to code management and defibrillation. Chapter 2 presents cardiovascular procedures, such as cardiopulmonary support — one of the newer procedures — and balloon valvuloplasty. Chapter 3 focuses on respiratory care, including inserting and caring for various types of airways, transtracheal oxygen therapy, and thoracic drainage.

In Chapter 4, you'll read about neurologic and musculoskeletal care, such as cerebrospinal fluid drainage and traction. Chapter 5 covers GI, renal, and urologic procedures, including nasogastric and esophageal tube insertion and removal and peritoneal dialysis. Chapter 6 discusses skin and wound care and contains entries on wound irrigation, burn care, and colostomy and ileostomy care. The final chapter addresses important diagnostic procedures, such as lumbar puncture and echocardiography.

For easier reading, each procedure in the seven chapters follows the same format. First, an introduction defines and describes the procedure and its purpose. Next comes a list of indications, followed by a discussion of contraindications and complications. An equipment inventory follows, along with steps for preparing the equipment and recommendations for physically—and psychologically—preparing the patient.

Then come the step-by-step directions for performing or assisting with the procedure. Illustrations or photographs accompany key steps so you can see exactly what to do. Cautions come next, so you know what to watch out for. Each entry concludes with a section on monitoring the patient and providing follow-up care. Here you'll also find special considerations, as well as guidelines for patient teaching and documenting the procedure.

After Chapter 7 comes the *Advanced skill-test,* a multiple-choice self-test designed to help you evaluate what you've learned and further build your skills. Answers and complete rationales follow the test.

Throughout *Performing Advanced Procedures,* special graphic devices, or logos, direct your attention to important recurring topics. The *Troubleshooting* logo highlights techniques you can use to detect and correct equipment problems. A detailed description of the newest equipment—frequently accompanied by a photograph or an illustration—carries the *Advanced Equipment* logo. A *Complications* logo alerts you to key information on detecting and treating critical complications. A *Home Care* logo presents the essentials of teaching the patient or a family member how to perform a procedure at home. And when you see the *Skill Tip* logo, you'll find concise directions and advice that can improve your care.

Performing Advanced Procedures contains many additional features. For instance, in Chapter 3, you'll find full-color photographs showing how to perform closed tracheal suctioning. Another series of photographs describes how to use a pulse oximeter.

No matter where you work, whether it's a hospital, an extended care facility, or some other setting, you'll find *Performing Advanced Procedures* indispensable. Its easy-to-use format, clear explanations, and instructional illustrations and photographs make it a must. I recommend this book highly. With it, you'll be able to perform advanced procedures with skill and confidence.

Beverly Ann McGuffin, RN, MS

Quality Assurance Nurse Coordinator
Community Mental Health
San Francisco
Member, Committee on Standards and Guidelines
ANA Congress of Nursing Practice

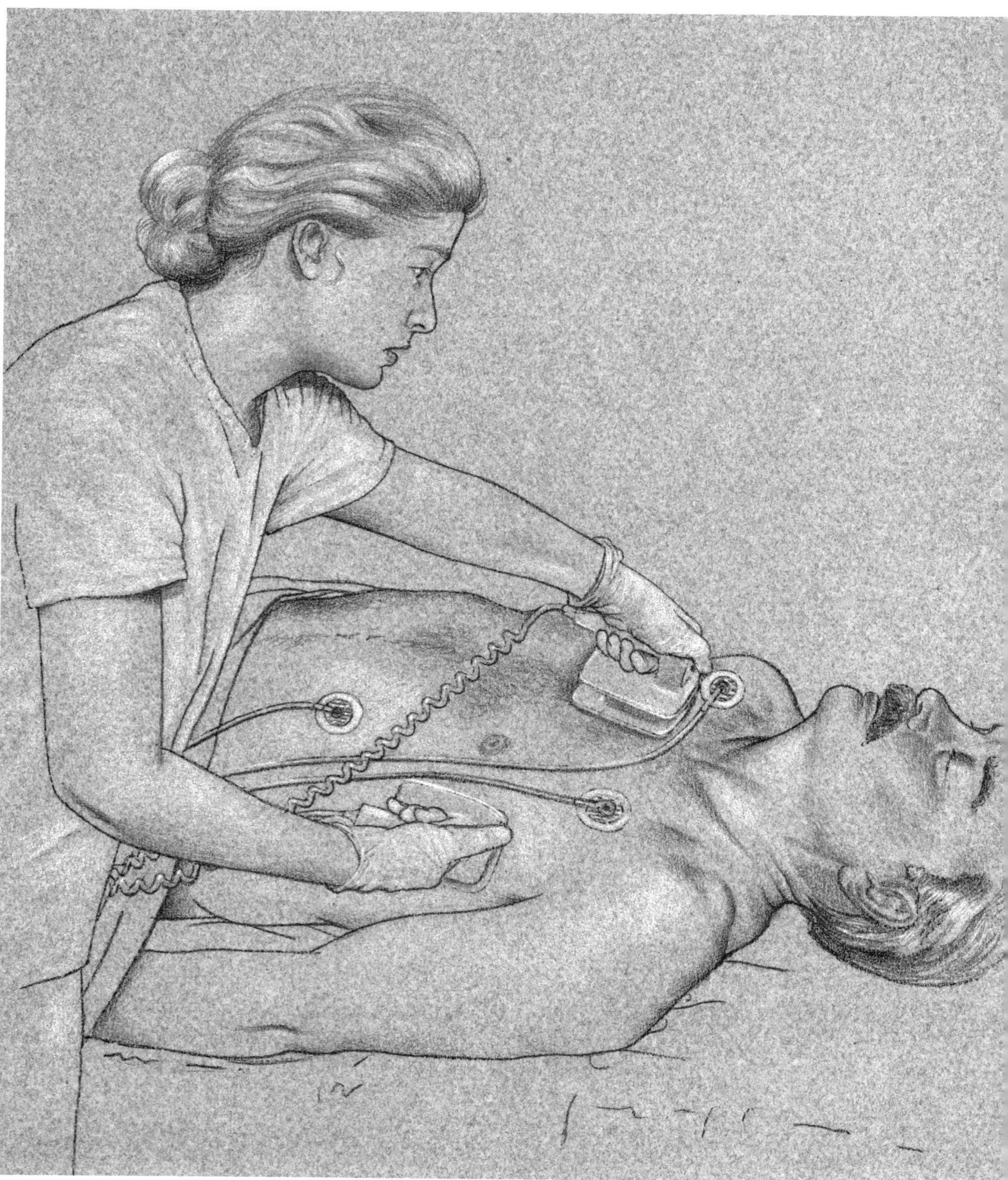

CHAPTER 1

Cardiopulmonary life support

A cardiopulmonary emergency can strike anytime, anywhere. Whether it results from a primary cardiac disorder or an unrelated accident or disorder, a cardiopulmonary emergency threatens your patient's life and challenges your nursing skills. Are you confident you'd know how to respond?

To respond quickly and effectively, you need to keep abreast of the latest advances in procedures, ranging from cardiopulmonary resuscitation (CPR) to temporary pacemaker insertion and monitoring. This chapter will help you do this. It describes the latest CPR and obstructed airway management techniques for adults as well as for infants and children. It also discusses the protocol for successfully managing a code, as well as temporary pacemakers. Finally, the chapter explains how to perform defibrillation and synchronized cardioversion.

CPR for adults

Knowing how to perform CPR effectively is a vital skill. An emergency procedure, CPR helps provide oxygenated blood to a patient's heart, brain, and other vital organs after his heartbeat and breathing have stopped.

Because brain damage begins within 4 minutes after circulation and breathing cease, you must initiate CPR as soon as possible after an arrest. If more than 10 minutes elapse from the time of an arrest until the beginning of adequate CPR, brain damage will almost certainly result. However, there are exceptions, such as a drowning victim who has been immersed in cold water or someone who has suffered hypothermia. If you have any doubt as to how long the victim's pulse and respirations have been absent, you should perform CPR. (See *Why CPR is effective.*)

Why CPR is effective

Experts currently have two theories as to why CPR is effective: the cardiac pump theory or the thoracic pump theory. These theories continue to be researched. Below is an explanation of each theory.

Cardiac pump theory

According to the cardiac pump theory, external chest compressions exert direct pressure on the heart, squeezing it between the sternum and vertebral column. This increases pressure within the ventricles, closing off the mitral and tricuspid valves. In turn, this increases stroke volume and coronary artery blood flow.

Thoracic pump theory

This theory holds that external chest compressions produce a rise in intrathoracic pressure that's transmitted to all intrathoracic vessels. The increased pressure on these vessels promotes blood flow to extrathoracic vessels, enhancing stroke volume and coronary artery blood flow. According to the thoracic pump theory, the heart serves merely as a passive conduit.

Debate over the theories

No one's quite sure which of these two mechanisms predominantly accounts for the effectiveness of CPR, and it's possible that both play equally effective roles. The current thinking among most researchers, however, is that the thoracic pump theory is the dominant mechanism. Those who hold this view believe that the cardiac pump mechanism is operative only in certain patients—for example, those who have cardiomegaly, narrow anteroposterior chest dimensions, or a compliant chest.

Indications

CPR may be used for conditions causing cardiopulmonary arrest, including:

- myocardial infarction or ventricular fibrillation
- trauma, such as drowning, electric shock, suffocation, poisoning, motor vehicle accident, burns, or smoke inhalation
- drug overdose or severe allergic reaction
- choking
- laryngospasm and edema from upper respiratory infections
- sudden infant death syndrome.

Contraindications and complications

CPR is contraindicated if the doctor has written a no-code order for the patient.

If you do perform CPR, keep in mind that the procedure commonly causes gastric distention—the result of overventilation. Other complications typically occur because of improper hand placement during cardiac compressions. These include rib fractures, liver lacerations, and lung punctures. (See *Potential hazards of CPR.*)

Equipment

CPR requires no special equipment, but you do need to place the patient on a hard surface to perform the procedure adequately.

You may also wish to use a mouth-to-mask device to perform rescue breathing. Although not required, a mouth-to-mask device may help prevent the transmission of certain diseases. In addition, if you'll be exposed to the patient's body fluids while performing CPR, you should wear protective equipment, including gloves, goggles, and a mask. In fact, it's a good idea to keep such equipment in a hanging bag on the crash cart for easy access during an emergency.

COMPLICATIONS

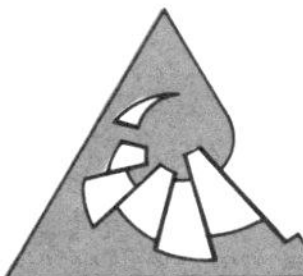

Potential hazards of CPR

HAZARD	CAUSES	ASSESSMENT FINDINGS	PREVENTIVE MEASURES
Sternal and rib fractures	• Osteoporosis • Malnutrition • Improper hand placement	• Paradoxical chest movement • Chest pain or tenderness that increases with inspiration • Crepitus • Palpation of movable bony fragments over the sternum • On palpation, sternum feels unattached to surrounding ribs	*While performing CPR:* • Place your hands correctly on the sternum. • Don't rest your hands or fingers on the patient's ribs. • Interlock your fingers. • Keep your bottom hand in contact with the chest, but release pressure after each compression. • Compress the sternum at the recommended depth for the patient's age.
Pneumothorax, hemothorax, or both	• Lung puncture from fractured rib	• Chest pain and dyspnea • Hypoxemia and central cyanosis • Decreased or absent breath sounds over the affected lung • Tracheal deviation from midline • Hypotension • Hyperresonance to percussion over the affected area along with shoulder pain (pneumothorax)	• Follow the measures listed for sternal and rib fractures.
Injury to the heart and great vessels (pericardial tamponade, atrial or ventricular rupture, vessel laceration, cardiac contusion, punctures of the heart chambers)	• Improperly performed chest compressions • Transvenous or transthoracic pacing attempts • Central line placement during resuscitation • Intracardiac drug administration	• Jugular vein distention • Muffled heart sounds • Pulsus paradoxus • Narrowed pulse pressure • Electrical alternans (decreased electrical amplitude of every other QRS complex) • Adventitious heart sounds • Hypotension • Electrocardiogram changes (arrhythmias, ST-segment elevation, T-wave inversion, and marked decrease in QRS voltage)	• Perform chest compressions properly.
Organ laceration (primarily liver and spleen)	• Forceful compression • Sharp edge of a fractured rib or xiphoid process	• Persistent right upper quadrant tenderness (liver injury) • Persistent left upper quadrant tenderness (splenic injury) • Increasing abdominal girth • Delayed capillary refill • Oliguria	• Follow the measures listed for sternal and rib fractures.
Complications from tracheal intubation	• Insertion of tracheal tube into the right or left mainstem bronchus • Intubation of the esophagus	• Absent breath sounds over one lung • Unilateral chest expansion • Auscultation of air movement in the stomach during ventilation • Gastric distention • Central cyanosis	• Auscultate breath sounds bilaterally; assess for equal chest expansion.
Aspiration of stomach contents	• Gastric distention and an elevated diaphragm from high ventilatory pressures	• Fever, hypoxia, and dyspnea • Auscultation of wheezes and crackles • Increased white blood cell count • Changes in color and odor of lung secretions	• Intubate early. • Insert a nasogastric tube and apply suction, if gastric distention is marked.

Essential steps

An easy way to remember basic CPR procedure is to follow the ABC guidelines: *airway* open, *breathing* restored, *circulation* restored. After these steps have been completed, drug therapy, electrocardiogram (ECG) evaluation, or defibrillation may follow.

The specific CPR techniques you'll use depend on whether or not you're the sole rescuer. You'll vary your technique if another rescuer arrives while you're giving CPR. The American Heart Association (AHA) currently recommends the following step-by-step guidelines for CPR.

One-person rescue

If you're the sole rescuer, expect to open the patient's airway, check for breathing, and assess for circulation before beginning compressions.

Open the airway. Perform these steps to open your patient's airway.

- First, assess the patient to determine if he's unconscious. Gently shake his shoulders and shout, "Are you okay?" This helps ensure that you won't start CPR on a conscious person. Also check to see if the patient has an injury, particularly to the head or neck. If you suspect a head or neck injury, move him as little as possible to reduce the risk of paralysis.
- Next, call out for help. Send someone to contact the emergency medical service (EMS), if appropriate and if possible. If nobody is available, you should contact the EMS and return to the patient quickly. Place the patient in the supine position on a hard, flat surface. When moving him, roll his head and torso as a unit. Avoid twisting or pulling his neck, shoulders, or hips.
- Kneel near the patient's shoulders. This position will give you easy access to his head and chest.
- Remember that the back of the tongue and the epiglottis commonly obstruct the airway of unconscious persons. If the patient doesn't appear to have a neck injury, use the head-tilt, chin-lift maneuver to open his airway. To do so, place the hand closest to the patient's head on the patient's forehead. Then apply enough pressure to tilt the patient's head back. Next, place the fingertips of your other hand under the bony part of his lower jaw near the chin. Now lift the patient's chin. At the same time, keep his mouth partially open.
- Avoid placing your fingertips on the soft tissue under the patient's chin because this maneuver may inadvertently obstruct the airway you're trying to open.
- If you suspect a neck injury, use the jaw-thrust maneuver instead of the head-tilt, chin-lift maneuver. To accomplish this, kneel at the patient's head with your elbows on the ground. Rest your thumbs on his lower jaw near the corners of the mouth, pointing your thumbs toward his feet. Then place your fingertips around the lower jaw. To open the airway, lift the lower jaw with your fingertips.
- Tilting the head back and moving the lower jaw (chin) forward lifts the tongue and the epiglottis from the back of the throat and usually opens the airway. (See *Two maneuvers to open a patient's airway.*)

Check for breathing. Evaluate your patient's breathing with the following steps.

- While maintaining the open airway, place your ear over the patient's mouth and nose. Now, listen for the sound of air moving, and note whether his chest rises and falls. You may also feel airflow on your cheek. If he starts to breathe, keep the airway open and continue checking his breathing until help arrives. If you don't suspect cervical trauma, place the patient in the recovery position. That is, roll him onto his side, moving his head, shoulders, and torso simultaneously. This position helps protect the airway.
- If the patient doesn't start breathing after you open his airway, begin rescue breathing. Pinch his nostrils shut with the thumb and index finger of the hand you've had on his forehead.
- Take a deep breath and place your mouth over the patient's mouth, creating a tight seal. Give two full ventilations, taking a deep breath after each to allow enough time for his chest to expand and relax and to prevent gastric distention. Each ventilation should last 1½ to 2 seconds.

Two maneuvers to open a patient's airway

Depending on the circumstances, you may use one of two methods to open a patient's airway. When performing CPR, you'll typically use the head-tilt, chin-lift maneuver, illustrated below.

However, if you suspect a neck injury, use the jaw-thrust maneuver, as shown below. This maneuver opens the patient's airway without moving his head.

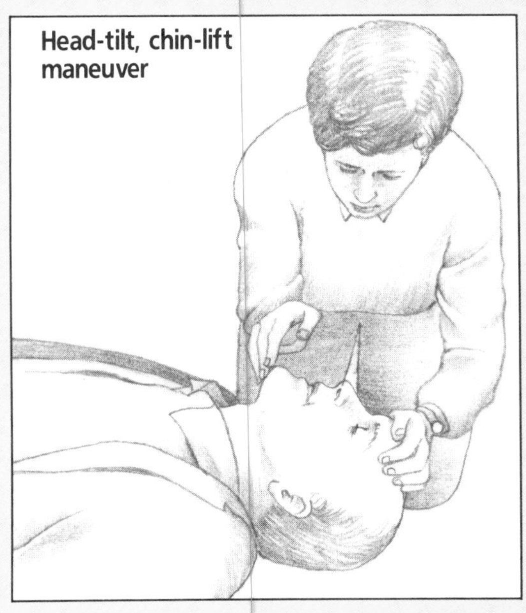
Head-tilt, chin-lift maneuver

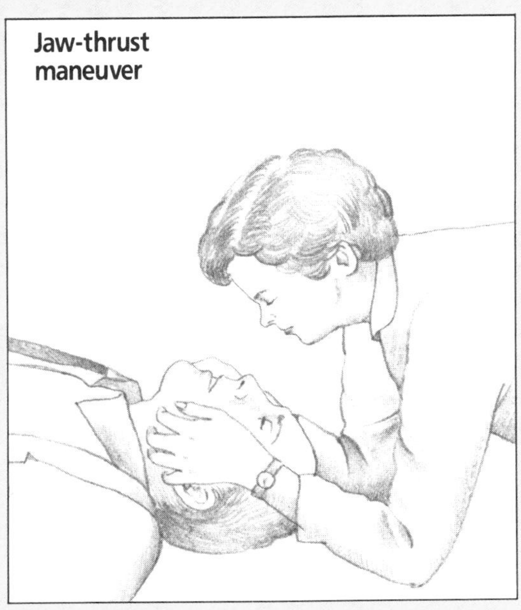
Jaw-thrust maneuver

• If the first ventilation isn't successful, reposition the patient's head and try again. If you're still not successful, he may have a foreign-body airway obstruction. Check for loose dentures. If dentures or any other objects are blocking the airway, follow the procedure for clearing an airway obstruction. (See the "Obstructed airway management" entry in this chapter.)

Assess circulation. Perform the following steps to evaluate your patient's circulation.

• Keep one hand on the patient's forehead so his airway remains open. With your other hand, palpate the carotid artery that's closer to you. To do this, place your index and middle fingers in the groove between the trachea and the sternocleidomastoid muscle. Palpate for 5 to 10 seconds.

• If you detect a pulse, don't begin chest compressions. Instead, perform rescue breathing by giving the patient 12 ventilations/minute (or one every 5 seconds). After every 12 ventilations, recheck his pulse.

• If there's no pulse, start giving chest compressions. Make sure your knees are apart for a wide base of support. Using the hand closer to the patient's feet, locate the lower margin of the rib cage. Then move your fingertips along the margin to the notch where the ribs meet the sternum.

• Place your middle finger on the notch and your index finger next to your middle finger. Your index finger will now be on the bottom of the sternum.

• Put the heel of your other hand on the sternum, next to the index finger. The long axis of

Cough CPR: An effective self-help technique

Some patients can recognize the symptoms of a potentially fatal arrhythmia before lapsing into unconsciousness. In these instances, the patient can perform cough CPR. This self-administered form of CPR can either convert the arrhythmia or delay unconsciousness, thus allowing the patient extra time to seek medical help. The major disadvantage of cough CPR is that the patient must start the process before losing consciousness. Also, the patient must have a strong cough.

Cough CPR occurs in two phases. The first phase, called *cough systole,* consists of the cough itself. Coughing increases intrathoracic and intra-abdominal pressure. This propels blood from the pulmonary vasculature through the left side of the heart and also increases arterial blood flow to the brain.

The next phase occurs after the cough, when the patient inhales sharply. In this phase, called *cough diastole,* intrathoracic and intra-abdominal pressure decreases, allowing blood to move through the right side of the heart and into the pulmonary vasculature. At the same time, venous return increases, the heart readies itself for further pumping with subsequent coughs, and air enters the lungs.

The American Heart Association is currently researching this form of CPR so that it can be taught with basic life support.

the heel of your hand will be aligned with the long axis of the sternum.
• Take the first hand off the notch and put it on top of the hand on the sternum. Make sure you have one hand directly on top of the other and your fingers aren't on his chest. This position will keep the force of the compression on the sternum and reduce the risk of a rib fracture, lung puncture, or liver laceration.
• With your elbows locked, arms straight, and your shoulders directly over your hands, you're ready to give chest compressions. Using the weight of your upper body, compress the patient's sternum 1½" to 2" (4 to 5 cm), delivering the pressure through the heels of your hands. After each compression, release the pressure and allow the chest to return to its normal position so that the heart can fill with blood. Don't change your hand position during compressions to avoid injuring the patient. If your hands move out of position, find your landmarks again to avoid injuring the patient.
• Give 15 chest compressions at a rate of 80 to 100 per minute. Count, "One and two and three and..." up to 15. Open the airway and give 2 ventilations. Then find the proper hand position again and deliver 15 more compressions. Do four complete cycles of 15 compressions and 2 ventilations.
• Palpate the carotid pulse again. If there's still no pulse, continue performing CPR in cycles of 15 compressions and 2 ventilations. Every few minutes, check for breathing and a pulse. If you detect a pulse but he isn't breathing, give 12 ventilations/minute and monitor his pulse.
• If he has a pulse and is breathing, monitor his respirations and pulse closely. You should stop performing CPR only when his respirations and pulse return, EMS personnel arrive and relieve you, or you're exhausted.

Two-person rescue

If another rescuer arrives while you're giving CPR, follow these steps.
• If you haven't contacted the EMS, tell the second rescuer to do so. He should then return to help with the rescue. If he's not a health care professional, ask him to stand by. Then, if you become fatigued, he can take over one-person CPR.
• Have him begin by checking the patient's pulse for 5 seconds after you've given two ventilations. If he doesn't feel a pulse, he should give two ventilations and begin chest compressions.
• If the rescuer is another health care professional, the two of you can perform two-person CPR. He should start assisting after you've finished a cycle of 15 compressions, 2 ventilations, and a pulse check.
• The second rescuer should get into place opposite you. While you're checking for a pulse, he should be finding the proper hand placement for delivering chest compressions.

• If you don't detect a pulse, say, "No pulse, continue CPR," and give one ventilation. Then the second rescuer should begin delivering compressions at a rate of 80 to 100 per minute. Compressions and ventilations should be administered at a ratio of five compressions to one ventilation. The compressor (at this point, the second rescuer) should count out loud so the ventilator can anticipate when to give ventilations. To ensure that the ventilations are effective, the rescuer performing the chest compressions should stop briefly or at least long enough to observe the patient's chest rise with the air supplied by the rescuer giving ventilations.
• As the ventilator, you must check for breathing and a pulse. Signal the compressor to stop giving compressions for 5 seconds so you can make these assessments.
• After a minimum of 10 cycles or when the compressor (second rescuer) becomes tired, the compressor may call for a switch. This should be stated clearly to allow for a smooth transition. The compressor can substitute the word "change" for the word "one" as he counts compressions. In other words, he'd say, "Change and two and three and four and five." You'd then give a ventilation and become the compressor by moving down to the patient's chest and placing your hands in the proper position.
• The second rescuer would become the ventilator and move to the patient's head. He'd check the pulse for 5 seconds. If he found no pulse, he'd say, "No pulse," and give a ventilation. You'd then give compressions at a rate of 80 to 100 per minute or five compressions for each ventilation. Both of you should continue giving CPR in this manner until the patient's respirations and pulse return, EMS personnel arrive and relieve you, or both of you are exhausted.
• A second rescuer may instinctively take the patient's pulse without waiting for the end of a cycle. This is not part of the AHA's recommendations and may confuse some rescuers. The recommendations aim to have all rescuers act in the same way so that time isn't wasted and all efforts help restore the patient's respirations and heartbeat.

Monitoring and aftercare

• Document why you initiated CPR, whether the patient suffered from cardiac or respiratory arrest, when you found the patient and started CPR, and how long he received CPR. Note the patient's response and any complications. Also include any interventions taken to correct complications.
• If the patient also received advanced cardiac life support, document which interventions were performed, who performed them, when they were performed, and what equipment was used.
• If appropriate, teach the patient to perform cough CPR. This self-administered technique can convert a potentially fatal arrhythmia or delay unconsciousness. (See *Cough CPR: An effective self-help technique.*)

CPR for infants and children

Because of the small size and physical immaturity of infants and small children, you'll need to vary your CPR technique. In children, cardiopulmonary arrest typically results from hypoxia, as opposed to the primary cause in adults, which is a cardiac abnormality. Therefore, a key aspect of educating parents and others about basic life support techniques for infants and children includes education about how to prevent accidents that could result in the need for CPR. Also, because cardiopulmonary arrest in children occurs after a slow decline in respiratory function, you need to be aware of the early signs of respiratory distress. Recognizing such signs early, and taking appropriate action, will increase the child's chances for survival.

Indications

CPR may be used for conditions causing cardiopulmonary arrest, including:
• injuries from motor vehicle accidents
• suffocation (from foreign bodies, such as toys or food), smoke inhalation, or drowning
• sudden infant death syndrome

• respiratory tract infections
• poisoning.

Equipment

Pediatric CPR requires no special equipment. As with adults, however, you need to place the patient on a hard surface to perform the procedure adequately.

Essential steps

If the child is over age 8, use the same CPR technique as you would for an adult. But if the patient is a small child (between ages 1 and 8) or an infant (less than age 1), modify your technique as described below.

One-rescuer CPR for a child

You'll perform CPR as you would for an adult or older child, but with several key differences.

Open the airway. Begin by attempting to open the child's airway.
• Assess the child to determine unresponsiveness. Gently shake the shoulder and shout, "Are you okay?" Call out for help. Send someone to contact the EMS. If you're alone and the child is obviously not breathing, perform CPR for 1 minute before calling for help.
• Position the child on his back on a hard, flat surface. Be careful when moving the child, especially if you suspect a head or neck injury. Evaluate the circumstances surrounding the arrest to determine how careful you need to be. For example, there's a greater risk that the child has a neck, spine, or bone injury if he's been in a motor vehicle accident or if he's fallen from a tree, than if you simply found him in bed not breathing.
• Turn the child as a unit, firmly supporting the head and neck so that the head doesn't roll, twist, or tilt backward.
• Next, open the airway using the head-tilt, chin-lift method. To accomplish this, place the hand closest to the child's head on his forehead and tilt his head gently back. Next, place the fingertips of your other hand under the bony part of the lower jaw near the chin. Lift the chin upward, keeping the mouth partially open.
• Avoid placing your fingertips on the soft tissue under the child's chin because this maneuver may inadvertently obstruct the airway.
• If you suspect a neck injury, use the jaw-thrust maneuver instead of the head-tilt, chin-lift maneuver. To do so, place two or three fingers under each side of the lower jaw at its angle and lift the jaw upward.

Check for breathing. Perform these steps to check the child's breathing.
• Keeping the airway open, place your ear over the child's mouth and nose. Observe the child's chest for movement; look, listen, and feel for breathing. If the child is breathing, keep the airway open and continue checking his breathing until help arrives.
• If the child is not breathing, begin rescue breathing by making a seal between your mouth and the mouth of the child. Pinch his nose tightly, using the thumb and forefinger of the hand that you had on his forehead.
• Give two breaths, each lasting 1 to 1½ seconds; then pause 1 to 1½ seconds between each breath. Giving the breaths slowly will help you deliver an adequate volume of air at a low pressure, which helps avoid gastric distention. Deliver enough air to make the child's chest rise and fall.
• If the first ventilation isn't successful, reposition the child's head and try again. If you're still not successful, the child may have a foreign-body airway obstruction. Follow the procedure for airway obstruction before continuing with CPR.

Assess circulation. To evaluate the child's circulation, perform these steps.
• While maintaining the head tilt with one hand on the forehead, use your other hand to palpate the carotid artery, just as you would for an adult.
• If you detect a pulse, don't begin chest compressions. Instead, perform rescue breathing once every 4 seconds, or 15 times a minute.
• If there is no pulse, and you haven't sent someone for help yet, tell a bystander to call the EMS. Then start giving chest compressions. Make sure your knees are apart for a wide base of support. Locate the lower margin of the rib cage. Then move your fingertips along

the margin to the notch where the ribs meet the sternum.

• Place your middle finger on the notch and your index finger next to your middle finger. Your index finger will now be on the bottom of the sternum.

• Place the heel of *one* hand next to the index finger and compress the chest with *one* hand to a depth of 1" to 1.5" (2.5 to 4 cm). (See *Correct hand placement in chest compression for CPR,* page 10.)

• Be sure to keep your fingers off the child's ribs. Perform smooth compressions, allowing the chest to return to its normal position between each compression. Doing so allows the heart to fill with blood. Perform 80 to 100 compressions/minute, giving one rescue breath for every five compressions.

• After 10 cycles of compressions and rescue breaths, stop and palpate the carotid pulse. If you don't detect a pulse, give one rescue breath and then continue the cycle of compressions and rescue breathing.

• Every few minutes, feel for a pulse. If the pulse returns, check for spontaneous breathing. If you detect a pulse but the child isn't breathing, give one rescue breath every 4 seconds (15 breaths/minute) and monitor his pulse.

• If the child has a pulse and is breathing, maintain an open airway and monitor his pulse and respirations closely. You should stop performing CPR only when his pulse and respirations return, EMS personnel arrive to relieve you, or you're exhausted.

Two-rescuer CPR for a child

If a second rescuer arrives, end a cycle with one breath. Then have the second rescuer check the child's pulse. If there is no pulse, the second rescuer should give one rescue breath and then begin one-rescuer CPR. Meanwhile, monitor the effectiveness of the CPR by watching for the rise and fall of the child's chest during rescue breaths and by checking the pulse during chest compressions.

One-rescuer CPR for an infant

When performing CPR on an infant, you'll modify your technique because of the infant's small size.

Open the airway. Begin by attempting to open the infant's airway.

• Determine unresponsiveness by tapping or gently shaking the infant's shoulder or flicking the infant's foot with your fingers. Call out for help. Send someone to contact the EMS. If you're alone, and the infant is obviously not breathing, perform CPR for 1 minute before calling for help.

• Position the infant on his back on a hard, flat surface. Be sure to turn the infant as a unit, firmly supporting the head and neck so that the head doesn't roll, twist, or tilt backward.

• Next, open the airway by using the head-tilt, chin-lift method. Place the hand closest to the infant's head on his forehead and tilt the head gently back. Then place the fingertips of your other hand under the bony part of the lower jaw near the chin. Lift the chin upward, keeping the mouth partially open. Take care not to tilt the head back too far.

• Avoid placing your fingertips on the soft tissue under the infant's chin because this maneuver may inadvertently obstruct the airway.

Check for breathing. To evaluate the child's breathing, perform these steps.

• While keeping the airway open, place your ear over the infant's mouth and nose. Observe the infant's chest for movement; look, listen, and feel for breathing. If the infant is breathing, keep the airway open and continue checking his breathing until help arrives.

• If the infant isn't breathing, begin rescue breathing by making a seal between your mouth and the mouth and nose of the infant.

• Give two slow, gentle rescue breaths, pausing 1 to 1½ seconds between each breath. Giving the breaths slowly will help you deliver an adequate volume of air at a low pressure, which helps avoid gastric distention. Deliver enough air to make the infant's chest rise and fall.

• If the first ventilation isn't successful, reposition the infant's head and try again. If you're still not successful, the infant may have a foreign-body airway obstruction. Follow the procedure for airway obstruction before continuing with CPR.

Correct hand placement in chest compression for CPR

Correct hand placement is crucial if you're to perform CPR safely and effectively. Study the following illustrations to learn how hand placement varies when performing CPR on an adult, a child, and an infant.

Adult

To locate the correct hand placement position on an adult, slide your fingers along the lower rib margin to the notch where the ribs and sternum meet.

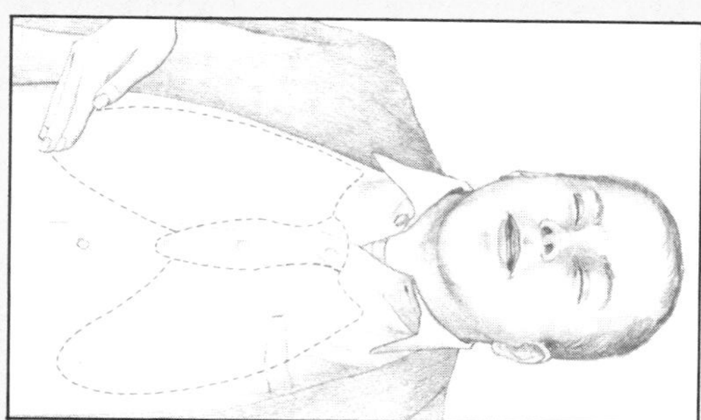

Place your middle finger on this spot.

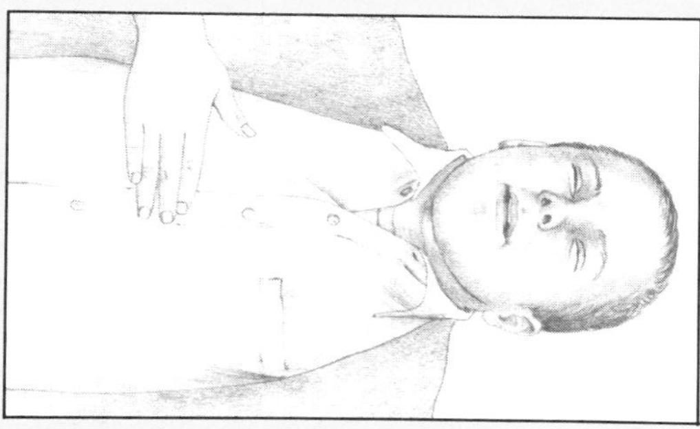

Then place the heel of your other hand on the sternum, one finger's width above the middle finger.

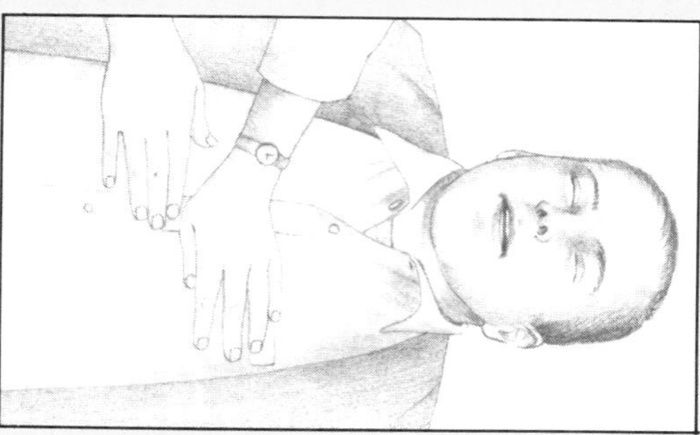

Child

For a child, move your fingertips along the lower rib margin to the notch where the ribs and sternum meet. Place your middle finger on the notch and your index finger next to your middle finger. Then place the heel of one hand next to the index finger.

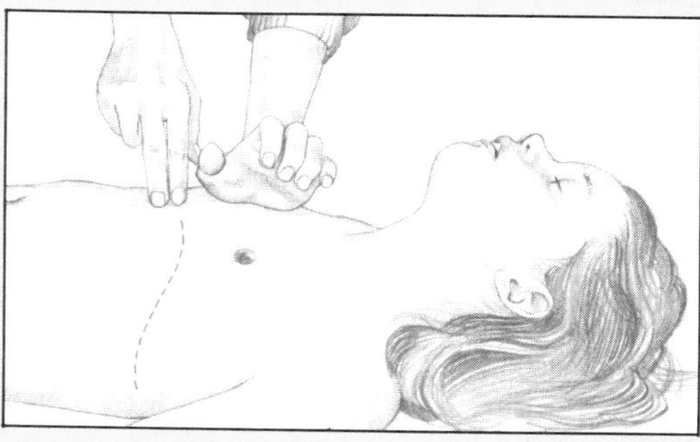

Infant

For an infant, place the index finger of your hand between the infant's nipples. The area of compression is one finger's width below this point, at the location of the middle and ring fingers.

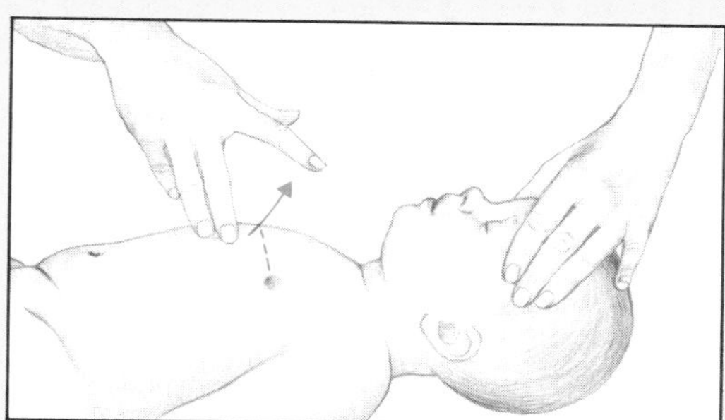

Assess circulation. Perform the following steps to assess the infant's circulation.

- While maintaining the head tilt with one hand on the forehead, use your other hand to feel for the brachial pulse.
- If you detect a pulse, don't begin chest compressions. Instead, perform rescue breathing once every 3 seconds, or 20 times a minute.
- If there's no pulse, and you haven't sent someone for help, tell a bystander to call the EMS.
- Then begin chest compressions. To start, draw an imaginary line connecting the infant's nipples. Place the index finger of the hand farthest from the infant's head at the center of this line. The area of compression is one finger's width below this spot, at the location of the middle and ring fingers. Using two or three fingers, compress the sternum to a depth of ½" to 1" (1 to 2.5 cm).
- Perform smooth compressions, allowing the chest to return to its normal position between each compression. Doing so allows the heart to fill with blood. Perform at least 100 compressions/minute, giving one rescue breath for every five compressions.
- After 10 cycles of compressions and rescue breaths, stop and check the brachial pulse. If there's still no pulse, give one rescue breath and continue compressions with rescue breaths.
- Every few minutes, feel for a pulse. If the pulse returns, check for spontaneous breathing. If you detect a pulse but the infant isn't breathing, give one rescue breath every 3 seconds (20 breaths/minute) and monitor his pulse.
- If the infant has a pulse and is breathing, maintain an open airway and monitor his respirations and pulse closely. You should stop performing CPR only when his respirations and pulse return, EMS personnel arrive to relieve you, or you're exhausted.

Obstructed airway management

A patient's obstructed airway, as demonstrated by an inability to speak, cough, or breathe, demands immediate action. If the patient is conscious, use the abdominal thrust maneuver to dislodge the obstruction. This maneuver creates enough diaphragmatic pressure in the static lung below the foreign body to expel the obstruction. If the patient is unconscious, perform an abdominal thrust followed by a finger sweep maneuver to manually remove the foreign body from the patient's mouth.

Indications

The only indication for these procedures is a foreign body lodged in the throat or bronchus.

Contraindications and complications

Don't perform these maneuvers if the patient has an incomplete or a partial airway obstruction or if he can breathe well enough to dislodge the foreign body by coughing. Also, don't perform the abdominal thrust if the patient is pregnant, markedly obese, or has recently undergone abdominal surgery. For such patients, use a chest-thrust maneuver, which forces air out of the lungs to create an artificial cough.

Complications related to these maneuvers include injuries such as ruptured or lacerated abdominal or thoracic viscera. These injuries may result from incorrect hand placement during the maneuver or because the patient has a condition, such as osteoporosis or metastatic cancer, which has increased his risk for a fracture. After the patient has regained consciousness and can breathe independently, he may also complain of nausea, regurgitation, and achiness.

Essential steps

- Determine the patient's degree of obstruction by tapping his shoulder and asking, "Are you choking?" If he has a complete airway obstruction, he won't be able to answer because the obstruction will block airflow to his vocal cords. If he makes crowing sounds, his airway

Clearing an obstructed airway

When trying to clear a patient's obstructed airway, it's crucial that you position your hands and body properly. Doing so will aid in efficient airway clearance and will also help prevent complications or injuries.

Conscious adult

To hold your hands correctly, make a fist with one hand and then grasp the fist with your other hand.

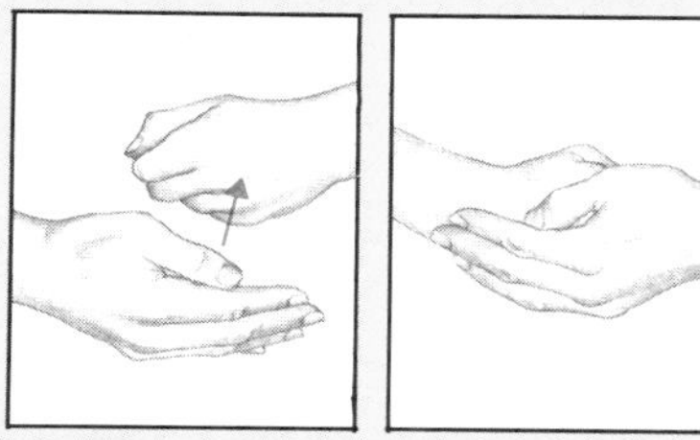

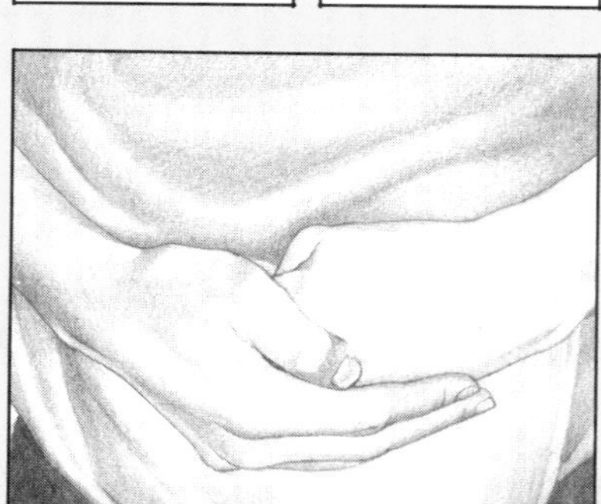

If the patient is conscious, stand behind her and place the thumb side of your fist against her abdomen, slightly above the umbilicus and well below the xiphoid process.

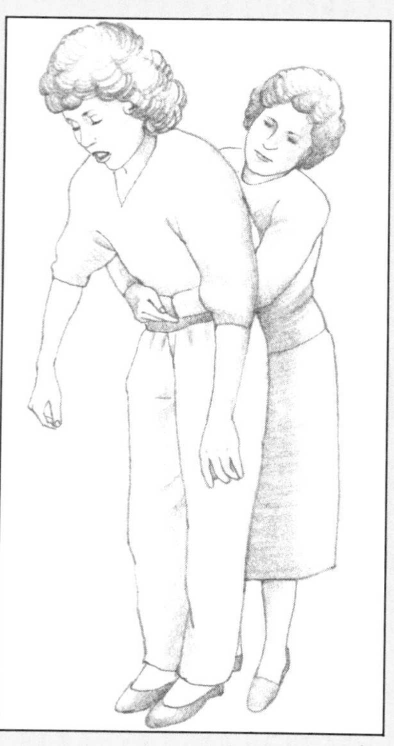

Unconscious adult

If the patient is unconscious, kneel astride her thighs. Place the heels of your hands, one on top of the other, between the patient's umbilicus and the tip of her xiphoid process.

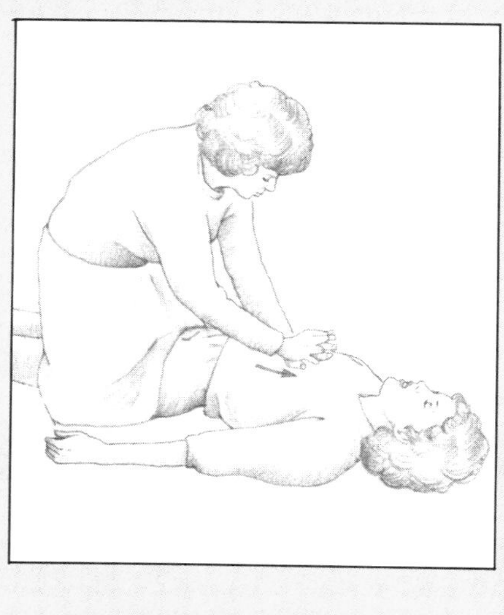

is partially obstructed, and you should encourage him to cough. This will either clear the airway or make the obstruction complete.

For a complete obstruction, your specific interventions will depend on the patient's age and degree of consciousness. You'll also need to vary your technique if the patient is pregnant or obese.

Conscious adult

- First, tell the patient that you'll try to dislodge the foreign body.
- Standing behind the patient, wrap your arms around his waist. Make a fist with one hand and place the thumb side against his abdomen, slightly above the umbilicus and well below the xiphoid process. Then grasp your fist with the other hand.
- Squeeze the patient's abdomen 6 to 10 times

with quick inward and upward thrusts. Make each thrust a separate and distinct movement, with each forceful enough to create an artificial cough that will dislodge an obstruction. (See *Clearing an obstructed airway.*)

• Make sure you have a firm grasp on the patient because he may lose consciousness and need to be lowered to the floor. Look around the floor for objects that may harm him. Then, if he does lose consciousness, lower him carefully to the floor. Support his head and neck to prevent injury, and continue as described below.

Unconscious adult

• If you come upon an unconscious adult, ask any witnesses what happened. Begin CPR and attempt to ventilate him. If you can't ventilate him, reposition his head and try again.

• If you still can't ventilate the patient, or if a conscious patient loses consciousness during abdominal thrusts, kneel astride his thighs.

• Place the heel of one hand on top of the other. Then place your hands between his umbilicus and the tip of his xiphoid process at the midline. Push inward and upward with 6 to 10 quick abdominal thrusts.

• After delivering the abdominal thrusts, open the patient's airway by grasping the tongue and lower jaw with your thumb and fingers. Lift the jaw to draw the tongue away from the back of the throat and away from any foreign body.

• If you can see the object, remove it by inserting your index finger deep into the throat at the base of the tongue. Using a hooking motion, remove the obstruction. (*Note:* Some clinicians object to a blind finger sweep when you can't see the obstruction because your finger acts as a second obstruction. They believe that, in most cases, the tongue-jaw lift described above should be enough to dislodge the obstruction.)

• After removing the object, try to ventilate the patient. Then assess for spontaneous respirations and check for a pulse. Proceed with CPR if necessary.

• If you can't remove the obstruction, attempt to ventilate the patient. If you can't, repeat the sequence of performing abdominal thrusts and mouth checks and attempting to ventilate until you clear the airway.

Obese or pregnant adult

• If the patient is conscious, stand behind her and place your arms under her armpits and around her chest.

• Place the thumb side of your clenched fist against the middle of the sternum, avoiding the margins of the ribs and the xiphoid process. Grasp your fist with your other hand and perform a chest thrust with enough force to expel the foreign body.

• Continue this maneuver until the patient expels the obstruction or loses consciousness.

• If the patient loses consciousness, carefully lower her to the floor.

• Kneel close to the patient's side and place the heel of one hand just above the bottom of the patient's sternum. The long axis of the heel of your hand should align with the long axis of the patient's sternum. Place the heel of your other hand on top of that, making sure your fingers don't touch the patient's chest. Deliver each thrust forcefully enough to remove the obstruction.

Conscious or unconscious child

• If the child is conscious and can stand, perform abdominal thrusts using the same technique as you would with an adult, but use less force.

• If he's unconscious or lying down, kneel at his feet; if he's a large child, kneel astride his thighs. If he's lying on an examination table, stand by his side. Deliver abdominal thrusts as you would for an adult patient, but use less force.

Conscious or unconscious infant

• Whether the infant is conscious or not, place him face down so that he's straddling your arm with his head lower than his trunk. Rest your forearm on your thigh and deliver four back blows with the heel of your hand between the infant's shoulder blades.

• If this maneuver doesn't remove the obstruction, place your free hand on the infant's back. Supporting his neck, jaw, and chest with your other hand, turn him over onto your thigh.

Clearing an infant's obstructed airway

When clearing an infant's airway, use both back blows and chest thrusts, as shown below.

Back blows
To deliver back blows, straddle the infant over your arm, keeping his head lower than his trunk. Deliver four back blows with the heel of your hand.

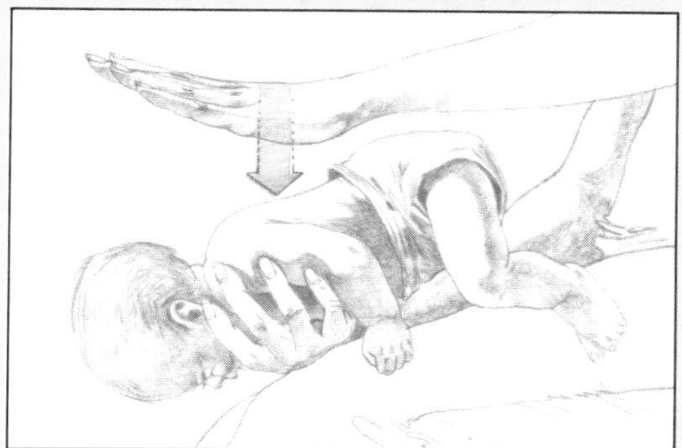

Chest thrusts
While resting the infant on your thigh and keeping his head lower than his trunk, administer four chest thrusts.

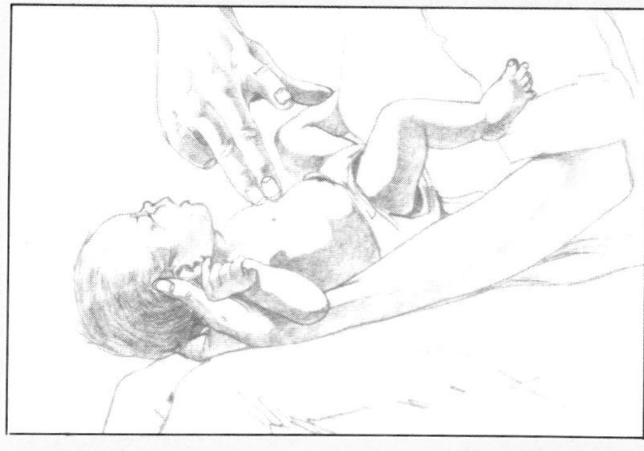

Keep his head lower than his trunk.
• Position your fingers. To do so, imagine a line between the infant's nipples and place the index finger of your free hand on his sternum, just below this imaginary line. Then place your middle and ring fingers next to your index finger and lift the index finger off his chest. Deliver four chest thrusts as you would for chest compression, but at a slower rate.
• If the patient vomits during abdominal thrusts, quickly wipe out his mouth with your fingers and resume the maneuver as necessary.
• Continue the sequence of performing back blows, chest thrusts, and mouth checks, and attempt to ventilate until successful. Even if your efforts to clear the airway don't seem to be effective, keep trying. As oxygen deprivation increases, smooth and skeletal muscles relax, making your maneuvers more likely to succeed. (See *Clearing an infant's obstructed airway.*)

Cautions
Never perform a blind finger sweep on an infant or child because you risk pushing the foreign body farther back into the airway.

Monitoring and aftercare
• Record the date and time of the procedure, the patient's actions before the obstruction (if known), the approximate length of time it took to clear the airway, and the type and size of the object removed.
• In your documentation, also note the patient's vital signs after the procedure, any complications that occurred and nursing actions taken, and his tolerance of the procedure.

Code management

The goals of any code are to restore the patient's spontaneous heartbeat and respirations and also to prevent hypoxic damage to the brain and other vital organs. Fulfilling these goals requires a team approach. Ideally, the team should consist of health care workers trained in advanced cardiac life support (ACLS), although nurses trained in basic life support (BLS) may also be a part of the team. Sponsored by the AHA, the ACLS course incorporates BLS skills with advanced resuscitation techniques.

In most hospitals, ACLS-trained nurses provide the first resuscitative efforts to cardiac arrest patients, often administering cardiac medications and performing defibrillation before the doctor's arrival. Because ventricular fibrillation commonly precedes sudden cardiac arrest, initial resuscitative efforts focus on rapid recognition of arrhythmias and, when indicated, defibrillation. If monitoring equipment isn't available, you should simply perform BLS measures. Of course, the scope of your responsibilities in any situation depends on your hospital's policies and procedures and your state's nurse practice act.

Indications

- Absent pulse
- Apnea
- Ventricular fibrillation
- Ventricular tachycardia
- Asystole

Contraindications and complications

Contraindications include a no-code order written by the patient's doctor or an advance directive from the patient or his family requesting that the patient not be resuscitated.

Complications of CPR, even when performed correctly, include fractured ribs, a lacerated liver, a punctured lung, and gastric distention.

Equipment

Oral, nasal, and endotracheal (ET) airways • one-way valve masks • oxygen source • oxygen flowmeter • intubation supplies • hand-held resuscitation bag • suction supplies • nasogastric (NG) tube • goggles, masks, and gloves • cardiac arrest board • peripheral I.V. supplies, including 14G and 18G peripheral I.V. catheters • central I.V. supplies, including an 18G thin-wall catheter, a 6-cm needle catheter, and a 16G 15- to 20-cm catheter • I.V. administration sets (including microdrip and minidrip) • I.V. fluids, including dextrose 5% in water (D_5W), 0.9% sodium chloride solution, and lactated Ringer's solution • ECG monitor • cardioverter or defibrillator • conductive medium • ECG leads • cardiac medications, including epinephrine, lidocaine, procainamide, bretylium, atropine, isoproterenol, dopamine, calcium chloride, and dobutamine • optional: external pacemaker, percutaneous transvenous pacer, cricothyrotomy kit, end-tidal carbon dioxide detector

Organizing your crash cart

When responding to a code, you can't waste time searching the drawers of your crash cart for the equipment you need. One way to make sure you know the precise location of everything is to follow the ABCD plan to an organized crash cart. Label the crash cart drawers with the letters A, B, C, and D and fill them as follows.

A: Airway control drawer
This drawer should contain all of the equipment necessary for maintaining a patient's airway. It should include oral, nasal, and endotracheal airways; an intubation tray containing a laryngoscope and blades; an extra laryngoscope; lidocaine ointment; tape; a 10-cc syringe to inflate the endotracheal balloon; extra batteries and light bulbs; and suction devices.

B: Breathing drawer
This drawer should contain all of the equipment needed to support the patient's ventilation and oxygenation. Oxygenation is maintained with nasal cannulas, face masks, and Venturi masks. Ventilation is supported by maintaining gastric compression with nasogastric tubes.

C: Circulation drawer
In this drawer, place anything needed to start a central or peripheral I.V. line, such as catheters, tubing, start kits, pump tubing, and 250-ml or 500-ml bags of I.V. solutions (dextrose 5% in water and 0.9% sodium chloride solution).

D: Drug drawer
This drawer should contain all medications needed for advanced cardiac life support.

Preparation

Because effective emergency care depends on reliable and accessible equipment, the equipment, as well as the personnel, must be ready for a code at any time. (See *Organizing your crash cart.*). You also should be familiar with the cardiac drugs you may have to administer. (See *Common emergency cardiac drugs.*)

Always be aware of your patient's code status as defined by the doctor's orders, the patient's advance directives, and family wishes. If the doctor has ordered a "no code," make sure the doctor has written and signed the order. If possible, have the patient or a responsible family member cosign the order.

For some patients, you may need to consider whether the family wishes to be present during a code. If the family wants to be present, and if a nurse or clergyman can remain with the family, consider allowing them to remain during the code.

Essential steps

• If you're the first to arrive at the site of a code, assess the patient's level of consciousness (LOC), airway, breathing, and circulation, and then begin CPR. (See *Treating lethal arrhythmias,* page 19.) Use a pocket mask, if available, to ventilate the patient.
• Call for help. When a second BLS provider arrives, have that person call a code and retrieve the emergency equipment.
• Once the emergency equipment arrives, have the second BLS provider place the cardiac arrest board under the patient and then assist with two-rescuer CPR. Meanwhile, have the nurse assigned to the patient relate the patient's medical history and describe the events leading to the arrest.
• A third person, either a nurse certified in BLS or a respiratory therapist, will then attach the hand-held resuscitation bag to the oxygen source and begin to ventilate the patient with 100% oxygen.
• When the ACLS-trained nurse arrives, she'll expose the patient's chest and apply defibrillator pads. She'll then apply the paddles to the patient's chest to obtain a "quick look" at the patient's cardiac rhythm. If the patient is in ventricular fibrillation, ACLS protocol calls for defibrillation as soon as possible with 200 joules. The ACLS-trained nurse will act as code leader until the doctor arrives.
• If not already in place, apply ECG electrodes and attach the patient to the defibrillator's cardiac monitor. Avoid placing electrodes on bony prominences or hairy areas. Also avoid the areas where the defibrillator pads will be placed and where chest compressions will be given.
• As CPR continues, you or an ACLS-trained nurse will then start two peripheral I.V. lines with large-bore I.V. catheters. Be sure to use only a large vein, such as the antecubital vein, to allow for rapid fluid administration and to prevent drug extravasation.
• As soon as the I.V. catheter is in place, begin an infusion of 0.9% sodium chloride solution or lactated Ringer's solution to help prevent circulatory collapse. D_5W continues to be acceptable but the recent ACLS guidelines encourage the use of 0.9% sodium chloride solution or lactated Ringer's solution because D_5W can produce hyperglycemic effects during a cardiac arrest.
• While one nurse starts the I.V. lines, the other nurse will set up portable or wall suction equipment, and suction the patient's oral secretions as necessary to maintain an open airway.
• The ACLS-trained nurse will then prepare and administer emergency cardiac drugs as needed. Keep in mind that drugs administered through a central line reach the myocardium more quickly than those administered through a peripheral line.
• If the patient doesn't have an accessible I.V. line, you may administer medications such as epinephrine, lidocaine, and atropine through an ET tube. To do so, dilute the drugs in 10 ml of 0.9% sodium chloride solution or sterile water and then instill them into the patient's ET tube. Afterward, manually ventilate the patient to distribute the drug throughout the bronchial tree, which aids in absorption.
• The ACLS-trained nurse will also prepare for, and assist with, ET intubation. During intubation attempts, take care not to interrupt CPR for longer than 30 seconds.
• Suction the patient as needed. After the patient has been intubated, assess the patient's breath sounds to ensure proper tube placement. If the patient has diminished or absent breath sounds over the left lung field, the doctor will pull back the ET tube slightly and reas-

Common emergency cardiac drugs

You may be called on to administer a variety of cardiac drugs during a code. The following chart lists the most common emergency cardiac drugs, along with their actions, indications, and dosage.

DRUG	ACTIONS	INDICATIONS	USUAL ADULT DOSAGE
adenosine (Adenocard)	• Allows conduction through atrioventricular (AV) node; may interrupt reentry through AV node • Shortens duration of atrial action potential during supraventricular tachycardia and produces atropine-resistant bradycardia • Premature ventricular contractions (PVCs), premature atrial contractions, sinus tachycardia, and AV blocks may occur, but typically resolve spontaneously	• Supraventricular tachycardia, including those associated with accessory bypass tracts (Wolff-Parkinson-White syndrome)	• 6 mg I.V. push over 1 to 2 sec initially; may be increased to 12 mg if conversion has not occurred • *Caution:* Slower than recommended administration decreases effectiveness.
atropine	• Accelerates AV conduction and heart rate by blocking vagal nerve	• Symptomatic bradycardia • Asystole • AV block	• For bradycardia, 0.5 to 1 mg I.V. push (for asystole, 1 mg); repeat every 3 to 5 min until heart rate >60 beats/min up to 2-mg total
bretylium (Bretylol)	• Causes initial release of norepinephrine, followed by adrenergic blockade • Raises ventricular fibrillation threshold	• Ventricular fibrillation unresponsive to lidocaine and defibrillation • Recurrent ventricular fibrillation (despite lidocaine) • Ventricular tachycardia with a pulse unresponsive to lidocaine and procainamide	• 5 mg/kg I.V. push initially; may be increased to 10 mg/kg and repeated every 5 min up to 35 mg/kg. • *Caution:* Hypotension occurs with administration; nausea and vomiting occur when the patient is awake.
dobutamine (Dobutrex)	• Increases myocardial contractility without raising oxygen demand • Decreases left ventricular diastolic pressure	• Congestive heart failure • Cardiogenic shock	• 2 to 20 μg/kg/min by continuous I.V. infusion
dopamine (Intropin)	• Produces inotropic effect, increasing cardiac output, blood pressure, and renal perfusion • May enhance myocardial automaticity, causing ventricular arrhythmias	• Hypotension (except when caused by hypovolemia)	• Continuous I.V. infusion at 2 to 5 μg/kg/min initially; can be increased to 20 μg/kg/min as needed to raise blood pressure (*Note:* Always dilute and give I.V. drip, never I.V. push.) • *Caution:* Don't administer in same I.V. line with alkaline solution.
epinephrine (Adrenalin)	• Increases heart rate, peripheral resistance, and blood flow to heart (enhancing myocardial and cerebral oxygenation) • Strengthens myocardial contractility • Increases coronary perfusion pressure during CPR	• Ventricular fibrillation • Pulseless ventricular tachycardia • Electromechanical dissociation • Asystole • Hypotension (secondary agent)	• 1 mg I.V. push initially; may be repeated every 3 to 5 min as needed • 1 mg (10 ml) of 1:10,000 solution endotracheally if no I.V. line is available (*Note:* 1:1,000 solution contains 1 mg/ml, so it must be diluted in 9 ml of 0.9% sodium chloride solution to provide 1 mg/10 ml.) • For hypotension, 1 mg/500 ml of D_5W by continuous infusion, starting at 1 μg/min and titrated to achieve desired effect • May be given by intracardiac injection (hazardous), but only by the doctor • *Caution:* Don't administer in same I.V. line with alkaline solutions. • Many reports have shown that doses of 10 mg I.V. or more achieved resuscitation, whereas lower doses failed to restore a pulse.

(continued)

Common emergency cardiac drugs *(continued)*

DRUG	ACTIONS	INDICATIONS	USUAL ADULT DOSAGE
isoproterenol (Isuprel)	• Enhances automaticity and accelerates conduction • Increases heart rate and cardiac contractility, but exacerbates ischemia and arrhythmias in patients with ischemic heart disease • Raises blood pressure by increasing cardiac output and decreasing peripheral resistance • Promotes bronchodilation	• Indicated only for temporary control of severe bradycardia unresponsive to atropine (while awaiting pacemaker insertion) • Not indicated for cardiac arrest	• Start I.V. drip of 1 mg in 500 ml of D_5W at 2 to 10 μg/min (30 ml/hr or 30 microdrops/min). Titrate to produce heart rate of 60 beats/min or systolic blood pressure of >90. • *Caution:* Don't give I.V. push and don't mix with another drug.
lidocaine (Xylocaine)	• Depresses automaticity and conduction of ectopic impulses in ventricles, especially in ischemic tissue • Raises fibrillation threshold, especially in an ischemic heart	• Frequent premature ventricular contractions • Ventricular tachycardia • Ventricular fibrillation	• 1 to 1.5 mg/kg (usually 50 to 75 mg) I.V. push initially; may be followed by 0.5 to 1.5 mg/kg bolus dose every 5 to 10 min up to total of 3 mg/kg (usually 225 mg) in 15 to 20 min • Continuous I.V. infusion of 2 g/500 ml D_5W at 2 to 4 mg/min (30 to 60 ml/hr or 30 to 60 microdrops/min) to prevent recurrence of lethal arrhythmias
magnesium sulfate	• Mechanism of action is unclear but may help in cardiac arrest associated with refractory ventricular tachycardia or ventricular fibrillation	• Cardiac arrest associated with refractory ventricular tachycardia or ventricular fibrillation	• For life-threatening arrhythmias, 1 to 2 g (approximately 8 to 16 mEq) I.V. in 100 ml of D_5W over 1 to 2 min; the dose may be repeated in 5 to 15 min if the patient fails to respond • In nonemergency situation, 2 to 4 g I.V. over 20 to 60 min • *Caution:* If hypotension develops, slow or stop infusion.
procainamide (Pronestyl)	• Depresses automaticity and conduction • Prolongs refraction in the atria and ventricles	• Suppresses PVCs and ventricular tachycardia unresponsive to lidocaine	• 50 mg I.V. push over 2½ min (20 mg/min) • Repeat every 5 minutes until one of the following events occurs: the patient's arrhythmia is suppressed; the patient develops hypotension; the QRS complex widens by 50% of its original width; or a total of 1 g of the drug has been given.
sodium bicarbonate	• May counteract metabolic acidosis	• Preexisting metabolic acidosis (may be used 10 min into cardiac arrest if patient is unresponsive to other treatment)	• 1 mEq/kg (50 to 75 mEq) I.V. push initially over 3 to 5 min; repeat half the initial dose every 10 min or as dictated by arterial blood gas levels • *Caution:* Don't mix with calcium chloride or epinephrine.
verapamil (Isoptin)	• Slows conduction through AV node • Causes vasodilation • Produces negative inotropic effect on heart, depressing myocardial contractility	• Paroxysmal atrial tachycardia (PAT) with narrow QRS complex unresponsive to carotid sinus massage	• 2.5 to 5 mg I.V. push over 2 to 3 min initially; may be increased to 5 to 10 mg and repeated in 15 to 30 min if PAT persists and the patient demonstrates no adverse reaction to the initial dose

sess. When the tube is correctly positioned, tape it securely. To serve as a reference, mark the point on the tube that's level with the patient's lips.

• Throughout the code, check the patient's carotid or femoral pulses before and after each defibrillation. Also check the pulses frequently during the code to evaluate the effectiveness of cardiac compressions.

• Meanwhile, other members of the code team

Treating lethal arrhythmias

As taught by the American Heart Association, the advanced cardiac life support (ACLS) course outlines a specific protocol for treating life-threatening arrhythmias. The ACLS course defines a lethal arrhythmia as having the following characteristics:

- ventricular rhythm rapid and chaotic, indicating varying degrees of depolarization and repolarization; QRS complexes not identifiable
- patient unconscious at onset
- absent pulses, heart sounds, and blood pressure
- dilated pupils
- rapid development of cyanosis.

The following chart outlines the steps an ACLS-certified nurse should take to treat such potentially lethal arrhythmias as ventricular fibrillation and pulseless ventricular tachycardia. Even if you're not ACLS certified, the chart will help you know what to expect in such an emergency.

Establish responsiveness.
▼
Check pulse. If no pulse, then:
▼
Perform CPR until a defibrillator is available.
▼
Check rhythm. If ventricular fibrillation or tachycardia appears, then:
▼
Defibrillate using 200 joules.
▼
Defibrillate using 200 to 300 joules.
▼
Defibrillate using 360 joules.
▼
If ventricular fibrillation or tachycardia persists, then:
▼
Continue CPR.
▼
Intubate as soon as possible.
▼
Establish I.V. access.
▼
Administer epinephrine, 1:10,000, 1 mg I.V. push every 3 to 5 minutes.
▼
Defibrillate using 360 joules, 30 to 60 seconds after epinephrine.
▼
Administer lidocaine 1.5 mg/kg I.V. push.
▼
Defibrillate using 360 joules.
▼
Administer bretylium 5 mg/kg I.V. push.
▼
Defibrillate using 360 joules.
▼
Administer bretylium 10 mg/kg I.V. push (consider sodium bicarbonate).
▼
Defibrillate using 360 joules.
▼
Repeat lidocaine or bretylium.
▼
Defibrillate using 360 joules.

should keep a written record of the events. Other duties include prompting participants about when to perform certain activities (such as when to check a pulse or take vital signs), overseeing the effectiveness of CPR, and keeping track of the time between therapies. Each team member should know what each participant's role is, to prevent duplicating effort. Finally, someone from the team should make sure that the primary nurse's other patients are reassigned to another nurse.

- If the family is at the hospital during the code, have someone, such as a clergy member or social worker, remain with them. Keep the family informed of the patient's status.
- If the family isn't in the hospital, contact them as soon as possible. Encourage them not

ADVANCED EQUIPMENT

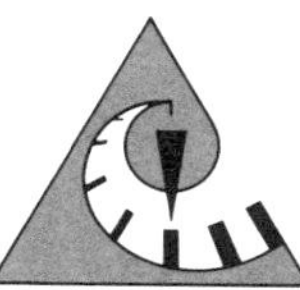

Monitoring end-tidal CO_2

End-tidal carbon dioxide (CO_2) monitoring has proved to be a valuable adjunct to arterial blood gas analysis during advanced cardiac life support (ACLS). If a patient is exhaling a normal amount of CO_2, then you know his lungs are being properly ventilated and his pulmonary circulation is adequately perfused. Without adequate ventilation and perfusion, end-tidal CO_2 values will be low to absent. Research studies have also correlated a rise in exhaled CO_2 with the return of spontaneous circulation in cardiac arrest victims.

To monitor a patient's end-tidal CO_2, attach an end-tidal CO_2 detector between the endotracheal tube and the bag-mask ventilator, as shown.

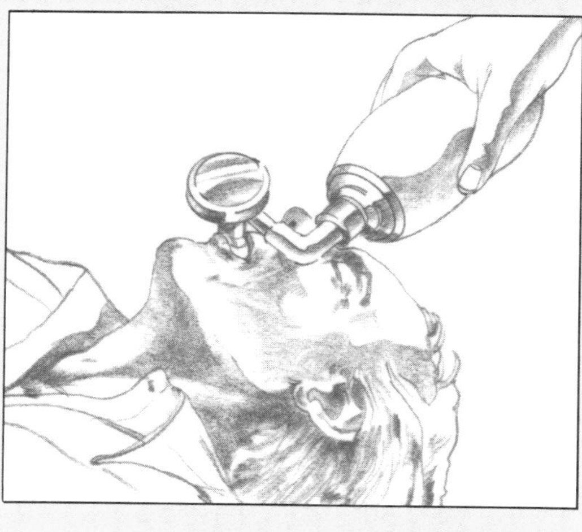

to drive to the hospital, but offer to call someone who can give them a ride.

Monitoring and aftercare

• During the code, document the events in as much detail as possible. Note whether the arrest was witnessed or unwitnessed, the time of the arrest, the time CPR was begun, the time the ACLS-trained nurse arrived, and the total resuscitation time. Also document the number of defibrillations, the times they were performed, the joule level, the patient's cardiac rhythm before and after the defibrillation, and whether or not the patient had a pulse.

• Document all drug therapy, including dosages, routes of administration, and patient response. You'll also want to record all procedures, such as peripheral and central line insertion, pacemaker insertion, and ET tube insertion with the time performed and the patient's tolerance of the procedure. Also keep track of all arterial blood gas results. (See *Monitoring end-tidal CO_2*.)

• Finally, document any complications and the measures taken to correct them. Once your documentation is complete, have the doctor and ACLS nurse review and then sign the document.

• When the patient's condition has stabilized, assess his LOC, breath sounds, heart sounds, peripheral perfusion, bowel sounds, and urine output. Take the patient's vital signs every 15 minutes and continuously monitor his cardiac rhythm.

• Make sure the patient receives an adequate supply of oxygen, whether through a mask or a ventilator.

• Check the infusion rates of all I.V. fluids, and use infusion pumps to deliver vasoactive drugs. So that you can evaluate the effectiveness of fluid therapy, insert an indwelling urinary catheter if the patient doesn't already have one. Also insert an NG tube to relieve or prevent gastric distention.

• If appropriate, reassure the patient and explain what is happening. Allow the patient's family to visit as soon as possible. If the patient dies, notify the family and allow them to see the patient as soon as possible.

• Be sure to document all of your findings. Record whether the patient is transferred to another unit or facility along with the condition of the patient at the time of transfer and whether the family was notified.

• To make sure your code team performs optimally, schedule a time to review the code.

Temporary pacemakers

Usually inserted in an emergency, a temporary pacemaker consists of an external battery-powered pulse generator and a lead or electrode system. Four types of temporary pacemakers exist: transcutaneous, transvenous, transthoracic, and epicardial.

In a life-threatening situation, when time is critical, a *transcutaneous pacemaker* is the best choice. This device works by sending an electrical impulse from the pulse generator to the patient's heart by way of two electrodes, which are placed on the front and back of the patient's chest. Transcutaneous pacing is quick and effective, but it's only used until the doctor can institute transvenous pacing.

Besides being more comfortable for the patient, a *transvenous pacemaker* is more reliable than a transcutaneous pacemaker. Transvenous pacing involves threading an electrode catheter through a vein into the patient's right atrium or right ventricle. The electrode then attaches to an external pulse generator. As a result, the pulse generator can provide an electrical stimulus directly to the endocardium. This is the most common type of pacemaker.

As an elective surgical procedure or as an emergency measure during CPR, a doctor may choose to insert a *transthoracic pacemaker.* To insert this type of pacemaker, the doctor performs a procedure similar to a pericardiocentesis, in which he uses a cardiac needle to pass an electrode through the chest wall and into the right ventricle. This procedure carries a significant risk of coronary artery laceration and cardiac tamponade.

During cardiac surgery, the surgeon may insert electrodes through the epicardium of the right ventricle and, if he wants to institute atrioventricular sequential pacing, the right atrium. From there, the electrodes pass through the chest wall, where they remain available if temporary pacing becomes necessary. This is called *epicardial pacing.*

Besides helping to correct conduction disturbances, a temporary pacemaker may help diagnose conduction abnormalities. For example, during a cardiac catheterization or electrophysiology study, a doctor may use a temporary pacemaker to localize conduction defects. In the process, he may also learn whether the patient risks developing an arrhythmia.

Indications

- Symptomatic bradycardia
- Tachyarrhythmias
- Electrolyte disturbances
- Digoxin or barbiturate overdose
- Diagnostic procedures to localize conduction defects

Contraindications and complications

Among the contraindications to pacemaker therapy are electromechanical dissociation and ventricular fibrillation.

Complications associated with pacemaker therapy include microshock, equipment failure, and competitive or fatal arrhythmias. *Transcutaneous pacemakers* may also cause skin breakdown and muscle pain and twitching when the pacemaker fires. *Transvenous pacemakers* may cause such complications as pneumothorax or hemothorax, cardiac perforation and tamponade, diaphragmatic stimulation, pulmonary embolism, thrombophlebitis, and infection. Also, if the doctor threads the electrode through the antecubital or femoral vein, venous spasm, thrombophlebitis, or lead displacement may result.

Complications of *transthoracic pacemakers* include pneumothorax, cardiac tamponade, emboli, sepsis, lacerations of the myocardium or coronary artery, and perforations of a cardiac chamber. *Epicardial pacemakers* carry a risk of infection, cardiac arrest, and diaphragmatic stimulation.

Equipment

Gather the equipment you'll need, depending on the device you're using.

Transcutaneous pacemaker

Transcutaneous pacing generator • transcutaneous pacing electrodes • cardiac monitor

Other temporary pacemakers

Temporary pacemaker generator with new battery • guide wire or introducer • electrode catheter • sterile gloves • sterile dressings • adhesive tape • povidone-iodine solution • nonconducting tape or rubber surgical glove • pouch for external pulse generator • emergency cardiac drugs • intubation equipment • defibrillator • cardiac monitor with strip-chart recorder • equipment to start a peripheral I.V. line, if appropriate • I.V. fluids • sedative • optional: elastic bandage or gauze strips, restraints

Transvenous pacemaker
(In addition to equipment listed for temporary pacemakers) bridging cable • percutaneous introducer tray or venous cutdown tray • sterile gowns • linen-saver pad • antimicrobial soap • alcohol sponges • vial of 1% lidocaine • 5-ml syringe • fluoroscopy equipment, if necessary • fenestrated drape • prepackaged cutdown tray (for antecubital vein placement only) • sutures • receptacle for infectious wastes

Transthoracic pacemaker
(In addition to equipment listed for temporary pacemakers) transthoracic/cardiac needle

Epicardial pacemaker
(In addition to equipment listed for temporary pacemakers) atrial epicardial wires • ventricular epicardial wires • sterile dressing materials (if the wires won't be connected to a pulse generator)

Preparation

For all temporary pacing, explain the procedure to the patient and his family. Ideally, the doctor will first explain the benefits and risks of the procedure and obtain the patient's written consent. In an emergency, however, this may not be possible. Regardless, keep the patient informed throughout the process of pacemaker insertion and tell his family when the patient's condition stabilizes.

You should be familiar with pacemaker polarity. For current to flow between the pulse generator and the heart, a pacemaker electrode must have a negative pole as well as a positive pole. The negative pole paces while the positive pole serves as the ground. There are two types of pacing electrodes: bipolar and unipolar.

Most pacing electrodes are bipolar, meaning that the internal electrode contains both poles. The tip of the electrode contains the negative pole; an exposed metal ring about 1" (2.5 cm) away contains the positive pole. When preparing to pace a patient, you'll attach the distal negative electrode wire to the negative terminal on the pulse generator. The current will then flow from the generator to the negative pole in the endocardium, then back to the proximal positive pole (ground) on the generator to complete the electrical circuit.

A bipolar electrode provides good contact with endocardial tissue. It produces short pacing spikes because the two poles are so close together.

Unipolar electrodes usually are reserved for permanent pacemakers, although some temporary pacemakers have one. The unipolar electrode gets its name from the single pole—the negative one—embedded in its tip. This pole both senses and stimulates electrical activity. The positive pole, or ground, is outside the heart.

Unipolar electrodes produce tall pacing spikes because of the distance between the two poles. Because of the electrode's large surface area, it is particularly sensitive to the patient's intrinsic rhythm.

Transcutaneous pacemaker
If necessary, clip the hair over the areas of electrode placement. However, don't shave the area. If you nick the skin, the current from the pulse generator could cause discomfort. Also, the nicks could become irritated or infected after the electrodes are applied.

Transvenous pacemaker
Check the patient's history for hypersensitivity to local anesthetics. Then, attach the cardiac monitor to the patient and obtain a baseline assessment, including vital signs, skin color, LOC, heart rate and rhythm, and the patient's emotional state. Next, insert a peripheral I.V. line if the patient doesn't already have one. Then begin an I.V. infusion of D_5W at a keep-vein-open rate.

Next, insert a new battery into the external pacemaker generator and then test it to make sure it has a strong charge. Connect the bridging cable to the generator, and align the positive and negative poles. This cable allows slack between the electrode catheter and the generator, reducing the risk of accidental catheter displacement.

Then place the patient in the supine position. If necessary, clip the hair around the insertion site. Next, open the supply tray while maintaining a sterile field. Using sterile technique, clean the insertion site with antimicrobial soap and then wipe the area with povidone-iodine solution. Cover the insertion site with a fenestrated drape. Because fluoroscopy may be used during the placement of leadwires, put on a protective apron.

Transthoracic pacemaker

Clean the skin to the left of the xiphoid process with povidone-iodine solution. Work quickly because CPR must be interrupted for the procedure.

Epicardial pacemaker

Because epicardial pacemaker wires may be placed during cardiac surgery, inform the patient about this possibility during your preoperative teaching.

Essential steps

The steps for pacemaker insertion vary with the type of pacemaker being inserted.

Transcutaneous pacemaker

- Attach monitoring electrodes to the patient in lead I, II, or III position. Do this even if the patient is already on telemetry monitoring because you'll need to connect the electrodes to the pacemaker. If you select the lead II position, adjust the LL electrode placement to accommodate the anterior pacing electrode and the patient's anatomy.
- Plug the patient cable into the ECG input connection on the front of the pacing generator. Set the selector switch to the MONITOR ON position.
- You should see the ECG waveform on the monitor. Adjust the R-wave beeper volume to a suitable level and activate the alarm by pressing the ALARM ON button. Set the alarm for 10 to 20 beats lower and 20 to 30 beats higher than the intrinsic rate.
- Press the START/STOP button for a printout of the waveform.
- Now you're ready to apply the two pacing electrodes. First, to ensure good skin contact, make sure the patient's skin is clean and dry.
- Pull off the protective strip from the posterior electrode (marked BACK) and apply the electrode on the left side of the back, just below the scapula and to the left of the spine.
- The anterior pacing electrode (marked FRONT) has two protective strips — one covering the jellied area and one covering the outer rim. Expose the jellied area and apply it to the skin in the anterior position — to the left side of the precordium in the usual V_2 to V_5 position. Move this electrode around to get the best waveform. Then expose the electrode's outer rim and firmly press it to the skin. (See *Proper electrode placement,* page 24.)
- Now you're ready to pace the heart. After making sure the energy output in milliamperes (mA) is on 0, connect the electrode cable to the monitor output cable.
- Check the waveform; look for a tall QRS complex in lead II.
- Next, turn the selector switch to PACER ON. Tell the patient that he may feel a thumping or twitching sensation. Reassure him that you'll give him medication if he can't tolerate the discomfort.
- Now set the rate dial to 10 to 20 beats higher than the patient's intrinsic rhythm. Look for pacer artifact or spikes, which will appear as you increase the rate. If the patient doesn't have an intrinsic rhythm, set the rate at 60.
- Slowly increase the amount of energy delivered to the heart by adjusting the OUTPUT MA dial. Do this until capture is achieved — you'll see a pacer spike followed by a widened QRS complex that resembles a premature ventricular contraction. This is the pacing threshold. To ensure consistent capture, increase output by 10%. But don't go any higher because you'd cause the patient needless discomfort.
- With full capture, the patient's heart rate should be approximately the same as the pacemaker rate set on the machine. The usual pacing threshold is between 40 and 80 mA.

Proper electrode placement

Place the electrodes for a noninvasive temporary pacemaker at heart level, with the heart lying between the two electrodes. This placement ensures the shortest distance the electrical stimulus must travel to the heart.

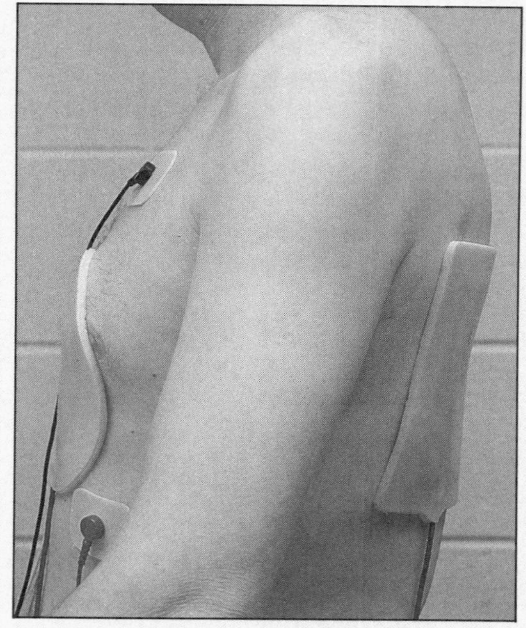

Transvenous pacemaker

• Provide the doctor with the local anesthetic.
• After anesthetizing the insertion site, the doctor will puncture the brachial, femoral, subclavian, or jugular vein. Then he'll insert a guide wire or an introducer and advance the electrode catheter.
• As the catheter advances, watch the cardiac monitor. When the electrode catheter reaches the right atrium, you'll notice large P waves and small QRS complexes. Then, as the catheter reaches the right ventricle, the P waves will become smaller while the QRS complexes enlarge. When the catheter touches the right ventricular endocardium, expect to see elevated ST segments or premature ventricular contractions, or both.
• Once in the right ventricle, the electrode catheter will send an impulse to the myocardium, causing depolarization. If the patient needs atrial pacing, either alone or with ventricular pacing, the doctor may place an electrode in the right atrium.
• Meanwhile, continuously monitor the patient's cardiac status and treat any arrhythmias as appropriate. Also assess the patient for jaw pain and earache, symptoms indicating that the electrode catheter has missed the superior vena cava and has moved into the neck instead.
• Once the electrode catheter is in place, attach the catheter leads to the bridging cable, lining up the positive and negative poles.
• Check the battery's charge by pressing the BATTERY TEST button.
• Set the pacemaker as ordered. (See *Using a temporary pacemaker.*)
• The doctor will then suture the catheter to the insertion site. Afterward, put on sterile gloves and apply a sterile dressing to the site. Label the dressing with the date and time of application.

Transthoracic pacemaker

• After interrupting CPR, the doctor will insert a transthoracic needle through the patient's chest wall to the left of the xiphoid process into the right ventricle. He'll then follow the needle with the electrode catheter.
• Connect the electrode catheter to the generator, lining up the positive and negative poles. Watch the cardiac monitor for signs of ventricular pacing and capture.
• After the doctor sutures the electrode catheter into place, use sterile technique to apply a sterile 4" × 4" gauze dressing to the site. Tape the dressing securely, and label it with the date and time of application.
• Check the patient's peripheral pulses and vital signs to assess cardiac output. If you can't palpate a pulse, continue performing CPR.
• If the patient has a palpable pulse, assess the patient's vital signs, ECG, and LOC.

ADVANCED EQUIPMENT

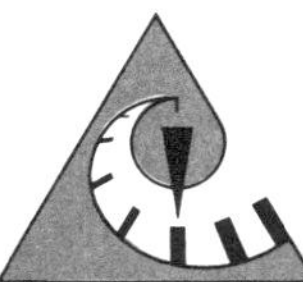

Using a temporary pacemaker

After attaching a pacemaker to a patient, you'll first adjust the rate dial as ordered by the doctor. The patient's underlying rhythm determines the rate. Typically, you'll set the rate for at least 60 beats/minute to ensure adequate cardiac output.

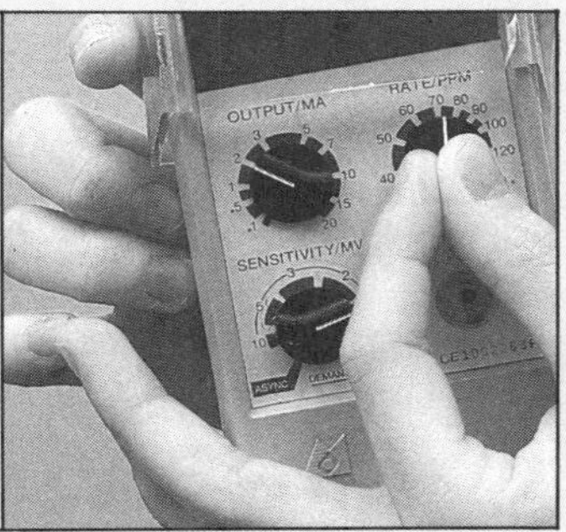

If the doctor orders and your hospital's protocol permits, you'll need to measure the pacing threshold: the minimum amount of energy (measured in milliamperes [mA]) that will stimulate an electrical response (P wave or QRS complex) in the heart. The pace indicator should flash each time you see a pacemaker spike on the electrocardiogram (ECG).

To measure pacing threshold, first verify 1:1 capture (a QRS complex for every pacemaker spike) on the ECG. If the patient is already 100% paced, gradually decrease the milliamperes by turning the dial counterclockwise until you no longer see a wide QRS complex after the pacemaker spike. That means 1:1 capture is lost. If the patient's intrinsic rhythm is greater than the rate set on the pulse generator (overriding the pacemaker), you'll first have to increase the rate to about 10 beats above the patient's rate to obtain a paced rhythm. Otherwise, you won't see any changes on the ECG.

Next, increase the milliamperes slowly by turning the dial clockwise to find the point at which capture is achieved. This is the pacing threshold. Reset the output/milliamperes control to two or three times this threshold. Then, document the threshold in your nurses' notes. A reliable pacemaker position will have a threshold of 2 mA or less.

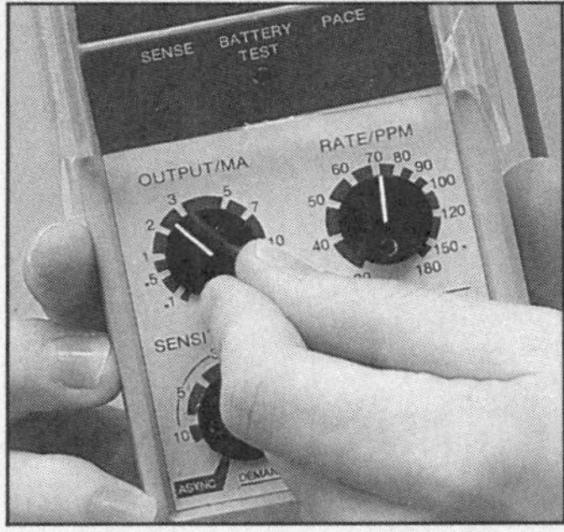

Now, consider the sensitivity threshold, which is the amount of millivolts (mV) needed to inhibit the pacemaker from firing. The higher numbers represent less-sensitive settings (fixed-rate, or asynchronous, mode). At the lowest sensitivity, the pacemaker will ignore intrinsic heart activity and pace at a fixed rate. At the greatest sensitivity—or lowest numbers—the pacemaker may interpret a small amount of voltage as heart activity (demand mode).

If hospital protocol allows you to determine the sensitivity threshold, set the rate control at least 10 impulses/minute below the patient's intrinsic rate. Turn the sensitivity dial clockwise to the most sensitive position (1.5 mV) and set the output control at 5 mA to ensure capture. Watch the ECG waveform; at these settings, the pacemaker should stop pacing and the sense indicator should start flashing as the pacemaker senses naturally occurring R waves.

Next, slowly move the sensitivity dial counterclockwise (which will decrease the pacemaker's ability to sense the patient's R waves) until the pacemaker begins firing pacing stimuli and the pace indicator begins flashing. Then, turn the dial clockwise again (which will increase the pacemaker's ability to detect an R wave). The sense indicator should start to flash. This is the sensitivity threshold, in millivolts.

Reset the sensitivity control so that it's two or three times more sensitive than the sensitivity threshold level. For example, if the sensitivity threshold is 6 mV, you'll set it on 2 mV. The pacemaker will then be more sensitive to a smaller amount of current. If the rate has been changed, remember to return it to the ordered rate and to document the sensitivity threshold in your notes.

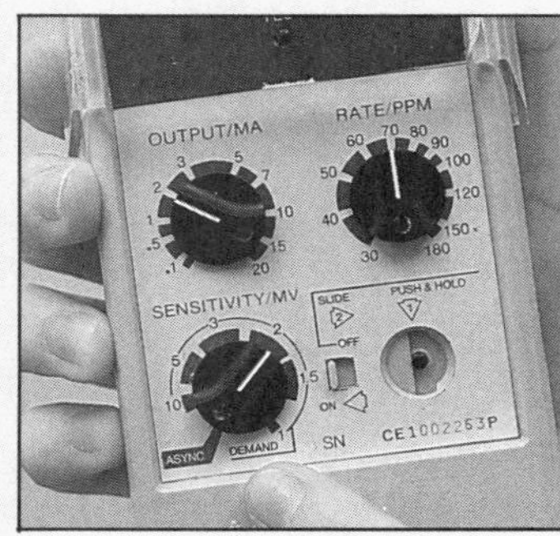

SKILL TIP

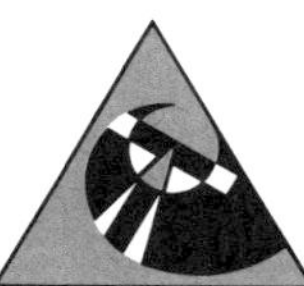

Preventing microshock

One of your primary goals with a patient is preventing injury. But it's especially important when the patient has a temporary pacemaker because he's at risk for microshock—minute electrical charges delivered to the heart through the pacing electrode. These charges can't be felt, but they can cause lethal ventricular fibrillation if delivered straight to the heart. Here's how you can prevent microshock:

- Protect the tips of the epicardial pacing electrode wires by covering them with finger cots or gloves if they aren't connected to the pulse generator. You could also insert them into plastic foam or needle caps.
- Wear gloves whenever you're touching the uninsulated ends of the pacing electrodes.
- Keep the dressing dry and intact.
- Make sure a defibrillator is close by when the pacemaker wire is inserted or connected to lead V of the electrocardiograph. The pacemaker lead may trigger ventricular ectopy or fibrillation.
- Do not let ungrounded, unchecked electrical equipment come in contact with the patient or be used in the immediate area of the patient (such as touching the patient's own radio).
- Do not forget to touch a grounded area when entering the patient's room. This will discharge static electricity before you touch the patient or lean against his bed.

Epicardial pacemaker

- During cardiac surgery, the doctor will hook epicardial wires into the epicardium just before the end of the surgery. Depending on the patient's condition, the doctor may insert either atrial or ventricular wires, or both.
- If indicated, connect the electrode catheter to the generator, lining up the positive and negative poles. Set the pacemaker as ordered.
- If the wires won't be connected to an external pulse generator, place them in a sterile rubber finger cot. Then cover both the wires and the insertion site with a sterile, occlusive dressing. This will help protect the patient from microshock as well as infection.

Cautions

Closely monitor the sensitivity setting on the pulse generator. Excessive sensitivity may cause the pulse generator to interpret P or T waves as QRS complexes and fail to pace. On the other hand, insufficient sensitivity may cause the generator to deliver a pacing stimulus at the wrong time, resulting in a lethal arrhythmia.

You'll also need to take care to prevent microshock. This includes warning the patient not to use any electrical equipment that isn't grounded, such as telephones, electric shavers, televisions, or lamps. (See *Preventing microshock*.)

Other safety measures you'll want to take include placing a plastic cover supplied by the manufacturer over the pacemaker controls to avoid an accidental setting change. Also, insulate the pacemaker by covering all exposed metal parts, such as electrode connections and pacemaker terminals, with nonconducting tape, or place the pacing unit in a dry, rubber surgical glove. If the patient is disoriented or uncooperative, use restraints to prevent accidental removal of pacemaker wires. If the patient needs emergency defibrillation, make sure the pacemaker can withstand the procedure. If unsure, disconnect the pulse generator to avoid damage.

When using a *transcutaneous pacemaker,* don't place the electrodes over a bony area because bone conducts current poorly. Keep in mind that, if the patient is diaphoretic, you'll need to change the electrodes frequently. Also, with female patients, place the anterior electrode under the patient's breast but not over her diaphragm. Placing the electrode over the diaphragm could cause the diaphragm to be paced, resulting in shortness of breath and increased patient anxiety.

During insertion of a *transvenous pacemaker,* expect to see temporary ventricular ectopy or tachyarrhythmias. Treat these arrhythmias, as indicated, with lidocaine. If bradyarrhythmias occur, administer atropine. If the doctor inserts the electrode through the brachial or femoral vein, immobilize the patient's arm or leg to avoid putting stress on the pacing wires.

Monitoring and aftercare

- After insertion of any temporary pacemaker, assess the patient's vital signs, skin color, LOC, and peripheral pulses to determine the effectiveness of the paced rhythm.
- Perform a 12-lead ECG to serve as a baseline, and then perform additional ECGs daily or with clinical changes. Also, if possible, obtain a rhythm strip before, during, and after pacemaker placement; anytime pacemaker settings are changed; and whenever the patient receives treatment because of a complication caused by the pacemaker.
- Continuously monitor the ECG reading, noting capture, sensing, rate, intrinsic beats, and competition of paced and intrinsic rhythms. If the pacemaker is sensing correctly, the sense indicator on the pulse generator should flash with each beat. (See *When a temporary pacemaker malfunctions,* page 28.)
- Record the date and time of pacemaker insertion, the type of pacemaker, the reason for insertion, and the patient's response. Note the pacemaker settings. Document any complications and the interventions taken.
- Also monitor all patients for signs and symptoms of infection, including redness and drainage at the insertion site, malaise, chills, and an increased white blood cell count. To help prevent infection, maintain sterile technique when changing the dressing.
- If the patient has received a transvenous or transthoracic pacemaker, secure the pulse generator to the patient's chest, waist, or upper arm with a strap or pacemaker pouch. Then arrange for a chest X-ray to check electrode placement and to rule out pneumothorax.
- Check pacemaker sensitivity and threshold every 8 hours.
- Also change the pacemaker's battery every 2 to 3 days if the pulse generator is being used continuously. After inserting new batteries, write the date and time on a piece of adhesive tape and attach it to the back of the pulse generator.
- If the patient has a transcutaneous pacemaker, record the reason for transcutaneous pacing, the time the pacing was started, and the locations of the electrodes.
- Every 1 to 2 hours, check to make sure the electrodes are firmly attached to the patient's chest. Poor electrode adherence may interfere with pacing. If the patient complains of pain with pacing, set the mA at the lowest possible setting and administer diazepam or oxazepam if necessary. However, if the patient is large, muscular, or obese, a higher mA setting may be necessary.
- Be aware that, because of muscle stimulation, patients with a transcutaneous pacemaker may have a falsely elevated blood pressure in the left arm. This typically occurs in patients who are asystolic and who are receiving 100 mA. To avoid falsely elevated readings, measure blood pressures in the patient's right arm.
- If the patient has epicardial pacing wires in place, clean the insertion site with povidone-iodine solution and change the dressing daily. At the same time, monitor the site for signs of infection. Always keep the pulse generator nearby in case pacing becomes necessary.
- Be aware that, over time, epicardial wires tend to lose their effectiveness. That's because, as the patient becomes mobile, the wires may pull away from the epicardium. What's more, the tissue at the site of electrode attachment becomes fibrotic over time, requiring higher output settings if pacing becomes necessary. After you remove epicardial wires, monitor the patient for cardiac tamponade for 24 hours.

Defibrillation

The standard treatment for ventricular fibrillation, defibrillation involves using electrode paddles to direct an electric current through the patient's heart. The current causes the myocardium to depolarize which, in turn, encourages the sinoatrial (SA) node to resume control of the heart's electrical activity. The electrode paddles delivering the current may be placed on the patient's chest or, during cardiac surgery, directly on the myocardium.

Because ventricular fibrillation will lead to death if not corrected, the success of defibrillation depends on the early recognition and quick treatment of this arrhythmia. Besides treating ventricular fibrillation, defibrillation may

TROUBLESHOOTING

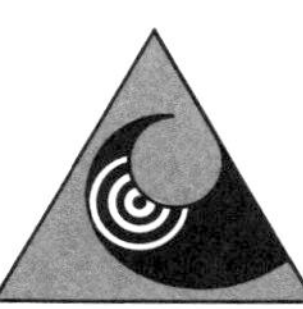

When a temporary pacemaker malfunctions

On occasion, a temporary pacemaker may fail to function appropriately. When this occurs, you'll need to take immediate action to correct the problem. Study the following chart to learn which steps to take when your patient's pacemaker malfunctions.

Failure to pace

This happens when the pacemaker either doesn't fire or fires too often. The pulse generator may not be working properly, or it may not be conducting the impulse to the patient.

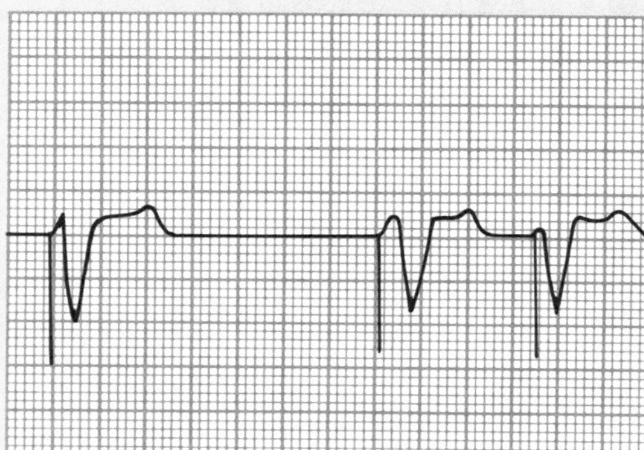

Nursing interventions

- If the pacing or sensing indicator flashes, check the connections to the cable and the position of the pacing electrode in the patient (by X-ray). The cable may have come loose, or the electrode may have been dislodged, pulled out, or broken.
- If the pulse generator is turned on but the indicators still aren't flashing, change the battery. If that doesn't help, use a different pulse generator.
- Check the settings if the pacemaker is firing too rapidly. If they're correct, or if altering them (according to hospital policy or the doctor's order) doesn't help, change the pulse generator.

Failure to capture

Here, you see pacemaker spikes but the heart isn't responding. This may be caused by changes in the pacing threshold from ischemia, an electrolyte imbalance (high or low potassium or magnesium), acidosis, an adverse reaction to a medication, a perforated ventricle, fibrosis, or the position of the electrode.

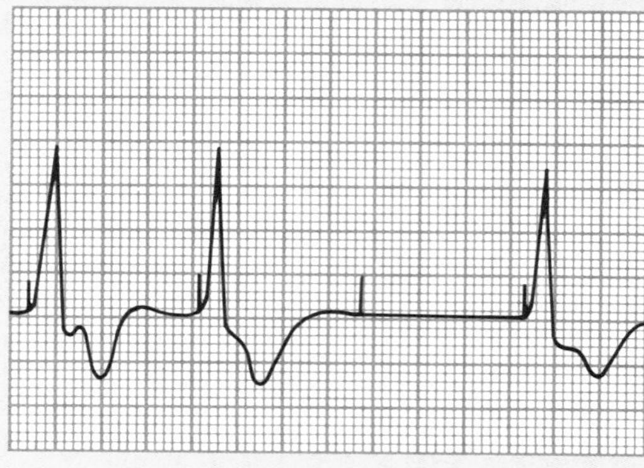

Nursing interventions

- If the patient's condition has changed, notify the doctor and ask him for new settings.
- If pacemaker settings are altered by the patient or others, return them to their correct positions. Then make sure the face of the pacemaker is covered with a plastic shield. Also, tell the patient or others not to touch the dials.
- If the heart is not responding, try any or all of these suggestions: Carefully check all connections; increase the milliamperes slowly (according to hospital protocol or the doctor's order); turn the patient on his left side, then on his right (if turning him to the left didn't help); reverse the cable in the pulse generator so the positive electrode wire is in the negative terminal and the negative electrode wire is in the positive terminal; schedule an anteroposterior or lateral chest X-ray to determine the position of the electrode.

TROUBLESHOOTING

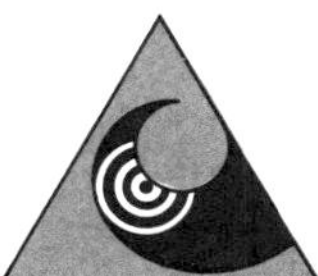

When a temporary pacemaker malfunctions *(continued)*

Failure to sense intrinsic beats

This could cause ventricular tachycardia or ventricular fibrillation if the pacemaker fires on the vulnerable T wave. This could be caused by the pacemaker sensing an external stimulus as a QRS complex, which could lead to asystole, or by the pacemaker not being sensitive enough, which means it could fire anywhere within the cardiac cycle.

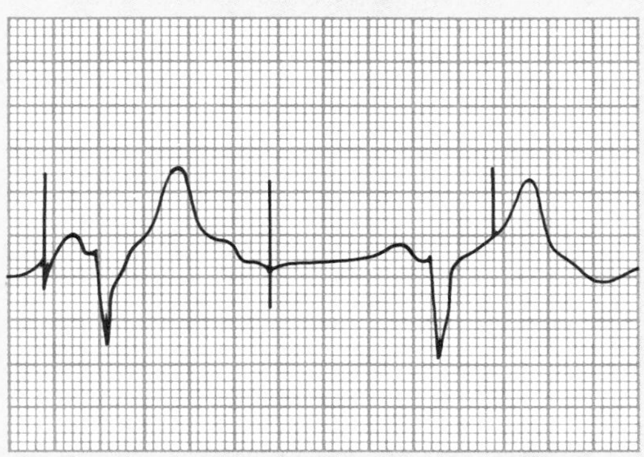

Nursing interventions

- If the pacemaker is undersensing, turn the sensitivity control completely to the right. If it's oversensing, turn it slightly to the left.
- If the pacemaker isn't functioning correctly, change the battery or the pulse generator.
- Remove things in the room causing electromechanical interference (razors, radios, cautery, and so on). Check the ground wires on the bed and other equipment for obvious damage. Unplug each piece and see if the interference stops. When you locate the cause, notify the hospital engineer and ask him to check it.
- If the pacemaker is still firing on the T wave and all else has failed, turn off the pacemaker. Make sure atropine is available in case the patient's heart rate drops. Be prepared to call a code and institute CPR if necessary.

also be used to treat ventricular tachycardia that doesn't produce a pulse.

Indications

- Ventricular fibrillation
- Ventricular tachycardia (without a pulse)

Contraindications and complications

Unless the patient has a no-code order or advance directive, defibrillation has no contraindications. The procedure, however, can cause accidental electric shock to those providing care. To avoid this, make sure that no one is touching the bed or the patient when defibrillation is performed.

To also help avoid accidental electric shock, clear paddles that have been charged but won't be used. Do this by turning the machine off, adjusting the energy selector dial, or by placing the paddles into their protective housing and discharging them into the machine. Never discharge paddles against each other or into the air.

Skin burns, which usually result from an insufficient amount of conductive medium, are another common complication.

Equipment

Defibrillator • external paddles • internal paddles (sterilized for cardiac surgery) • conductive medium pads • ECG monitor with recorder • oxygen therapy equipment • hand-held resuscitation bag • airway equipment • emergency pacing equipment • emergency cardiac medications

Preparation

Assess the patient to determine the lack of a pulse. Call for help, and perform CPR until the defibrillator and emergency equipment arrive.

Placing defibrillator paddles correctly

When positioning defibrillator paddles, place one paddle to the right of the upper sternum, just below the right clavicle. Place the other paddle at the fifth or sixth intercostal space in the left anterior axillary line. This position is known as the standard or anterolateral position.

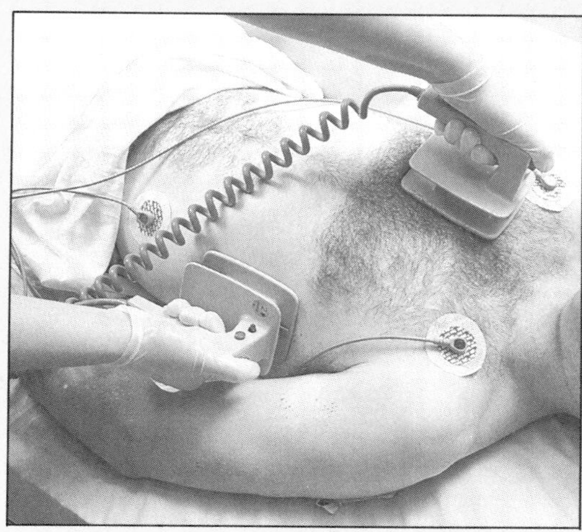

Essential steps

• If the defibrillator has "quick look" capability, place the paddles on the patient's chest to quickly view the cardiac rhythm. Otherwise, connect the monitoring leads of the defibrillator to the patient and assess the patient's cardiac rhythm.
• Expose the patient's chest and apply conductive pads at the paddle placement positions. (See *Placing defibrillator paddles correctly.*)
• Turn on the defibrillator and, if performing external defibrillation, set the energy level for 200 joules for an adult patient.
• Charge the paddles by pressing the charge buttons, located either on the machine or on the paddles themselves.
• Place the paddles over the conductive pads and press firmly against the patient's chest, using 25 lb of pressure.
• Reassess the patient's cardiac rhythm.
• If the patient remains in ventricular fibrillation or pulseless ventricular tachycardia, instruct all personnel to stand clear of the patient and the bed.
• Discharge the current by pressing both paddle charge buttons simultaneously.
• Leaving the paddles in position on the patient's chest, reassess the patient's cardiac rhythm and have someone else assess the pulse.
• If necessary, prepare to defibrillate a second time. Instruct someone to reset the energy level on the defibrillator to 200 to 300 joules. Announce that you are preparing to defibrillate, and follow the procedure as described above.
• Reassess the patient. If defibrillation is again necessary, instruct someone to reset the energy level to 360 joules. Then follow the same procedure as before.
• Perform the three countershocks in rapid succession, reassessing the patient's rhythm before each defibrillation.

Cautions

Before defibrillation, disconnect any telemetry or bedside monitors to prevent the electric shock from damaging those units. During defibrillation, don't lean on the paddles. Doing so may cause them to slip out of position.

Monitoring and aftercare

• If the patient remains without a pulse after three initial defibrillations, resume CPR, give supplemental oxygen, and begin administering appropriate medications, such as epinephrine. Also consider possible causes for failure of the patient's rhythm to convert, such as acidosis or hypoxia.
• If defibrillation restores a normal rhythm, check the patient's central and peripheral pulses and obtain a blood pressure reading, heart rate, and respiratory rate. Assess the patient's LOC, cardiac rhythm, breath sounds, skin color, and urine output. Obtain baseline blood gases and a 12-lead ECG. Provide supplemental oxygen, ventilation, and medications, as needed. Check the patient's chest for electrical burns and treat them, as ordered, with

ADVANCED EQUIPMENT

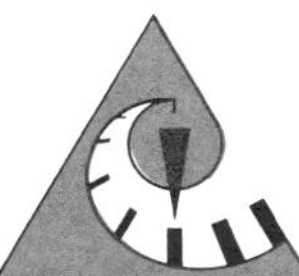

Understanding the AICD

An automatic implantable cardioverter defibrillator (AICD) has a pulse generator and lead systems to monitor the heart's activity and deliver shocks as necessary. It's useful for patients who have survived at least one episode of sudden cardiac death resulting from ventricular tachycardia or ventricular fibrillation, but not associated with an acute myocardial infarction. The device can also help patients who have had recurrent, life-threatening ventricular arrhythmias that don't respond to conventional drug therapy.

To insert the AICD, the surgeon will first position a bipolar lead transvenously in the endocardium of the right ventricle. Or he may place two leads 3/8" (1 cm) apart on the epicardium of the left ventricle. These leads record the heart rate.

The shocks are delivered by two patch leads sewn onto the heart as shown or by one patch lead and a lead (not shown) placed in the right atrium via the superior vena cava.

These devices can be programmed to fire during any type of tachyarrhythmia, such as supraventricular tachycardia or a nonmalignant wide-complex arrhythmia.

External defibrillation can be safely performed on these patients without damaging the device. However, try to avoid placing the paddles directly over the AICD.

The AICD is usually used in conjunction with drug therapy. Antiarrhythmics actually keep the patient's heart rhythm within the AICD's programmed parameters.

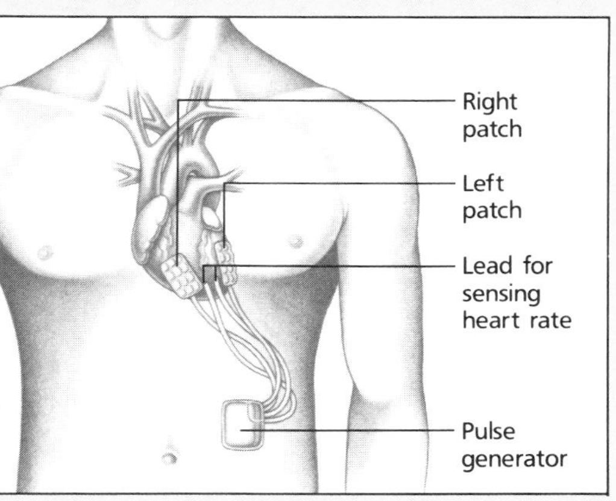

corticosteroid or lanolin-based creams. Also prepare the defibrillator for immediate reuse.

• Document the procedure, including the patient's predefibrillation and postdefibrillation ECG rhythms; the number of times defibrillation was performed; the voltage used with each attempt; whether a pulse returned; the dosage, route, and time of administration of medications; whether CPR was used; how the airway was maintained; and the patient's outcome. (See *Understanding the AICD.*)

Synchronized cardioversion

Used to treat tachyarrhythmias, cardioversion delivers an electrical charge to the myocardium at the peak of the R wave. This causes immediate depolarization, interrupting reentry circuits and allowing the SA node to resume control. Synchronizing the electrical charge with the R wave ensures that the current won't be delivered on the vulnerable T wave and thus disrupt repolarization.

Synchronized cardioversion is the treatment of choice for arrhythmias, such as atrial tachycardia, atrial flutter, atrial fibrillation, and symptomatic ventricular tachycardia that don't respond to vagal massage or drug therapy.

Cardioversion may be an elective or urgent procedure, depending on how well the patient tolerates the arrhythmia. For example, if the patient is hemodynamically unstable, he would require urgent cardioversion. Remember that, when preparing for cardioversion, the patient's condition can deteriorate quickly, necessitating immediate defibrillation.

Indications

- Stable paroxysmal atrial tachycardia
- Unstable paroxysmal supraventricular tachycardia
- Atrial fibrillation
- Atrial flutter
- Ventricular tachycardia

Contraindications and complications

Cardioversion enhances the effects of digitalis and may result in lethal arrhythmias. Patients on maintenance doses of digitalis usually have the dose withheld 24 hours prior to elective cardioversion. Urgent cardioversion is usually not indicated for digitalis toxicity arrhythmias. However, if the doctor decides to use cardioversion with digitalis toxicity, he premedicates the patient with lidocaine. Hypokalemia and hypomagnesemia may also cause arrhythmias after cardioversion, making these conditions further contraindications.

Common complications following cardioversion include transient, harmless arrhythmias such as atrial, ventricular, and junctional premature beats. Serious ventricular arrhythmias such as ventricular fibrillation may also occur. However, this type of arrhythmia is more likely to result from high amounts of electrical energy, digitalis toxicity, severe heart disease, electrolyte imbalance, or improper synchronization with the R wave.

Patients with mitral or aortic valve disease or left ventricular dysfunction may develop pulmonary edema after cardioversion. Also, 1.2% to 1.5% of the patients receiving cardioversion for atrial fibrillation suffer systemic embolization following the procedure. This complication can be minimized if the patient receives anticoagulant therapy.

Although rare, patients may also suffer unexplained hypotension that lasts for hours and then spontaneously resolves. Other complications include skin burns because of insufficient conductive medium and respiratory depression because of oversedation.

Equipment

Cardioverter/defibrillator • conductive medium pads • anterior, posterior, or transverse paddles • ECG monitor with recorder • sedative • oxygen therapy equipment • airway • hand-held resuscitation bag • emergency pacing equipment • emergency cardiac medications • automatic blood pressure cuff (if available) • pulse oximeter (if available)

Preparation

Explain the procedure to the patient, and make sure he has signed a consent form. Check the patient's recent serum potassium and magnesium levels and arterial blood gas results. Also check recent digoxin levels. Although digitalized patients may undergo cardioversion, they tend to require lower energy levels to convert. If the patient takes digoxin, withhold the dose the day of the procedure.

Withhold all food and fluids for 6 to 12 hours before the procedure. If the cardioversion is urgent, withhold the previous meal. Obtain a 12-lead ECG to serve as a baseline. Check to see if the doctor has ordered administration of any cardiac drugs before the procedure. Also verify that the patient has a patent I.V. site in case drug administration becomes necessary. Connect the patient to a pulse oximeter and automatic blood pressure cuff, if available. Consider administering oxygen for 5 to 10 minutes before the cardioversion to promote myocardial oxygenation. If the patient wears dentures, evaluate whether they support the patient's airway or may cause an airway obstruction. If they may cause an obstruction, remove them.

Place the patient in the supine position and assess his vital signs, LOC, cardiac rhythm, and peripheral pulses. Remove any oxygen delivery device just before cardioversion to avoid possible combustion. Have epinephrine, lidocaine, and atropine at the patient's bedside.

Essential steps

- Administer a sedative, as ordered. The patient should be heavily sedated but still able to breathe adequately.
- Carefully monitor the patient's blood pressure and respiratory rate until he recovers.
- Press the POWER button to turn on the defibrillator. Next, push the SYNC button to synchronize the machine with the patient's QRS complexes. Make sure the SYNC button flashes with each of the patient's QRS complexes. You should also see a bright green flag flash on the monitor.
- Turn the energy SELECT dial to the ordered amount of energy. ACLS protocols call for 50 to 360 joules for a patient with stable paroxysmal atrial tachycardia; 75 to 360 joules for a patient with unstable paroxysmal supraventricular tachycardia; 100 joules for a patient with atrial fibrillation; 50 joules for a patient with atrial flutter; 100 to 360 joules for a patient who has ventricular tachycardia with a pulse; and 200 to 360 joules for a patient with ventricular tachycardia with no pulse.
- Remove the paddles from the machine and prepare them as you would if you were defibrillating the patient. Place the conductive gel pads or paddles in the same positions as you would to defibrillate.
- Make sure everyone is away from the bed; then, push the discharge buttons. Hold the paddles in place and wait for the energy to be discharged—the machine has to synchronize the discharge with the QRS complex.
- Check the waveform on the monitor. If the arrhythmia fails to convert, repeat the procedure two or three more times at 3-minute intervals. Gradually increase the energy level with each additional countershock.

Cautions

If the patient is attached to a bedside monitor or telemetry, disconnect the units before cardioversion. The electric current it generates could damage the equipment.

Be aware that improper synchronization may result if the patient's ECG tracing contains artifact-like spikes, such as peaked T waves or bundle-branch blocks when the R′ wave may be taller than the R wave.

Although cardioversion is not recommended for patients with digitalis toxicity, it may, at times, be necessary. If so, administer a bolus of 50 to 100 mg of lidocaine immediately before cardioversion.

If the patient develops ventricular fibrillation or ventricular tachycardia and doesn't have a pulse, turn off the synchronizer switch on the cardioverter and defibrillate the patient. Have emergency medications available.

Hypokalemia, hypomagnesemia, acute myocardial ischemia, and digitalis or quinidine toxicity may increase the risk of ventricular fibrillation following cardioversion.

Although the electric shock of cardioversion won't usually damage an implanted pacemaker, avoid placing the paddles directly over the pacemaker. If the paddles have been recharged but you're not going to use them, clear the charge by turning the machine off, adjusting the energy selector dial, or placing the paddles in their protective housing and discharging them into the machine—never against each other or into the air.

Monitoring and aftercare

After the cardioversion, frequently assess the patient's LOC and respiratory status including airway patency, respiratory rate and depth, and need for supplemental oxygen. Because the patient will be heavily sedated, he may require airway support.

Record a postcardioversion 12-lead ECG and monitor the patient's ECG rhythm for 2 hours. Check the patient's chest for electrical burns.

Document the procedure, including the voltage delivered with each attempt, rhythm strips before and after the procedure, and how the patient tolerated the procedure.

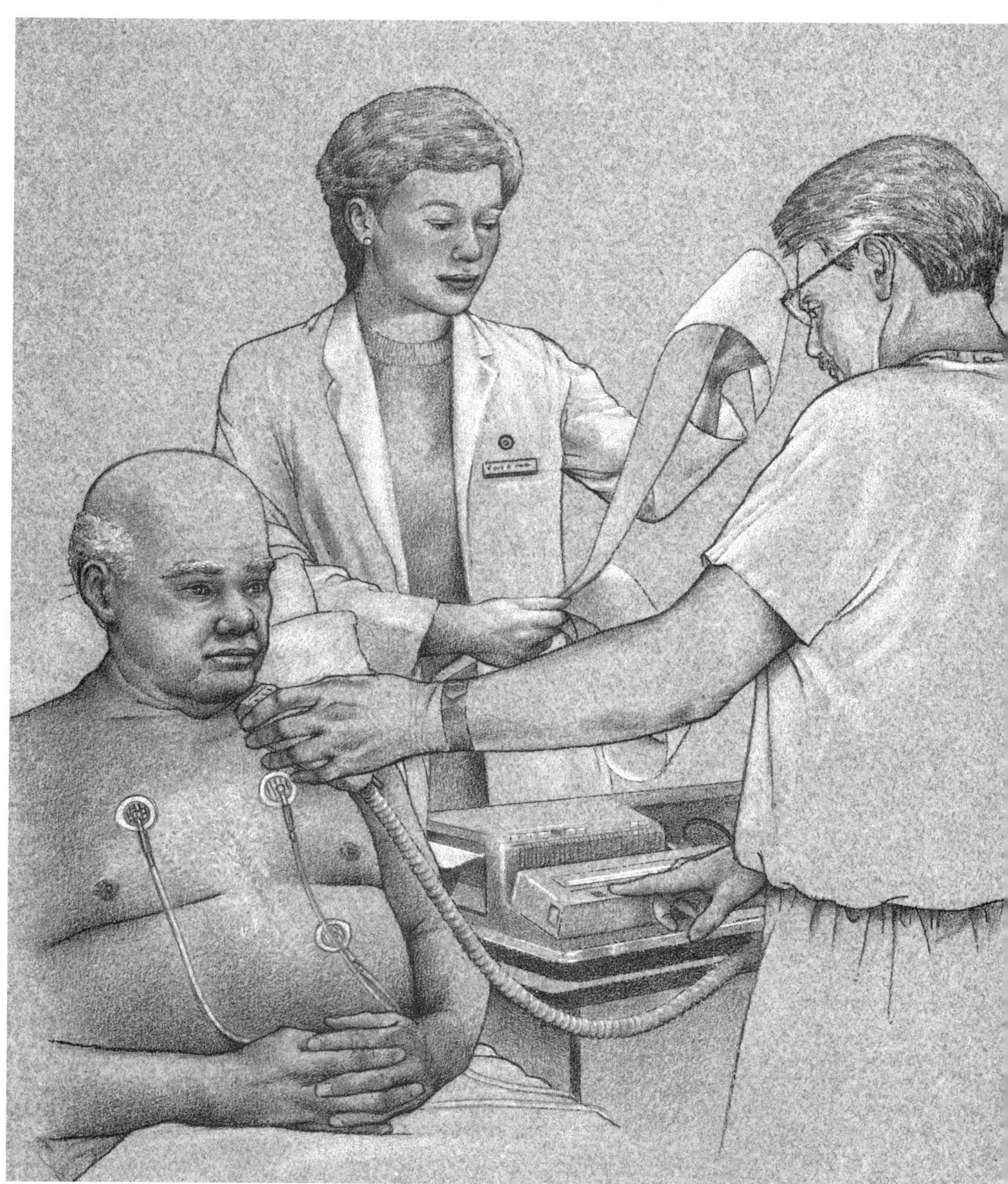

CHAPTER

Cardiovascular procedures

Until the 1970s, mortality from myocardial ischemia and its complications increased each decade in North America. But since then, it has declined dramatically. Although the reasons aren't entirely clear, this decline probably stems from better detection methods, improved medical and surgical care, and growing public awareness of preventive measures. Even so, cardiovascular disease kills more Americans today than any other cause.

Because cardiovascular disease is so pervasive, nurses in every area care for affected patients. And the procedures used to care for these patients seem to grow in number and complexity. This chapter will prepare you for these advanced procedures. It covers your role in caring for the patient undergoing permanent pacemaker implantation, pericardiocentesis, vagal maneuvers, ventricular assist device insertion, percutaneous transluminal coronary angioplasty, balloon valvuloplasty, application of a cardiopulmonary support system, autologous transfusion, and application of a pneumatic antishock garment.

Permanent pacemakers

Electronic devices implanted in a pocket beneath the skin, permanent pacemakers stimulate the heart into beating regularly when its natural pacemakers aren't functioning correctly. Unlike temporary pacemakers, they're used for long-term management of arrhythmias and bradycardia. Permanent pacemakers are usually inserted in the operating room under local anesthesia. They're usually implanted transvenously into the axilla or epicardium.

The self-contained, permanent pacemaker is small—about 1¾" × 1½" × ¼" (4.5 cm × 3.8 cm × 0.6 cm)—and light—weighing about 1 oz (28 g). It consists of two parts: a pulse generator, which contains the battery (energy source) and the circuitry, and the lead, containing an insulated wire and electrode. The battery's lithium electrochemical cells provide the power to produce electrical impulses and initiate depolarization of the myocardium. The timing of the impulses is controlled by the circuitry. A unipolar or bipolar lead transmits the electrical impulses from the generator to the heart, making contact with the endocardium through the electrode at the end of the lead. The electrode creates the electrical stimuli that cause the heart to contract and also senses beats originating from the heart's natural pacemaker. Pacing electrodes can be placed in the atria, in the ventricles, or in both chambers (atrioventricular [AV] sequential, dual-chamber pacemaker). (See *Pacemaker lead placement.*)

Most pacemakers implanted today are demand pacemakers; that is, they're triggered only when the patient's intrinsic heart rate drops below a preset level. Newer pacemakers are also programmable, so you can noninvasively change the rate, sensitivity, current output, or pacing mode as the patient's needs change.

A coding system developed by the Inter-Society Commission for Heart Disease Resources uses letters to describe pacemaker functions. (See *Understanding pacemaker codes.*)

When caring for the patient with a permanent pacemaker, your responsibilities are mainly monitoring and teaching. Preoperatively, you'll need to monitor the patient to prevent complications arising from arrhythmias. You'll also need to help him prepare psychologically for the insertion procedure and for living with a pacemaker. Postoperatively, you'll direct your care at relieving pain, monitoring to prevent complications, educating the patient about the pacemaker's function, and stressing the importance of follow-up care.

Pacemaker lead placement

In a dual-chamber pacemaker, leads are placed in the right ventricle and in the right atrium. The illustration below shows lead placement.

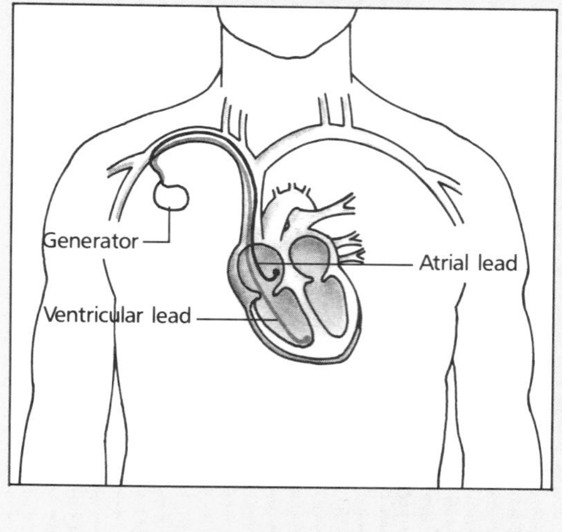

Indications

- Persistent, symptomatic bradycardia
- Sick sinus syndrome
- Second-degree AV block (Mobitz II)
- Third-degree AV block
- Sensitive carotid sinus syndrome (Stokes-Adams attacks) causing severe sinus bradycardia or AV block

Understanding pacemaker codes

A permanent pacemaker's three- to five-letter code refers to its capabilities.

First letter
(chamber that's paced)
A = atrium
V = ventricle
D = dual (both chambers)
O = not applicable

Second letter
(chamber that's sensed)
A = atrium
V = ventricle
D = dual (both chambers)
O = not applicable

Third letter
(how pulse generator responds)
I = inhibited
T = triggered
D = dual (inhibited and triggered)
O = not applicable

Fourth letter
(programmability functions)
P = programmable
M = multiprogrammable
C = communicating
R = rate modulation
O = none

Fifth letter
(pacemaker's antitachycardia and antiarrhythmia capabilities)
P = pacing
S = shock
D = dual (pacing and shock)
O = none

Common programming codes

DDD
Pace: atrium and ventricle
Sense: atrium and ventricle
Response: inhibited and triggered
This is a fully automatic, or universal, pacemaker.

VVIR
Pace: ventricle
Sense: ventricle
Response: inhibited
Programmability: rate modulation
This is a rate-adaptive pacemaker.

DVICO
Pace: atrium and ventricle
Sense: ventricle
Response: inhibited
Programmability: communicating
Antitachycardia and antiarrhythmia capabilities: none
This is a demand pacemaker.

Contraindications and complications

Complications of transvenous insertion include thrombus and embolus formation and cardiac tamponade, caused by perforation of the ventricular wall. Complications of epicardial placement are the same as those for thoracotomy and general anesthesia.

Other complications are related to the pacemaker itself. For example, many patients develop "frozen shoulder syndrome" from decreased movement on the side where the generator is implanted. Patients with VVI pacemakers (single-chamber units that pace and sense only the ventricle) may develop "pacemaker syndrome" months to years after insertion. This syndrome results from loss of AV synchrony (because only the ventricle is paced) with a reduction in cardiac output. Symptoms include dizziness, fatigue, syncope, palpitations, and neck vein pulsations. To correct pacemaker syndrome, the VVI pacemaker can be reprogrammed as a dual-chamber unit such as a DVI or DDD pacemaker, which restores AV synchrony, increasing cardiac output and relieving symptoms.

Pacemaker malfunction can also cause complications. For example, an electrode wire may dislodge, or a battery may fail in the unit, causing failure to discharge (pace), capture, or sense.

Equipment

Sphygmomanometer • stethoscope • electrocardiogram (ECG) monitor (with oscilloscope and strip-chart recorder) • sterile dressing tray • povidone-iodine ointment • shaving supplies or depilatory cream • sterile gauze dressing • nonallergenic tape • antibiotics • analgesics • sedatives • local anesthetic • alcohol sponges • emergency resuscitation equipment • sterile gown and mask • sterile drape • I.V. line for emergency medications • fluoroscope • pacemaker generator and electrode • pacing systems analyzer

Preparation

- Explain the procedure to the patient. Provide literature from the pacemaker manufacturer or the American Heart Association to help him learn about the pacemaker and how it works. Use visual aids, including a model of the pacemaker. Emphasize that the device will augment his natural heart rate.
- Ensure that the patient or a responsible family member signs a consent form. Ask whether the patient is allergic to anesthetics or iodine.
- Familiarize the patient with operating room procedure. Explain that he'll be awake but sedated, and will be able to hear the monitors beeping and people talking. Tell him that he'll receive a local anesthetic so he won't feel any pain.
- Tell him that the pacemaker won't limit his physical activity.
- Reassure him that electrical appliances, such as microwave ovens, won't affect pacemaker operation.
- Ask the patient if he shoots a rifle or shotgun. If so, the doctor will probably place the pacemaker on the side opposite where the gun is held. This prevents damaging the pacemaker during recoil.
- Ask the patient if he wears a hearing aid. If so, the doctor will place the pacemaker battery on the side opposite the hearing aid.
- Remove hair from the axilla to the midline and from the clavicle to the nipple line on the side selected by the doctor. For epicardial placement, shave from the nipple line to the umbilicus.
- Establish an I.V. line at a keep-vein-open rate to administer emergency drugs if an arrhythmia develops.
- Take vital signs and perform an ECG to establish a baseline.
- Provide sedation, as ordered.

Essential steps

- If you'll be present to monitor for arrhythmias during the insertion procedure, put on a gown and mask.
- Help the patient into a supine position. Have emergency resuscitation equipment on hand.
- Connect the ECG monitor to the patient, and run a baseline rhythm strip. Make sure that the machine has enough paper to run additional rhythm strips during the procedure. Leave the monitor screen on throughout the procedure.
- Drape the patient for surgery.
- Help the doctor anesthetize the insertion area.
- During transvenous placement, the doctor first makes an incision to insert the lead and uses the same site to create a pocket for the pulse generator.
- Guided by a fluoroscope, he passes the electrode catheter through the cephalic, external jugular, or subclavian vein and positions it under the trabeculae in the apex of the right ventricle.
- After the lead is in the proper position, he connects it to a pacing systems analyzer to check the stimulation and sensing thresholds. The stimulation threshold is the minimum stimulation needed to elicit atrial or ventricular contraction, and the sensing threshold is the minimum signal from the heart needed to prevent the pacer from discharging.
- The doctor then attaches the catheter to the pulse generator and checks the cardiac monitor for appropriate pacing and sensing. (See *Detecting pacemaker problems.*)
- If everything is functioning correctly, the doctor inserts the unit into the pocket created earlier and sutures it closed, leaving a small outlet for a drainage tube.
- During epicardial placement, the doctor first performs a thoracotomy; then he may apply the electrodes directly to the myocardium. In

TROUBLESHOOTING

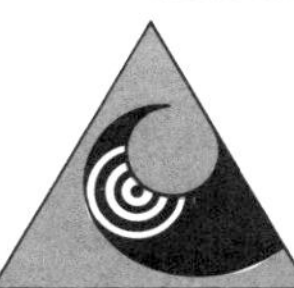

Detecting pacemaker problems

After the doctor attaches the catheter to the pulse generator, check the cardiac monitor to see if the pacemaker is pacing and sensing appropriately. If it's not, you may see one of the following problems on the monitor screen.

Loss of atrial capture (DDD mode)
A DDD (or AV sequential) pacemaker senses the atrium and ventricle and delivers an impulse when normal electrical activity doesn't occur. In this rhythm strip, the atrial (A) and ventricular (V) pacer spikes are initially followed by atrial and ventricular capture. Suddenly, atrial capture is lost. The pacemaker's atrial electrode still senses that normal atrial activity isn't occurring and continues to deliver an impulse. But the impulse doesn't cause atrial activity or capture as it should. The ventricular electrode is still sensing and pacing properly.

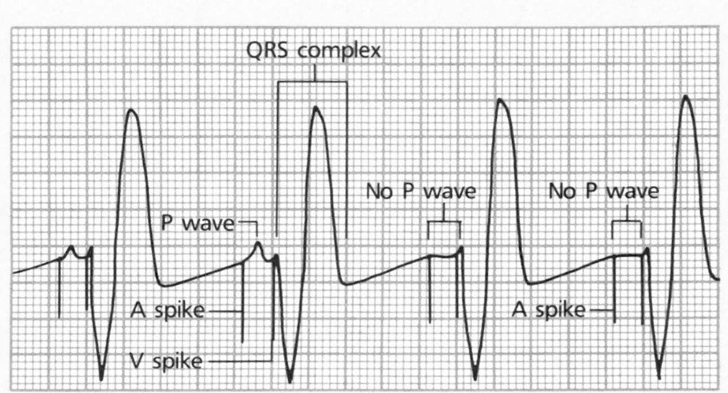

Loss of ventricular capture and sensing (VVI mode)
A VVI (or ventricular demand) pacemaker delivers an impulse to the ventricle when it doesn't sense a normal ventricular impulse. In this rhythm strip, the pacemaker delivers an impulse but doesn't capture the myocardium. So you see a ventricular (V) pacer spike but not a QRS complex. Also, the pacemaker isn't sensing normal ventricular activity and it's inappropriately delivering an impulse. So you see the QRS complex, then a pacer spike.

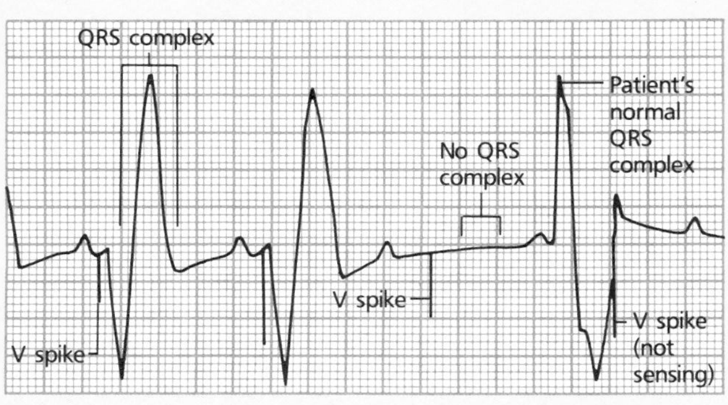

this procedure, he inserts the generator beneath the skin in the subcostal area. If the patient has a temporary pacemaker, the doctor will probably leave it in for 24 hours after inserting the permanent implant, in case the new pacemaker doesn't function correctly.

Cautions

When the patient returns from the operating room, watch for signs and symptoms of a perforated ventricle with resultant cardiac tamponade: persistent hiccups, distant heart sounds, pulsus paradoxus, hypotension with narrow pulse pressure, increased venous pressure, cyanosis, distended neck veins, decreased

HOME CARE

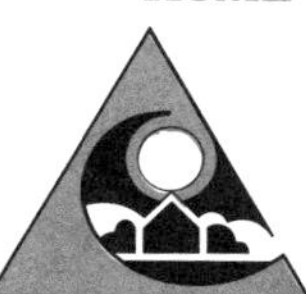

Teaching the patient with a permanent pacemaker

Begin your patient teaching when the decision for pacemaker insertion is made. The teaching methods you'll use and the amount of information you'll cover should depend on the patient's age, attention span, interest in learning, and even his eyesight. Clear up misconceptions about pacemakers by asking the patient what he already knows about them. Stress the positive aspects of living with a pacemaker – especially if the patient is having trouble accepting the idea. The topics below should be covered in your patient teaching. Teach them before, during, or after pacemaker insertion, depending on the patient's readiness.

Medical rationale

Discuss the medical reasons that the pacemaker is necessary and how it will improve the patient's quality of life. Also discuss the pacemaker's limitations, and dispel any misconceptions.

Physical activity

Explain passive range-of-motion exercises. Tell the patient that they'll be performed on the arm nearest the generator and will probably be started 24 to 48 hours postoperatively. They'll be discontinued when the patient stops having discomfort throughout all ranges of motion.

Tell the patient that he can return to work when the doctor gives his permission. Reassure him that touching the insertion site or performing normal activities such as bathing won't harm the pacemaker. But caution him to avoid activities that put stress or pressure on the insertion site – for example, contact sports. Because the pacemaker lead takes a few weeks to become secure within the endocardium, tell the patient not to lift anything heavier than 5 lb (2.3 kg) for 2 to 3 weeks.

Wound care

Instruct the patient to keep the incision clean and dry and to watch for signs of infection (redness, swelling, drainage, warmth, or tenderness). Recommend that he wear loose-fitting clothing directly over the incision until it's fully healed.

Medications

Teach the patient the importance of taking medications exactly as prescribed. Explain that these medications, along with the pacemaker, ensure optimum cardiac function. Provide written instructions whenever possible. Include such information as the name of the medication, the dose, the frequency of administration, the adverse effects, and how the drug supports cardiac function.

Pacemaker malfunction

Teach the patient about the signs and symptoms of pacemaker malfunction: dizziness, light-headedness, syncope, chest pain, shortness of breath, undue fatigue, and fluid retention. Instruct him to take his pulse daily on awakening. He should call the doctor if his pulse rate is 7 to 10 beats/minute below the preset rate or if his resting heart rate is 120 beats/minute or more. If he has a demand pacemaker, an irregular rhythm without accompanying physical symptoms may be normal because the intrinsic rate and the pacer rate are working together to maintain adequate cardiac output.

Pulse generator replacement

Inform the patient about the life expectancy of the pacemaker battery. Explain that battery replacement requires hospitalization but that the entire generator is usually replaced. Reassure the patient that the generator doesn't stop functioning abruptly; rather, the heart rate begins to slow gradually, so the patient has time to seek appropriate medical treatment.

Safety precautions

Tell the patient to inform all future health care providers that he has a pacemaker and is taking medications. He should always carry a pacemaker identification card that states the type of pacemaker, manufacturer, serial number, date of insertion, programmed settings, and doctor's name. Also, advise the patient to wear a medical identification bracelet.

Reassure the patient that pacemakers are now adequately shielded from the effects of common household electrical devices, such as microwave ovens. However, he should keep these devices in

HOME CARE

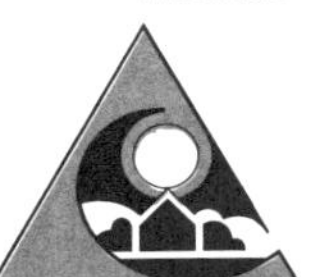

Teaching the patient with a permanent pacemaker *(continued)*

good working order. Although the pacemaker shouldn't activate airport security devices, advise the patient to show his pacemaker identification card to airport security personnel.

Follow-up care

Stress the importance of follow-up care. Explain that many pacemaker clinics can evaluate pacemaker function by phone, reducing the necessity for patient travel.

Precautions

Warn the patient that a few medical procedures are dangerous for patients with pacemakers. Magnetic resonance imaging (MRI) is contraindicated because the large magnetic field can produce asynchronous pacing (the pacemaker paces but doesn't sense). High-rate pacing (up to 400 beats/minute) can also occur when the radio frequency of the MRI interferes with the pacemaker.

During surgery, electrocautery can inhibit the pacemaker, causing it to sense the signals and mistake them for cardiac signals. It can also change the pacemaker's programming or cause it to lose its ability to deliver a stimulus. So patients undergoing electrocautery must be monitored closely.

Radiation therapy can have a cumulative effect on the pulse generator's circuitry, changing the molecular structure of the silicone chip and causing pacemaker failure. So the pacemaker should be covered with a lead shield and checked for proper functioning afterward.

urine output, restlessness, or complaints of chest fullness. If any of these develops, notify the doctor immediately.

Monitoring and aftercare

- Monitor the patient's ECG to detect arrhythmias and to check for correct pacemaker functioning.
- Also monitor the I.V. flow rate. The I.V. line is usually kept in place for 24 to 48 hours postoperatively for possible emergency treatment of arrhythmias.
- Check the dressing for signs of bleeding and infection (swelling, redness, or exudate). The doctor may order prophylactic antibiotics for up to 7 days after the implantation.
- Remind the patient to keep his arm immobile until told otherwise.
- Change the dressing and apply povidone-iodine ointment at least once every 24 to 48 hours, or according to the doctor's orders and hospital policy. If the dressing becomes soiled or the site is exposed to air, change the dressing immediately, regardless of when you last changed it.
- Check the patient's vital signs and level of consciousness (LOC) every 15 minutes for the first hour, every hour for the next 4 hours, every 4 hours for the next 48 hours, and then once every shift. (Confused elderly patients with second-degree heart block won't show immediate improvement in LOC.)
- Relieve patient discomfort with analgesics, as ordered.
- Teach the patient how to take his pulse, and tell him to do this every day at home. He should take it at the same time every day, after resting at least 5 minutes first (resting pulse rate), and count the beats for a full minute. Explain what constitutes an acceptable and unacceptable discrepancy between his pulse and the pacemaker's pulse generator setting, and whom to call if the discrepancy is unacceptable. The lower rate limit is usually 5 beats/minute below the pulse generator setting; the upper limit is usually 90 to 100 beats/minute. (See *Teaching the patient with a permanent pacemaker.*)
- Tell the patient to report dizziness, fainting spells, prolonged weakness or fatigue, palpitations, excessive hiccuping, chest pain, difficulty breathing, or swelling of legs, ankles, arms, or wrists.

• Show him how to inspect the surgical area for signs and symptoms of infection: redness, swelling, warmth, pain, and discharge. Tell him to report these findings to the doctor at once.
• About the third postoperative day, teach the patient range-of-motion exercises for the shoulder on the affected side.
• Advise the patient to wear a medical identification bracelet and to carry an identification card at all times. The card should contain the patient's name; the doctor's name, address, and phone number; the pacemaker type, model, and serial number; the pacing rate; and the date implanted.
• Stress the importance of follow-up care. Explain that the sensing and capturing functions of the pacer and battery can be evaluated by telephone. A transmitter relays an ECG signal to a receiver in the doctor's office or the pacemaker clinic.
• Document the type of pacemaker used, the serial number, the manufacturer's name, the pacing rate, the date of implantation, and the doctor's name. Note whether the pacemaker successfully treated the patient's arrhythmias, and include other pertinent observations, such as the condition of the incision site.

Pericardiocentesis

In pericardiocentesis, blood or fluid that has accumulated in the pericardium is aspirated by a needle inserted into the subxiphoid or left parasternal area, relieving pressure on the heart. The extracted fluid is then studied to help diagnose the underlying disease. This procedure is commonly performed as an emergency in the intensive care unit (ICU), when the accumulation is sudden and dramatic, causing hemodynamic compromise.

Normally, the pericardial sac has limited stretching ability and contains only 10 to 20 ml of fluid, which helps protect the myocardium. Intrapericardial pressure can increase drastically with the sudden addition of as little as 50 to 100 ml of fluid. Because the atria, ventricles, and coronary arteries are compressed from the increased pressure, the chambers can't hold their usual volume. This causes decreased cardiac output and poor tissue perfusion.

Your role in pericardiocentesis is to prepare the patient for the procedure, to gather the essential equipment, and to monitor for complications before, during, and after the procedure.

Indications

• Pericarditis
• Malignant neoplasm
• Life-threatening cardiac tamponade caused by chest trauma, cardiac surgery, or cardiac catheterization
• Hemorrhage following anticoagulant therapy
• Myocardial infarction (MI)

Contraindications and complications

Although it's often a lifesaving procedure, needle aspiration of the pericardial sac may cause several complications. The most common, cardiac arrhythmia, results from the needle touching the myocardium. Hemorrhage can occur if the myocardium or a coronary artery is lacerated, causing increased heart rate and decreased blood pressure.

Puncture of the lung, liver, or stomach can also occur. Signs and symptoms include chest or epigastric pain, dyspnea, or decreasing blood pressure. If the lung is punctured, the patient will also develop a pneumothorax. Finally, infection can result from pericardiocentesis if sterile technique isn't used. Signs include an elevated white blood cell count, fever, chills, and drainage or redness at the insertion site.

Equipment

Cardiac monitor with strip chart recorder • sterile specimen container • shaving supplies or depilatory cream • sterile 4" × 4" drain dressings • sterile gloves, gowns, and masks • povidone-iodine solution • vial of 1% or 2% lidocaine • adhesive tape • sterile 4" × 4" gauze pads • inside-the-needle I.V. catheter • sterile I.V. tubing • alcohol sponges • sterile drainage container • dextrose 5% in water (D_5W) • 50-ml syringe • three-way stopcock • intracardiac needle • hemostat • sedative (optional)

Many hospitals use prepackaged pericardiocentesis trays that contain most, but not all, of the equipment needed for the procedure.

Preparation

• Check the patient's history for hypersensitivity to the local anesthetic and the povidone-iodine solution.
• If the patient isn't already in the ICU, be prepared to transport him there for the procedure and for cardiac monitoring afterward.
• Obtain baseline vital signs, and administer a sedative if ordered. Connect a cardiac monitor to the patient.
• If the patient doesn't have a patent I.V. line for emergency medications, insert one and administer D_5W at a keep-vein-open rate.
• Explain the procedure to the patient, and assure him that you'll be nearby to monitor him and to assist the doctor.
• Put on gloves. Shave the patient's chest, or remove hair with a depilatory, from midsternum to below the xiphoid process. If the patient is unstable, skip this step.
• Clean the entire area with alcohol sponges, then with povidone-iodine. Wipe with a circular motion, moving away from the insertion site to help prevent infection.
• If the patient's condition allows, elevate his head 60 degrees and support his arms with pillows. This position makes needle placement easier.
• Put on a sterile gown and mask. Open the pericardiocentesis tray, using the outer wrapper to create a sterile field.
• Clean the rubber stopper of the lidocaine vial with an alcohol sponge, and invert it so that the doctor can withdraw the anesthetic.

Essential steps

• The doctor anesthetizes the insertion site. Then he connects the 50-ml syringe to a three-way stopcock and attaches the intracardiac needle. He inserts the needle to the left of the xiphoid process and advances it until he obtains a blood or fluid return. (See *Needle placement in pericardiocentesis.*)
• He attaches a hemostat to the needle at the chest wall to keep it from slipping out of position. Then he turns the three-way stopcock to keep air out of the pericardial sac.

Needle placement in pericardiocentesis

An intracardiac needle, connected to a 50-ml syringe and a three-way stopcock, is inserted to the left of the xiphoid process and advanced until a blood or fluid return is obtained.

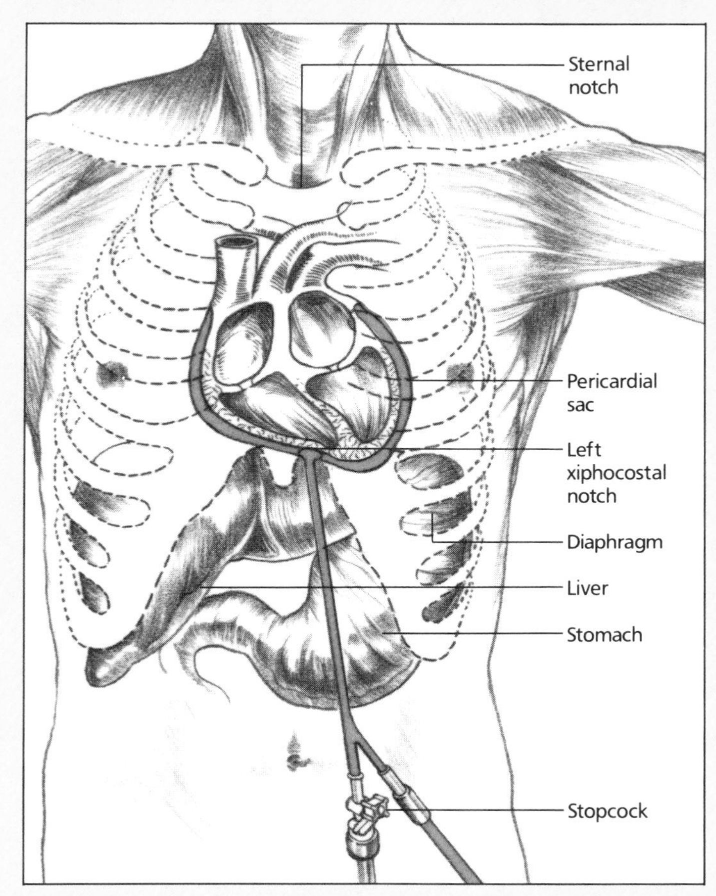

• If he needs a specimen, he withdraws the fluid and turns off the stopcock to the patient. Have the sterile specimen container ready for the specimen.
• If the patient has a lot of fluid in the pericardial sac, the doctor may insert an inside-the-needle (or "pigtail") catheter and leave it in place for several days. The catheter removes fluid gradually—about 100 ml every 4 to 6 hours. After insertion, attach the catheter to sterile tubing and a sterile drainage container. Put on sterile gloves, apply povidone-iodine ointment to the site, and cover the site with sterile drain dressings. Tape the dressings securely, and note the date and time on the dressing.

Cautions
Strict aseptic technique is essential for preventing infection. Be sure to clean the entire area thoroughly in case the myocardium tears during the procedure and the doctor needs to perform a thoracotomy to suture the tear. Monitor the patient's ECG during needle insertion. If the ECG pattern changes, notify the doctor; the needle may have touched or penetrated the ventricle.

Because pericardiocentesis can cause life-threatening complications, the patient should recover in the ICU. Despite pericardiocentesis, cardiac tamponade may recur. So be alert for signs indicating that fluid has reaccumulated in the pericardial sac: tachycardia, decreased blood pressure, shock, pallor, confusion, restlessness, dyspnea, oliguria, and thready pulse.

Monitoring and aftercare
• Using sterile techninue, cover the needle insertion site with sterile 4″ × 4″ gauze pads and tape them securely, noting the date and time on the dressing.
• After the procedure, monitor the patient closely. Report any changes that suggest perforation of the right ventricle or decreasing cardiac output.
• Continue ECG monitoring, especially if the catheter remains in place, because it can migrate and touch the ventricle.
• Record the reason for pericardiocentesis, who performed it, and the outcome. Note the type of fluid aspirated, the presence of clots, and any specimens taken. Record the patient's response during the procedure and his status afterward, noting any complications and subsequent interventions.

Vagal maneuvers

Known as vagal maneuvers, Valsalva's maneuver and carotid sinus massage are used to slow an accelerated heart rate. These maneuvers stimulate nerve endings, which respond as they would to an increase in blood pressure. They send this message to the brain stem, which in turn stimulates the autonomic nervous system to increase vagal tone and decrease the heart rate.

In Valsalva's maneuver, the patient holds his breath and bears down, raising his intrathoracic pressure. When this pressure increase is transmitted to the heart and great vessels, venous return, stroke volume, and systolic blood pressure decrease. Within seconds, the baroreceptors respond to these changes by increasing the heart rate and causing peripheral vasoconstriction. When the patient exhales at the end of the maneuver, his blood pressure rises to its previous level. This increase, combined with the peripheral vasoconstriction caused by bearing down, stimulates the vagus nerve, decreasing the heart rate.

In carotid sinus massage, manual pressure applied to the left or right carotid sinus slows the heart rate. The patient's response depends on the type of arrhythmia. If he has sinus tachycardia, his heart rate will slow gradually during the procedure and speed up again afterward. If he has atrial tachycardia, the arrhythmia may stop and the heart rate may remain slow because the procedure increases AV block. With atrial fibrillation or flutter, the ventricular rate may not change; in fact, AV block may even worsen. With paroxysmal atrial tachycardia, reversion to sinus rhythm occurs 20% of the time. Nonparoxysmal supraventricular tachycardia and ventricular tachycardia won't respond to carotid sinus massage.

Vagal maneuvers are usually performed at the bedside, either by a specially trained nurse or a doctor. If you don't perform the maneuver, your job is to prepare the patient, gather the necessary equipment, assist the doctor, and monitor for complications.

Indications

- Sinus tachyarrhythmias
- Atrial tachyarrhythmias
- Junctional tachyarrhythmias

(*Note:* Carotid sinus massage is used to diagnose and treat tachyarrhythmias.)

Contraindications and complications

Valsalva's maneuver and carotid sinus massage are contraindicated for patients with severe coronary artery disease (CAD), acute MI, or hypovolemia. Carotid sinus massage is contraindicated for patients with cardiac glycoside toxicity or cerebrovascular disease and for patients who've had carotid surgery.

Complications of Valsalva's maneuver include bradycardia accompanied by a decrease in cardiac output, possibly leading to syncope. This maneuver can also mobilize venous thrombi and cause bleeding.

Complications of carotid sinus massage include ventricular fibrillation, ventricular tachycardia, and ventricular standstill as well as worsening AV block that leads to junctional or ventricular escape rhythms. This maneuver can also cause cerebral damage from inadequate tissue perfusion, especially in elderly patients. Another possible neurologic complication is cerebrovascular accident (CVA) from decreased perfusion caused by total carotid artery blockage or from migrating endothelial plaque loosened by carotid sinus compression.

Equipment

Crash cart with emergency medications and airway equipment • ECG monitor and electrodes • I.V. catheter and tubing • D_5W • stethoscope • optional: shaving supplies, cardiotonic drugs

Preparation

- Assemble the appropriate equipment.
- Explain the procedure to the patient to ease his fears and promote cooperation. Ask him to tell you if he feels light-headed.
- Help the patient into a supine position.
- Insert an I.V. line if necessary. This line will be used if emergency drugs are necessary. Then administer D_5W at a keep-vein-open rate, as ordered.
- Prepare the patient's skin, shaving it if necessary. Attach ECG electrodes. Adjust the size of the ECG complexes on the monitor so that you can see the arrhythmia clearly.

Essential steps

For Valsalva's maneuver

- Ask the patient to take a deep breath, hold it, and then bear down, as if he were trying to defecate. If he doesn't feel light-headed or dizzy, and if no new arrhythmias occur, have him hold his breath and bear down for 10 seconds.
- If he does feel dizzy or light-headed, or if you see a new arrhythmia on the monitor, asystole for more than 6 seconds, frequent premature ventricular contractions (PVCs), or ventricular tachycardia or ventricular fibrillation, tell the patient to exhale and stop bearing down.
- After 10 seconds, ask the patient to exhale and breathe normally. If the maneuver was successful, the monitor will show his heart rate slowing before he exhales.

For carotid sinus massage

- Obtain a rhythm strip, using the lead that shows the strongest P waves.
- Auscultate both carotid sinuses. If you detect bruits, don't perform carotid sinus massage; if you don't hear bruits, perform the maneuver. (See *How to perform carotid sinus massage,* page 46.)
- Monitor the patient's ECG throughout the procedure. Inform the doctor when the ventricular rate slows sufficiently to permit diagnosis of the rhythm. He'll stop the massage then or as soon as any evidence of a rhythm change appears.
- If the procedure has no effect within 5 seconds, the doctor will stop massaging the right carotid sinus and start massaging the left. If this also fails, he'll administer a cardiotonic

How to perform carotid sinus massage

Before applying manual pressure to the patient's right carotid sinus, locate the bifurcation of the carotid artery on the right side of the neck. Turn the patient's head slightly to the left and hyperextend the neck. This brings the carotid artery closer to the skin and moves the sternocleidomastoid muscle away from the carotid artery.

Then, using a circular motion, gently massage the right carotid sinus between your fingers and the transverse processes of the spine for 3 to 5 seconds. Don't massage for more than 5 seconds to avoid risking life-threatening complications.

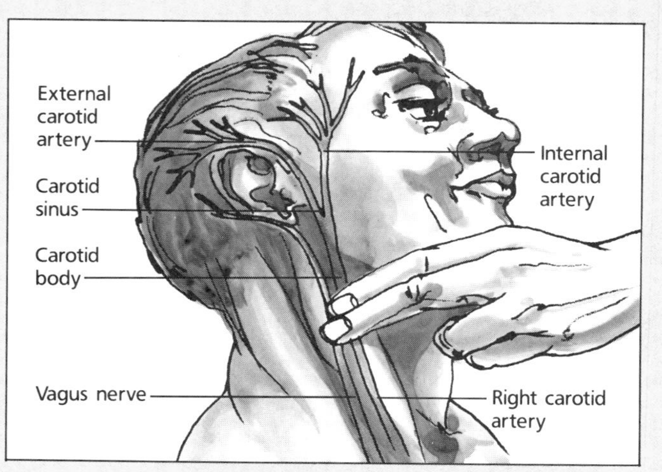

drug. Remember that a brief period of asystole—from 3 to 6 seconds—and several PVCs may precede conversion to normal sinus rhythm.

Cautions

Use caution when performing carotid sinus massage on elderly patients, patients receiving cardiac glycosides, and those with heart block, hypertension, CAD, diabetes mellitus, or hyperkalemia. The procedure may cause arterial pressure to plummet in these patients, although it usually rises quickly afterward. This is particularly true of elderly patients with heart disease. Have the crash cart handy to give emergency treatment if a dangerous arrhythmia occurs.

Vagal maneuvers occasionally cause bradycardia or complete heart block, so monitor the patient's cardiac rhythm closely. Bradycardia will usually pass quickly. If it doesn't, or if it advances to complete heart block or asystole, begin basic life support and, if necessary, advanced cardiac life support.

Monitoring and aftercare

- If the vagal maneuver slowed the patient's heart rate and converted the arrhythmia, continue monitoring him for several hours.
- Monitor the patient for signs and symptoms of vascular occlusion, including chest discomfort and dyspnea. Report such problems at once, and prepare the patient for diagnostic testing or transfer to the ICU, as ordered.
- Monitor the patient's ECG closely. If it indicates complete heart block or asystole, start basic life support at once, followed by advanced cardiac life support. If emergency medications don't convert the complete heart block, the patient may need a temporary pacemaker.
- Watch carefully during and after the procedure for changes in neurologic status. If you detect any, tell the doctor and prepare the patient for further diagnostic tests or transfer to the ICU, as ordered.
- Record the date and time of the procedure, who performed it, and why it was necessary. Note the patient's response, any complications, and the interventions performed. If possible, obtain an ECG rhythm strip before, during, and after the procedure to document changes.

Ventricular assist device

Although great strides have been made in cardiac surgery, a few patients still require unconventional methods of circulatory support afterward. A ventricular assist device (VAD) can temporarily sustain the life of a patient with acute ventricular failure despite maximum medical and surgical intervention.

Unlike the intra-aortic balloon pump, which increases cardiac output by only up to 15%, a VAD provides total support to the heart and circulation, allowing the heart to recover from any type of insult. With its pump, the device augments cardiac output just enough to allow tissue and organ perfusion while allowing the heart to rest and recover. Although a VAD is usually used to assist the left ventricle, it may also assist the right ventricle or both ventricles. (See *Helping the heart,* page 48.)

Caring for the patient with a VAD is complex and challenging. Besides being familiar with how the device works, your responsibilities include careful observation of the patient's status; continuous monitoring and interpretation of vital signs, hemodynamic pressures, and arterial blood gas values; and coordination of efforts with the pump perfusionist and other members of the interdisciplinary team.

Indications

- Cardiogenic shock after MI
- Irreversible cardiomyopathy
- Acute myocarditis
- Inability to be weaned from cardiopulmonary bypass support
- Valvular disease
- Bacterial endocarditis
- Heart transplant rejection
- Heart failure in patients awaiting a heart transplant

Contraindications and complications

A VAD is contraindicated in patients with central nervous system damage from prolonged cardiac arrest, in patients who would probably be impossible to wean from the VAD because of irreversible myocardial damage, in patients with sepsis, in those with severe renal failure, and in those with chronic liver disease.

Patients with a VAD are at high risk for complications, including hemolysis, thrombus formation, and subsequent pulmonary embolism or CVA. Other complications include respiratory and ventricular failure; renal insufficiency from decreased perfusion; bleeding from anticoagulation; air embolism if the catheters disconnect; and local or systemic infection.

Equipment

Shaving supplies or depilatory cream • povidone-iodine solution • ECG monitor • heparin • pulmonary artery catheter • arterial line catheter • cannulae • VAD • soft restraints

Preparation

- Tell the patient that the doctor will insert the VAD in the operating room and that he'll be transferred to the ICU afterward.
- Inform him that food and fluid intake will be restricted for several hours before the procedure.
- Explain that you'll continuously monitor his cardiac function with an ECG, a pulmonary artery catheter, and an arterial line. Offer reassurance.
- Review with the patient and family why the VAD is necessary. Also tell them what to expect in the ICU after insertion: continuous monitoring of vital signs, frequent observation and measurement of hemodynamic and pulmonary pressures, and continuous manipulation of the VAD.
- Make sure that the patient has signed a consent form before sending him to the operating room.
- If necessary, and the patient is stable enough, shave the patient's chest or remove hair with a depilatory cream. Scrub the chest with an antiseptic solution.
- The pump perfusionist primes the pump circuit and filter.

Essential steps

The steps for inserting the VAD will differ, depending on whether the device is inserted immediately after surgery in a patient who can't come off bypass support or if it's inserted in an emergency in a patient with heart failure

ADVANCED EQUIPMENT

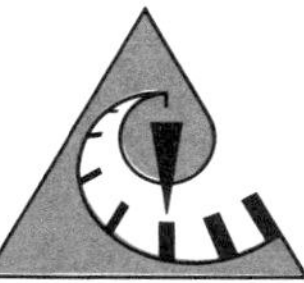

Helping the heart

The ventricular assist device (VAD) functions somewhat like an artificial heart. The major difference is that the VAD assists the heart, whereas the artificial heart replaces it. The VAD is designed to aid one or both ventricles. The pumping chambers themselves aren't usually implanted in the patient.

Inserted in the operating room, the permanent VAD is implanted in the patient's chest cavity, but it still provides only temporary support. The device receives power through the skin by a belt of electrical transformer coils (worn externally as a portable battery pack). It can also operate off of an implanted rechargeable battery for up to 1 hour at a time.

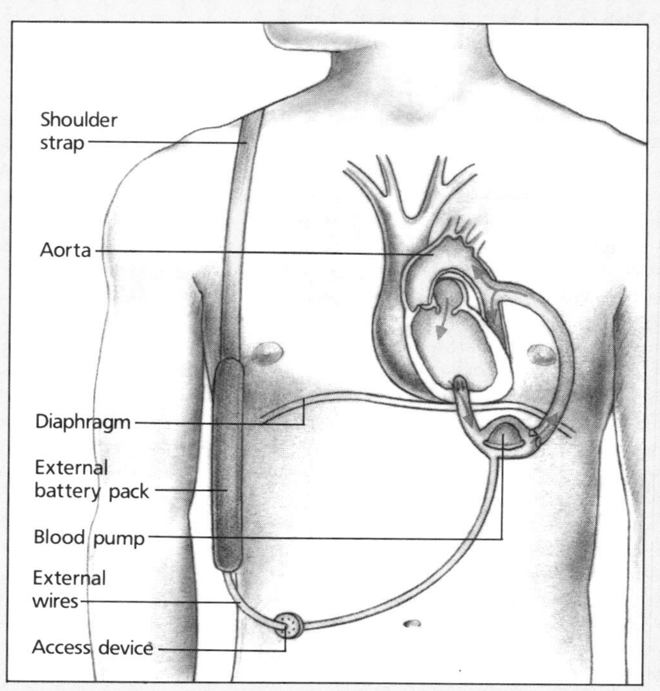

who's awaiting a heart transplant. Obviously, VADs are easier to connect during surgery, when the patient's chest is already open.

- After thoracotomy, the doctor inserts the two cannulae and sutures them in place.
- He begins administering heparin.
- He connects the pump circuit and gradually initiates pumping.
- He removes the cannulae from the sternal incision or separate parasternal incisions and closes the chest.

Cautions

Staff members caring for the patient should have a thorough knowledge of how the VAD works as well as an understanding of the complex physiologic and psychological needs of the patient and family. Experienced nurses and pump perfusionists must be in attendance 24 hours a day. When obtaining hemodynamic measurements, remember that cardiac output is accurate only with left VADs, not right VADs. To prevent air embolism, be sure to remove all air from the pump before connecting it to the patient's cannulae, and maintain all connections as long as the device is in use.

Monitoring and aftercare

- Monitor vital signs and intake and output frequently.
- Keep the patient immobile to prevent accidental extubation, contamination, or disconnection of the VAD. If necessary, use soft restraints.
- Monitor pulmonary artery pressures. If you've been taught how to adjust the pump, maintain cardiac output at 5 to 8 liters/minute, central venous pressure at 8 to 16 mm Hg, pulmonary

capillary wedge pressure at 10 to 20 mm Hg, mean arterial pressure at more than 60 mm Hg, and left arterial pressure between 4 and 12 mm Hg.

• Monitor the patient for signs and symptoms of poor perfusion and ineffective pumping, including arrhythmias, hypotension, slow capillary refill, cool skin, decreased peripheral pulses, oliguria or anuria, confusion, anxiety, and restlessness.
• Give inotropics and vasodilators, as ordered, and adjust dosages as necessary to maintain parameters.
• Work closely with the pump perfusionist, who's usually responsible for the pump's functioning.
• Administer heparin, as ordered, to prevent clotting in the pump head and thrombus formation. Check for bleeding, especially at the operative sites. Monitor laboratory studies, as ordered, especially complete blood count and coagulation studies.
• Assess the patient's incisions and the cannula insertion sites for signs of infection. Use strict aseptic technique. Monitor the patient's white blood cell count and differential daily, and take his rectal or core temperature every 4 hours. Administer antibiotics, as ordered.
• Check the pump tubing frequently for signs of disconnection.
• Change the dressings over the cannula sites daily or according to hospital policy.
• Provide supportive care, including range-of-motion exercises and mouth and skin care.
• If ventricular function fails to improve within 4 days, the patient may need a heart transplant. If so, provide psychological support for the patient and his family during the referral process. You may also initiate the transplant process by contacting the appropriate agency.
• The psychological effects of VAD insertion can produce stress in the patient, his family, and his close friends. If appropriate, refer them to other support resources.
• Note the patient's condition after VAD insertion. Document any pump adjustments as well as any complications and subsequent interventions.

Percutaneous transluminal coronary angioplasty

A nonsurgical approach to opening coronary vessels narrowed by arteriosclerosis, percutaneous transluminal coronary angioplasty (PTCA) uses a balloon-tipped catheter that's inserted into a narrowed coronary artery. It relieves pain due to angina and myocardial ischemia. The procedure is performed in the cardiac catheterization laboratory under local anesthesia. Cardiac catheterization usually accompanies PTCA to assess the stenosis and the efficacy of the angioplasty.

Catheterization is used as a visual tool to direct the balloon-tipped catheter through the vessel's area of stenosis. As the balloon is inflated, the plaque is compressed against the vessel wall, allowing coronary blood to flow more freely. (See *Performing PTCA,* page 50.)

A newer procedure, laser-enhanced angioplasty, is having promising results in vaporizing occlusions in atherosclerosis. (See *Laser-enhanced angioplasty,* page 51.)

Your responsibilities include teaching the patient and family about the procedure and assessing for complications after the angioplasty.

Indications

• Patients with chronic medical problems who are poor surgical risks
• Total coronary occlusion and plaque buildup in several areas
• Unstable or chronic angina
• Poor left ventricular function
• Angina following coronary artery bypass grafting
• Patients with acute MI who still have myocardial ischemia after thrombolysis

The ideal candidate for PTCA has single- or double-vessel disease excluding the left main coronary artery with at least 50% proximal stenosis. The lesion should be discrete, uncalcified, concentric, and not located near a bifurcation.

Performing PTCA

Percutaneous transluminal coronary angioplasty (PTCA) is a procedure that opens an occluded coronary artery without opening the chest. It's performed in the cardiac catheterization laboratory after coronary angiography confirms the presence and location of the occlusion. Once the occlusion is located, the doctor threads a guide catheter through the patient's femoral artery and into the coronary artery under fluoroscopic guidance, as shown in the first illustration.

When the guide catheter's position at the occlusion site is confirmed by angiography, the doctor carefully introduces into the catheter a double-lumen balloon that is smaller than the catheter lumen. He then directs the balloon through the lesion, where a marked pressure gradient will be obvious. The doctor alternately inflates (as shown in the second illustration) and deflates the balloon until an angiogram verifies successful arterial dilation and the pressure gradient has decreased.

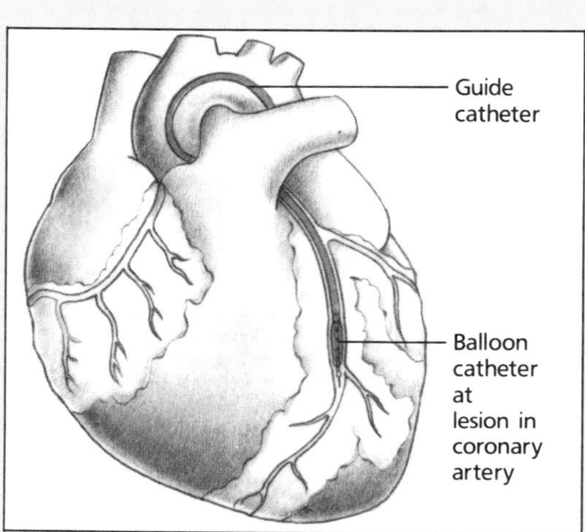

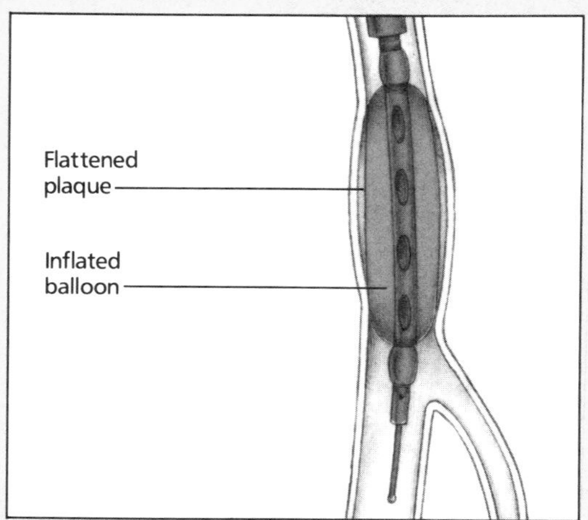

Contraindications and complications

PTCA is contraindicated in left main coronary artery disease, especially when the patient is a poor surgical risk; in patients with variant angina or critical valvular disease; and in patients with vessels occluded at the aortic wall orifice.

The most common complication of PTCA is prolonged angina. PTCA can also cause coronary artery perforation, balloon rupture, reocclusion (necessitating a coronary artery bypass graft), MI, pericardial tamponade, hematoma, hemorrhage, reperfusion arrhythmias, and closure of the vessel. (See *Vascular stents,* page 52.)

Equipment

Povidone-iodine solution • local anesthetic • I.V. solution and tubing • ECG and electrodes • oxygen • nasal cannula • shaving supplies or depilatory cream • sedative • pulmonary artery catheter • contrast medium • emergency medications • heparin for injection • 5-lb (2.3-kg) sandbag • introducer kit for PTCA catheter • sterile gown, gloves, and drapes • optional: nitroglycerin, soft restraints

Preparation

• Explain the procedure to the patient and family to reduce the patient's fear and promote cooperation.

• Inform the patient that the procedure lasts from 1 to 4 hours and that he may feel some discomfort from lying on a hard table for that long.
• Tell him that a catheter will be inserted into an artery or a vein in his groin and that he may feel pressure as the catheter moves along the vessel.
• Reassure him that although he'll be awake during the procedure, he'll be given a sedative. Explain that the doctor or nurse may ask him how he's feeling and that he should tell them if he experiences any angina.
• Explain that the doctor will inject a contrast medium to outline the lesion's location. Warn the patient that he may feel a hot, flushing sensation or transient nausea during the injection.
• Check the patient's history for allergies; if he's had allergic reactions to shellfish, iodine, or contrast media, notify the doctor.
• Administer 650 mg of aspirin the evening before the procedure to prevent platelet aggregation, as ordered.
• Make sure that the patient signs a consent form.
• Restrict food and fluids for at least 6 hours before the procedure or as ordered.
• Ensure that the results of coagulation studies, complete blood count, serum electrolyte studies, and blood typing and crossmatching are available.
• Insert an I.V. line in case emergency medications are needed.
• Shave hair from the insertion site (groin or brachial area), or use a depilatory cream. Then clean the area with povidone-iodine solution.
• Give the patient a sedative, as ordered.
• Take baseline peripheral pulses in all extremities.
• When the patient arrives at the cardiac catheterization laboratory, apply ECG electrodes and ensure I.V. line patency.
• Administer oxygen through a nasal cannula.

Essential steps

• Help the doctor put on a sterile gown and gloves. Open the sterile supplies.
• The doctor prepares the site and injects a local anesthetic. If the patient doesn't already have a pulmonary artery catheter in place, the doctor may insert one now.
• The doctor inserts a large guide catheter into the artery and sutures it in place. Then he threads an angioplasty catheter through the guide catheter. An angioplasty catheter is thinner and longer and has a balloon at its tip. Using a thin, flexible guide wire, he then threads the catheter up through the aorta and into the coronary artery to the area of stenosis.
• He injects a contrast medium through the angioplasty catheter and into the obstructed coronary artery to outline the lesion's location and help assess the blockage. He also injects heparin to prevent the catheter from clotting,

Laser-enhanced angioplasty

Laser-enhanced angioplasty shows great potential for vaporizing occlusions in patients with atherosclerosis. The procedure achieves its best results with thrombotic occlusions, but it may also be used to remove calcified plaques. New lasers that deliver energy in brief pulses have helped solve the problem of thermal or acoustic damage to local tissues. Using the pulsed beam, doctors can dispatch the blockage without destroying the vessel wall.

To perform the procedure, the doctor threads a laser-containing catheter into the diseased artery. When the catheter nears the occlusion, the doctor triggers the laser to emit rapid bursts. Between bursts he rotates the catheter, advancing it until the occlusion is destroyed. The procedure takes about an hour and requires only a local anesthetic. Clearing a completely occluded coronary artery requires ten 1-second bursts of laser energy, followed by balloon angioplasty. After the procedure, angiography may be used to document vessel patency.

Recently, cardiologists have successfully used laser techniques to open totally blocked right main coronary arteries, thereby avoiding bypass surgery. Cardiologists have also used combinations of direct laser energy, fiber optics, and balloon angioplasty catheters to open totally blocked right main coronary arteries. These advances may make it possible to perform angioplasty in community hospitals in nonsurgical settings.

ADVANCED EQUIPMENT

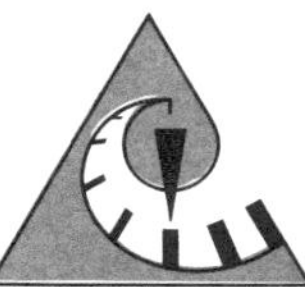

Vascular stents

Two serious complications of percutaneous transluminal coronary angioplasty (PTCA) are acute vessel closure and late restenosis. To prevent these problems, doctors are performing a new procedure called *stenting.* The stent currently being used—the Palmaz balloon-expandable stent—consists of a stainless steel tube, the walls of which have a rectangular design. When the stent expands, each rectangle stretches to a diamond shape. The expanded stent supports the artery and helps prevent restenosis.

The stent is used in patients at risk for abrupt clotting after PTCA. Stents may also be inserted after failed PTCA to keep the patient stable until he can undergo coronary artery bypass surgery; a stent also may be used as an alternative to this surgery.

For insertion, the stent is put on a standard balloon angioplasty catheter and positioned over a guide wire. Fluoroscopy verifies correct placement; then the stent is expanded and the catheter is removed, as shown below.

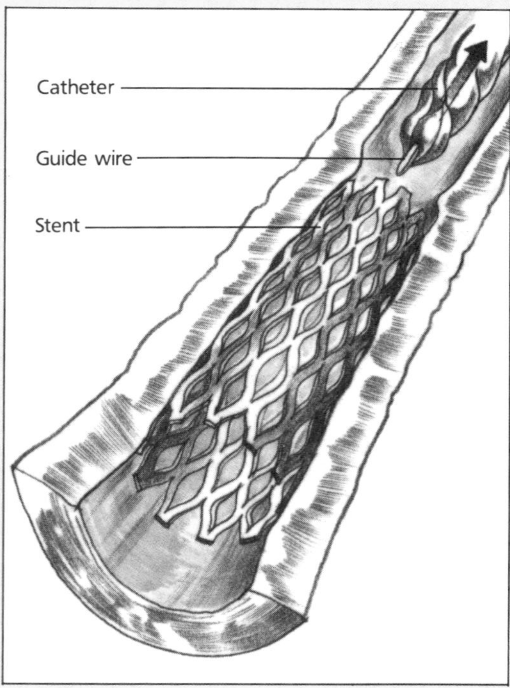

and intracoronary nitroglycerin to dilate coronary vessels and prevent spasm, if needed.
• He inflates the catheter's balloon for a gradually increasing amount of time and pressure. The expanding balloon compresses the atherosclerotic plaque against the arterial wall, expanding the arterial lumen. Because balloon inflation deprives the myocardium distal to the inflation area of blood, the patient may experience angina at this time. If balloon inflation fails to decrease the stenosis, a larger balloon may be used.
• After angioplasty, serial angiograms help determine the effectiveness of treatment.
• The doctor removes the angioplasty catheter while leaving the guide catheter in place, in case the procedure needs to be repeated because of vessel occlusion. The guide catheter is usually removed 8 to 24 hours after the procedure.

Cautions

Coronary spasm may occur during or after PTCA. For this reason, monitor the ECG for ST and T wave changes, and take vital signs frequently. Coronary artery dissection may occur with no early symptoms, but it can cause restenosis of the vessel. Be alert for symptoms of ischemia, which requires emergency coronary revascularization.

Monitoring and aftercare

• When the patient returns to the unit, he may be receiving I.V. heparin or nitroglycerin. If there is bleeding at the catheter insertion site, he may also have a sandbag on the insertion site to prevent a hematoma.
• Assess the patient's vital signs every 15 minutes for the first hour, then every 30 minutes for 4 hours, unless the patient's condition warrants more frequent checking.
• Assess peripheral pulses distal to the catheter insertion site as well as the color, sensation, temperature, and capillary refill of the affected extremity.
• Monitor ECG rhythm and arterial pressures.
• Instruct the patient to remain in bed for 8 hours and to keep the affected extremity straight; if the patient is restless and moving his extremities, apply soft restraints if neces-

sary. Elevate the head of the bed 15 to 30 degrees.

- Assess the catheter site for hematoma, ecchymosis, and hemorrhage. If an area of expanding hematoma appears, mark the site and alert the doctor. If bleeding occurs, locate the artery and apply manual pressure; then notify the doctor.
- Administer I.V. fluids as ordered — usually 100 ml/hour — to promote excretion of the contrast medium. Be sure to assess for signs of fluid overload (distended neck veins, atrial and ventricular gallops, dyspnea, pulmonary congestion, tachycardia, hypertension, and hypoxemia).
- After the doctor removes the catheter, apply direct pressure for at least 10 minutes and monitor the site frequently.
- Note the patient's tolerance of the procedure and his condition after it, including vital signs and the condition of the extremity distal to the insertion site. Document any complications and interventions.

Balloon valvuloplasty

Although the treatment of choice for valvular heart disease is surgery, balloon valvuloplasty is an alternative to valve replacement in patients with critical stenoses. This relatively new technique enlarges the orifice of a heart valve that has been narrowed by a congenital defect, calcification, rheumatic fever, or aging. It evolved from PTCA and uses the same balloon-tipped catheters for dilatation.

Balloon valvuloplasty was first performed successfully on pediatric patients, then on elderly patients who had stenotic valves complicated by other medical problems, such as chronic obstructive pulmonary disease. The procedure is done in the cardiac catheterization laboratory under local anesthesia. The doctor inserts a balloon-tipped catheter through the patient's femoral vein or artery, threads it into the heart, and repeatedly inflates it against the leaflets of the diseased valve. This increases the size of the orifice, improving valvular function and helping prevent complications from decreased cardiac output. (See *Balloon valvuloplasty,* page 54.)

Your role includes teaching the patient and family about valvuloplasty and monitoring for potential complications, both during and after the procedure.

Indications

- Patients who face a high risk from surgery
- Patients who refuse surgery
- Elderly patients, especially those older than age 80

Contraindications and complications

Severe complications, such as MI or calcium emboli (embolization of debris released from the calcified valve), are rare. Other complications include bleeding or hematoma at the insertion site, arrhythmias, circulatory disorders distal to the insertion site, guide wire perforation of the ventricle leading to tamponade, disruption of the valve ring, restenosis of the valve, and valvular insufficiency, which can contribute to congestive heart failure and reduced cardiac output. Infection and an allergic reaction to the contrast medium can also occur.

Equipment

Povidone-iodine solution • local anesthetic • valvuloplasty or balloon-tipped catheter • I.V. solution and tubing • ECG and electrodes • pulmonary artery catheter • contrast medium • oxygen • nasal cannula • sedative • emergency medications • shaving supplies or depilatory cream • heparin for injection • introducer kit for balloon catheter • sterile gown, gloves, mask, cap, and drapes • 5-lb (2.3-kg) sandbag • nitroglycerin (optional)

Preparation

- Reinforce the doctor's explanation of balloon valvuloplasty to the patient and his family, including its risks and alternatives.
- Reassure the patient that although he'll be awake during the procedure, he'll receive a sedative and a local anesthetic beforehand.
- Teach the patient what to expect. For example, inform him that his groin area will be shaved and cleaned with an antiseptic; he'll feel a brief, stinging sensation when the local

Balloon valvuloplasty

In balloon valvuloplasty, the doctor inserts a balloon-tipped catheter through the femoral vein or artery and threads it into the heart. After locating the stenotic valve, he inflates the balloon, increasing the size of the valve opening.

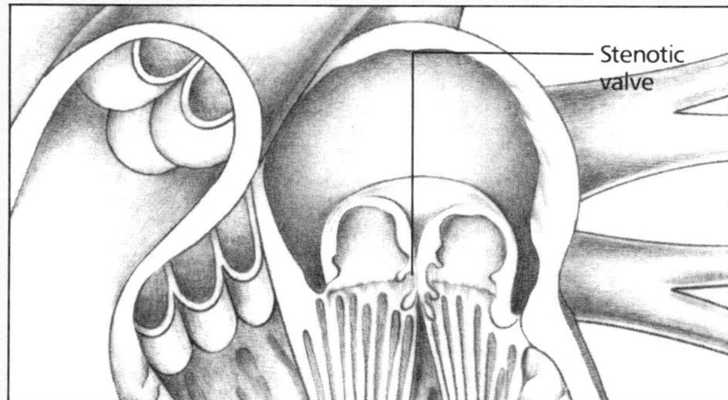

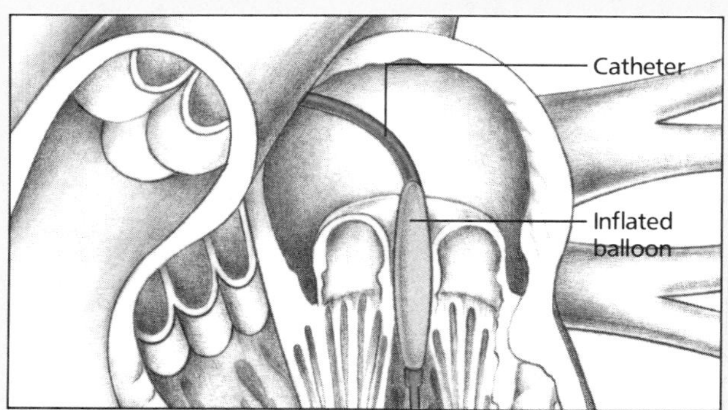

anesthetic is injected; and he may feel pressure as the catheter moves along the vessel. Describe the warm, flushed feeling he's likely to experience from injection of the contrast medium.
• Tell him that the procedure may last up to 4 hours and that he may feel discomfort from lying on a hard table for that long.
• Make sure that the patient has no allergies to shellfish, iodine, or contrast media, and that he or a family member has signed a consent form.
• Keep the patient off food and fluids (except for medications) for at least 6 hours before valvuloplasty or as ordered (usually after midnight the night before the procedure).
• Ensure that the results of routine laboratory studies and blood typing and crossmatching are available.
• Insert an I.V. line to provide access for medications.
• Take baseline peripheral pulses in all extremities.
• Shave the insertion sites or use a depilatory cream; then clean the sites with povidone-iodine solution.
• Give the patient a sedative, as ordered.
• Have the patient void.
• When the patient arrives at the cardiac catheterization laboratory, apply ECG electrodes and ensure I.V. line patency.
• Administer oxygen by nasal cannula.

Essential steps

• Help the doctor put on a sterile gown, gloves, mask, and cap and open the sterile supplies.
• The doctor prepares and anesthetizes the catheter insertion site (usually at the femoral artery). He may insert a pulmonary artery catheter if one is not already in place.
• He then inserts a large guide catheter into the site and threads a valvuloplasty or balloon-tipped catheter up into the heart.
• The doctor injects a contrast medium to visualize the heart valves and assess the stenosis. He also injects heparin to prevent the catheter from clotting.
• Using low pressure, he inflates the balloon on the valvuloplasty catheter for a short time, usually 12 to 30 seconds, gradually increasing the time and pressure. If the stenosis isn't reduced, a larger balloon may be used.
• After completion of valvuloplasty, a series of angiograms are taken to determine the effectiveness of the treatment.
• The doctor sutures the guide catheter in

place. He'll remove it after the effects of the heparin have worn off.

Cautions

Assess the patient's vital signs constantly during the procedure, especially if it's an aortic valvuloplasty. During balloon inflation, the aortic outflow tract is completely obstructed, causing blood pressure to fall dangerously low. Ventricular ectopy is also common during balloon positioning and inflation. Start treatment for ectopy when symptoms develop or when ventricular tachycardia is sustained. Carefully assess the patient's respiratory status—changes in rate and pattern can be the first sign of a complication, such as embolism.

Assess pedal pulses with a Doppler stethoscope. They'll be difficult to detect, especially if the catheter sheath remains in place. Also assess for complications: embolism, hemorrhage, chest pain, and cardiac tamponade. Using heparin and a large-bore catheter can lead to arterial hemorrhage. This complication can be reversed with protamine sulfate when the sheath is removed, or the sheath can be left in place and removed 6 to 8 hours after the heparin is discontinued. Chest pain can result from obstruction of blood flow during aortic valvuloplasty, so assess for symptoms of myocardial ischemia. Also be alert for symptoms of cardiac tamponade (decreased or absent peripheral pulses, pale or cyanotic skin, hypotension, and paradoxical pulse), which requires emergency surgery.

Monitoring and aftercare

- When he returns to the unit, the patient may be receiving I.V. heparin or nitroglycerin. He may also have a sandbag on the insertion site to prevent hematoma formation.
- Monitor ECG rhythm and arterial pressures.
- Monitor the insertion site frequently for signs of hemorrhage because exsanguination can occur rapidly.
- To prevent excessive hip flexion and migration of the catheter, keep the affected leg straight and elevate the head of the bed no more than 15 degrees. If necessary, use a soft restraint.
- Monitor vital signs every 15 minutes for the first hour, every 30 minutes for the next 2 hours, and then hourly for the next 5 hours. If vital signs are unstable, notify the doctor and continue to check them every 5 minutes.
- When you take vital signs, assess peripheral pulses distal to the catheter insertion site as well as the color, sensation, temperature, and capillary refill time of the affected extremity.
- Assess the catheter site for hematoma, ecchymosis, and hemorrhage. If a hematoma expands, mark the site and alert the doctor.
- Auscultate regularly for murmurs, which may indicate worsening valvular insufficiency. Notify the doctor if you detect a new or worsening murmur.
- Provide I.V. fluids at a rate of at least 100 ml/hour to help the kidneys excrete the contrast medium. Assess the patient for signs of fluid overload: distended neck veins, atrial and ventricular gallops, dyspnea, pulmonary congestion, tachycardia, hypertension, and hypoxemia. Monitor intake and output closely.
- Encourage the patient to perform deep-breathing exercises to prevent atelectasis. This is especially important in elderly patients.
- After the guide catheter is removed (usually 6 to 12 hours after valvuloplasty), apply direct pressure for at least 10 minutes and monitor the site frequently.
- Note the patient's tolerance for the procedure and his condition afterward. Document any complications and interventions.

Cardiopulmonary support system

A portable, percutaneous cardiopulmonary support system (CPS) provides rapid, temporary, complete support of cardiac and pulmonary function in critically ill patients who are unresponsive to conventional therapy. Developed in 1985 for bedside use in critical care units, the CPS perfuses vital organs until other, definitive measures can be initiated.

The CPS removes circulating venous blood by a large-bore cannula placed in the femoral or internal jugular vein. The pump carries blood through the membrane oxygenator,

ADVANCED EQUIPMENT

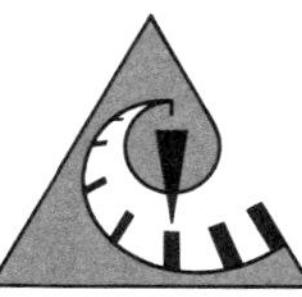

Cardiopulmonary support system

A cardiopulmonary support system (CPS) provides quick, temporary support of cardiac and pulmonary function in critically ill patients who don't respond to conventional treatment.

Bard system

The Bard CPS, shown below, is a full-support device that uses a Bio-Medicus pump to remove venous blood from a femoral cannula and move it through a membrane oxygenator. The blood is then warmed and returned to the patient through another femoral cannula. The extra lines shown provide pressure monitoring, a recirculation loop, and a purging circuit.

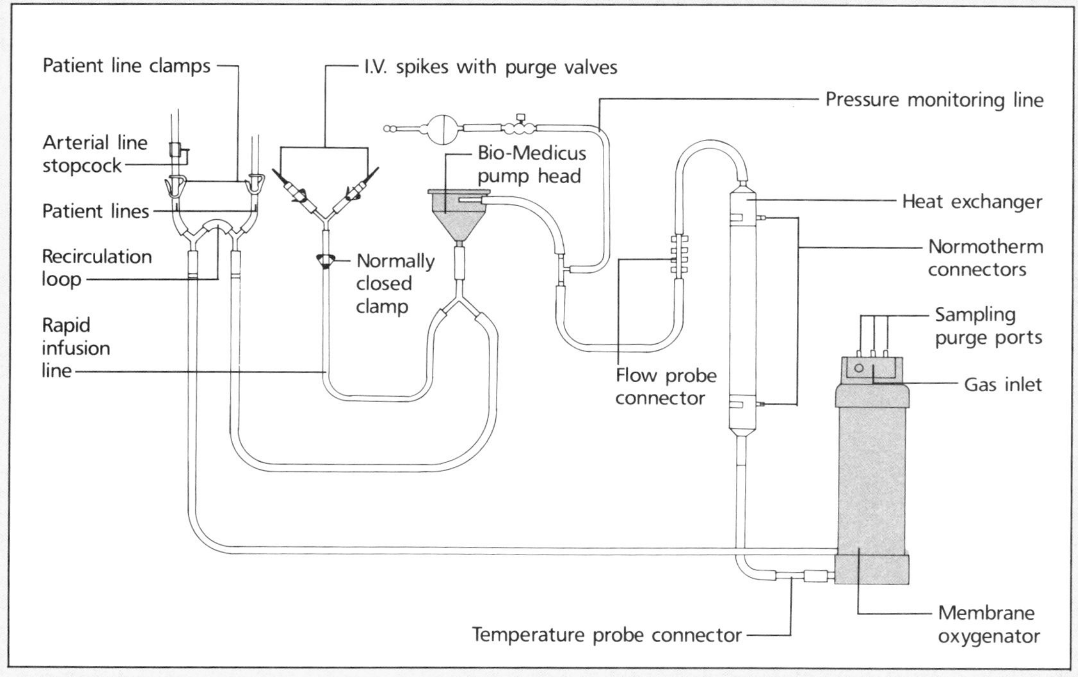

where the blood is oxygenated and carbon dioxide is removed. The blood is then heated and returned to the patient through another cannula inserted in the femoral artery. (See *Cardiopulmonary support system.*)

Another type of CPS, the hemopump, is less complicated than the Bard CPS and provides less support. (See *Hemopump,* page 58.)

Nurses are an integral part of the CPS team. You'll need to be experienced in critical care and have expertise in hemodynamic monitoring, pharmacologic support, and the principles of bypass. You'll be responsible for minute-to-minute observations and monitoring as well as for offering psychological support to patients and families.

Indications

- Cardiac arrest
- MI
- Cardiogenic shock
- Pulmonary embolus

- Septic shock
- Pulmonary edema
- Adult respiratory distress syndrome
- Smoke inhalation
- Drowning
- Hypothermia
- Drug overdose

Contraindications and complications

The CPS isn't recommended for trauma victims because the need for systemic anticoagulation could cause massive hemorrhage.

The most common complication of CPS use is bleeding, which can range from minor oozing to severe hemorrhage. Bleeding is caused by anticoagulation, hemolysis of red blood cells by the system's centrifugal pump, and damage to blood vessels during cannulation.

Thromboembolism may occur from inadequate anticoagulation, damage to the lining of the blood vessels by the cannulae, dislodged plaque during cannulation, or hemostasis. Infection, which is common, can be caused by poor sterile technique used in cannulation or by contamination of the CPS circuit.

Multisystem organ failure can occur during or after treatment with a CPS. It can result from massive blood transfusions, causing reactions or fluid overload. Capillary leakage is common with CPS or other bypass devices and results in third-spacing. Air embolism can occur if air remains in the circuitry during the priming or if air enters the system from a disconnection of any of the components.

Equipment

Heparin • priming solution • shaving supplies or depilatory cream • povidone-iodine solution • arterial line • pulmonary artery catheter • ECG monitor • sterile vascular cutdown trays • fluoroscopy equipment • CPS system with centrifugal pump, hollow-fiber membrane oxygenator, water-based heat exchanger, arterial and venous cannulae, and connecting tubes • arterial and venous sampling ports • recirculation loop • rapid volume infuser • portable oxygen

Preparation

- If time permits, provide the patient and family with information about the CPS. Explain what it is, what it can accomplish, and what the patient can expect in the ICU during the procedure (such as frequent monitoring of vital signs and continuous observation).
- Shave the insertion sites (usually in the groin), or use a depilatory cream for hair removal.
- Clean the area with povidone-iodine solution.
- If the patient doesn't already have an arterial line and a pulmonary artery catheter in place, set them up and help the doctor insert them.
- As ordered, give the patient a bolus of heparin (usually 300 units/kg of body weight) to prevent coagulation. Add 2,500 units of heparin to each 1-liter bag of priming solution.
- Set up the CPS circuitry and prime the system to remove all air from all system components.
- Reset and calibrate the centrifugal pump.
- Set the heat exchanger at an appropriate temperature.
- Connect the membrane oxygenator to a portable oxygen source.

Essential steps

- The doctor establishes vascular access by cannulating the femoral artery and vein percutaneously, if possible, or by performing a surgical cutdown. The internal jugular vein is another possible insertion site.
- To facilitate cannula insertion at either femoral site, rotate the patient's hip onto a firm surface, such as a cardiac board or a backboard.
- The doctor advances the cannulae until their tips are at the level of the superior vena cava and the right atrium.
- Connect the CPS circuit to the cannulae.
- Gradually increase the pump speed until you can no longer obtain a blood flow, as evidenced on the arterial waveform.

Cautions

To prevent an air embolism, be sure to remove all air from all components of the system. Do this by priming the circuit with an electrolyte solution to displace the air. Ensure that all connections are secure and that all lines are closed at all times.

When you're assessing hemodynamic status, remember that the thermal dilution car-

ADVANCED EQUIPMENT

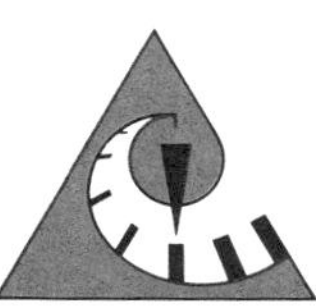

Hemopump

The hemopump is much less complicated than the Bard system because it isn't a full-support device. A temporary left ventricular assist device, the hemopump is used to treat patients in cardiogenic shock and those who've failed to be weaned from the cardiopulmonary bypass.

The pump has three main components: the purge assembly, the cannula and pump, and the control console. The purge assembly (shown at right) delivers lubricating fluid to the pump and the drive cable. A motor connected to the drive cable (bottom left) supplies power to the pump. A control console (not shown) is used to adjust the pump's rate and speed.

To insert the pump, the doctor performs a cutdown under local anesthesia over the femoral artery, then guides the cannula into the left ventricle. The pump draws blood from the left ventricle into the descending aorta and distributes it throughout the body. The section of cannula housing the pump is located in the descending aorta (bottom right).

Purge assembly

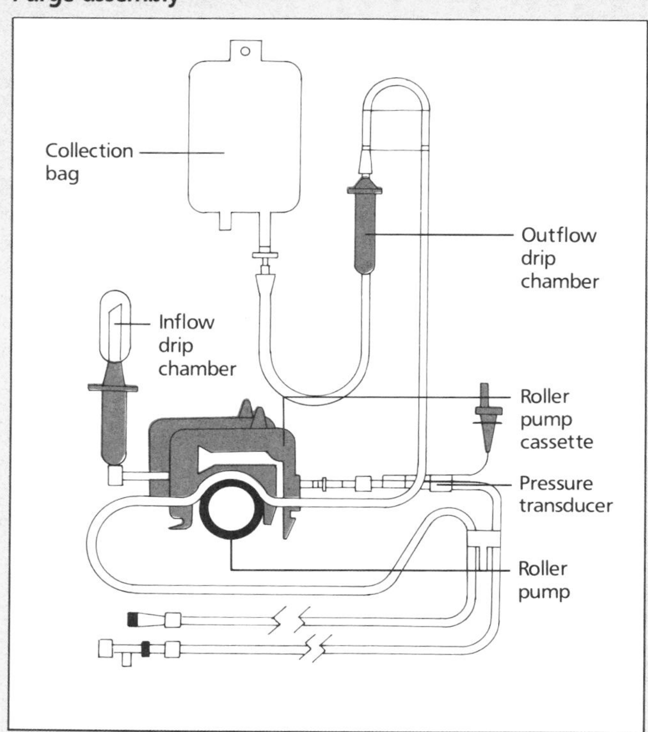

Motor and drive cable placement

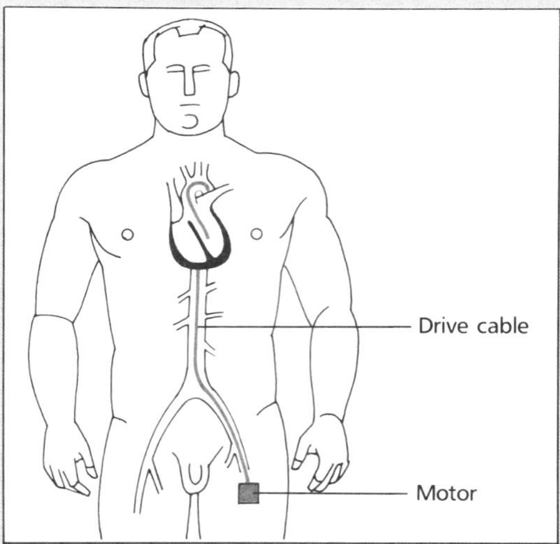

Cannula and pump placement

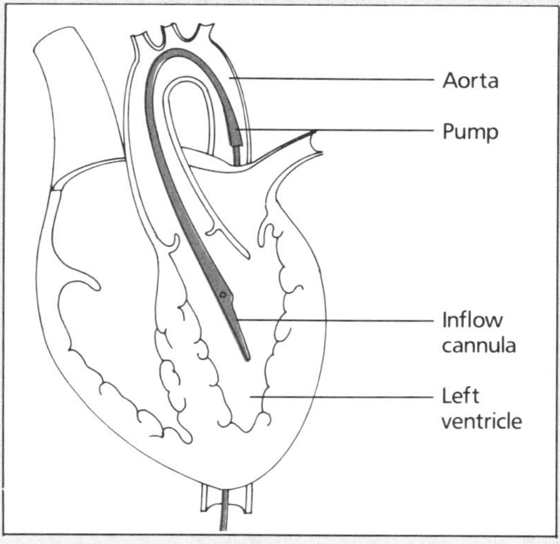

diac output will be inaccurate because the cannula removes the injectate from the right atrium. Use the pump flow to measure cardiac output. Frequent assessment of the patient's clinical status (not just hemodynamic status) is critical in detecting potential complications. Maintain adequate anticoagulation to prevent thromboembolism, a significant complication of CPS use.

Monitoring and aftercare

- To ensure adequate perfusion, assess the patient's hemodynamic and clinical status continuously. This includes cardiac output (blood flow), mean arterial pressure (MAP), and systemic vascular resistance (SVR).
- Watch for shuddering, or chattering, of the venous tubing, which indicates inadequate circulating blood volume. It can cause the vena cava at the tip of the venous cannula to collapse. To prevent this from occurring, provide adequate amounts of replacement fluid.
- Monitor vital signs every 15 minutes or as needed.
- Maintain blood flow at 50 to 60 ml/kg/minute. Inotropic agents usually aren't used during full CPS support. Administer fluid volume, if necessary. Use peripheral vasoactive drugs to improve SVR, if needed.
- Maintain SVR between 800 and 1,200 dynes/liter/second. On full CPS, this equals MAP divided by pump flow.
- Monitor intake and output.
- Observe the arterial waveform to ensure that no systolic-diastolic deflections occur, indicating that the heart isn't fully bypassed. You should see only MAP.
- Monitor the patient's clinical status, including LOC, urine output, and skin temperature. Take the patient's temperature frequently.
- Assess his ECG pattern frequently.
- Monitor arterial blood gas levels to ensure adequate tissue oxygenation. Also check the color of the mucous membranes as well as the color of blood returning to the patient by the arterial cannula.
- Administer anticoagulants continuously. Monitor activated clotting time (ACT) every 20 minutes, and adjust heparin as ordered to maintain ACT greater than 480 seconds.
- Assess the patient's breath sounds and breathing pattern. A decrease in sounds or respiratory distress can indicate pulmonary embolism.
- Observe for bleeding by checking all invasive sites, secretions, and body fluids.
- Assess all invasive sites for redness, pain, swelling, and drainage. If you see signs of infection, discontinue the line, culture the site, and administer antibiotics as ordered. Monitor the white blood cell count and differential.
- Document the time and date that CPS was initiated, the sites used, the patient's reaction to the procedure, his vital signs, his hemodynamic status, and all other pertinent observations.

Autologous transfusion

Also called autotransfusion, autologous transfusion is the collection, filtration, and reinfusion of the patient's own blood. Although the technique was developed in the 1920s, it wasn't used widely until the 1960s, when cardiac surgery became common. Today, with the concern over acquired immunodeficiency syndrome and other blood-borne diseases, autologous transfusion is on the rise.

Autologous transfusion has several advantages over transfusion of bank blood. Transfusion reactions don't occur, diseases aren't transmitted, anticoagulants aren't added (except in postoperative autotransfusion, when acid citrate dextrose [ACD] or citrate phosphate dextrose [CPD] is added), and the blood supply isn't depleted. And unlike bank blood, autologous blood contains normal levels of 2,3-diphosphoglycerate, which is helpful in tissue oxygenation.

Autologous transfusion is performed before, during, or after surgery and after traumatic injury. The three techniques used are preoperative blood donation, perioperative blood donation, and acute normovolemic hemodilution.

Preoperative blood donation is commonly recommended for patients scheduled for orthopedic surgery, which causes large blood loss. The donation period begins 4 to 6 weeks before surgery.

Perioperative blood donation (sometimes called intraoperative or postoperative) is used in vascular and orthopedic surgery and in treatment of traumatic injury. Blood may be collected during surgery or up to 12 hours afterward. (There may be a lot of bleeding following vascular and orthopedic surgery.) It's transfused immediately after collection or processed (washed) before infusion. Blood obtained postoperatively may be collected from chest tubes, mediastinal drains, or wound drains (placed in the surgical wound during surgery). Commonly inserted during orthopedic surgery, wound drains can be used when enough uncontaminated blood is recovered from a closed wound to reinfuse.

Acute normovolemic hemodilution is used mainly in open-heart surgery. One or 2 units of blood are drawn immediately before or after anesthesia induction. The blood is replaced with a crystalloid or colloid solution, such as lactated Ringer's solution or 5% dextran, to produce normovolemic anemia. The blood is reinfused right after surgery. The combination of reduced hemoglobin and the replacement solution causes the patient to lose fewer red blood cells during surgery.

The equipment and procedures presented here are for preoperative and perioperative blood donation only. Acute normovolemic hemodilution is performed the same way as preoperative blood donation, and blood collected this way is reinfused the same way as any other transfusion.

Your responsibilities for these techniques include patient teaching before the procedure, monitoring laboratory data during and after the procedure, collecting and reinfusing the blood in a preoperative donation, and observing the patient for complications.

Indications

• Elective surgery (blood donated over time)
• Nonelective surgery (blood withdrawn immediately before surgery)
• Perioperative and emergency blood salvage during and after thoracic or cardiovascular surgery, hip or knee resection, or liver resection; and during surgery for ruptured ectopic pregnancy and hemothorax
• Perioperative and emergency blood salvage for traumatic injury of the lungs, liver, chest wall, heart, pulmonary vessels, spleen, kidneys, inferior vena cava, or iliac, portal, or subclavian veins

Contraindications and complications

Autologous transfusion is contraindicated in patients with malignant neoplasms, coagulopathies, excessive hemolysis, and active infections. It's also contraindicated in patients taking antibiotics and in those whose blood becomes contaminated by abdominal contents. In addition, patients who've recently lost weight because of illness or malnutrition shouldn't donate blood.

Complications include hemolysis, air and particulate emboli, coagulation, thrombocytopenia, vasovagal reactions (from transient hypotension and bradycardia), and hypovolemia (especially in elderly patients). (See *Managing problems of autologous transfusion.*)

Equipment

For preoperative blood donation

Ferrous sulfate • povidone-iodine solution • alcohol • tourniquet • rubber ball • large-bore needle for venipuncture • collection bags • I.V. line • in-line filter for reinfusion

For perioperative blood donation

Autologous transfusion system, such as the Davol or Pleur-evac systems (see *Davol system,* page 62) • ACD or CPD • collection bottles • vacuum source regulator • suction tubing • 18G needle • blood administration set • 500 ml of 0.9% sodium chloride solution • Hemovac and another autologous transfusion system (optional)

Preparation

For preoperative blood donation

• Explain autologous transfusion to the patient, including what it is, how it's performed, how often he can donate blood (every 7 days), and how much he can donate (one unit every week until 3 to 7 days before surgery).

COMPLICATIONS

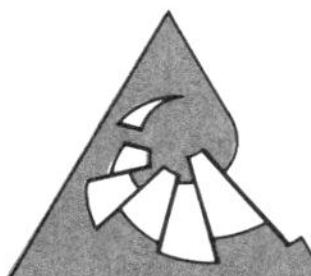

Managing problems of autologous transfusion

PROBLEM	CAUSE	INTERVENTION
Citrate toxicity (rare, unpredictable)	• Chelating effect on calcium of citrate in the citrate phosphate dextrose (CPD) • Predisposing factors, including hyperkalemia, hypocalcemia, acidosis, hypothermia, myocardial dysfunction, and liver or kidney problems.	• Watch for hypotension, arrhythmias, and myocardial contractility. • Prophylactic calcium chloride may be administered if more than 2,000 ml of CPD-anticoagulated blood is given over 20 minutes. • Stop infusing CPD and correct acidosis. Measure arterial blood gas and serum calcium levels frequently to assess for toxicity.
Coagulation	• Not enough anticoagulant • Blood not defibrinated in mediastinum	• Add CPD or another regional anticoagulant at a ratio of 7 parts blood to 1 part anticoagulant. Keep blood and CPD mixed by shaking collection bottle regularly. • Check for anticoagulant reversal. Strip chest tubes as needed.
Coagulopathies	• Reduced platelet and fibrinogen levels • Platelets caught in filters • Enhanced levels of fibrin split products	• Patients receiving autologous transfusions of more than 4,000 ml of blood may also need transfusion of fresh frozen plasma or platelet concentrate.
Emboli	• Microaggregate debris • Air	• Don't use equipment with roller pumps or pressure infusion systems. Before reinfusion, remove air from blood bags. • Reinfuse with a 20- to 40-unit microaggregate filter.
Hemolysis	• Trauma to blood caused by turbulence or roller pumps	• Don't skim operative field or use equipment with roller pumps. When collecting blood from chest tubes, keep vacuum below 30 mm Hg; when aspirating from a surgical site, keep vacuum below 60 mm Hg.
Sepsis	• Lack of aseptic technique • Contaminated blood	• Give broad-spectrum antibiotics. Use strict aseptic technique. Reinfuse patient within 4 hours. • Don't infuse blood from infected areas or blood with feces, urine, or other contaminants.

• At least 1 week before the first donation, give the patient ferrous sulfate or another iron preparation to take three times a day.
• To prevent hypovolemia, tell the patient to drink plenty of fluids before donating blood.
• Warn him that he may feel light-headed during the donation but that the problem can be treated without further compromise.
• Check the patient's hemoglobin level. It must be 11 g/dl or above to donate blood.

For perioperative blood donation
• If you know that the patient will leave surgery with a drain to the autologous transfusion device, tell him this beforehand.

Essential steps

For preoperative blood donation
• Check vital signs before blood donation.
• Help the patient into a supine position.
• Clean the needle insertion site (usually the antecubital fossa) with povidone-iodine solution, then with alcohol.
• Apply a tourniquet.

ADVANCED EQUIPMENT

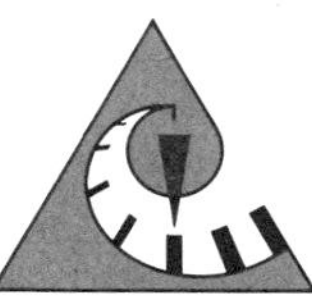

Davol system

Several perioperative autologous transfusion systems are available, including the Davol, illustrated below.

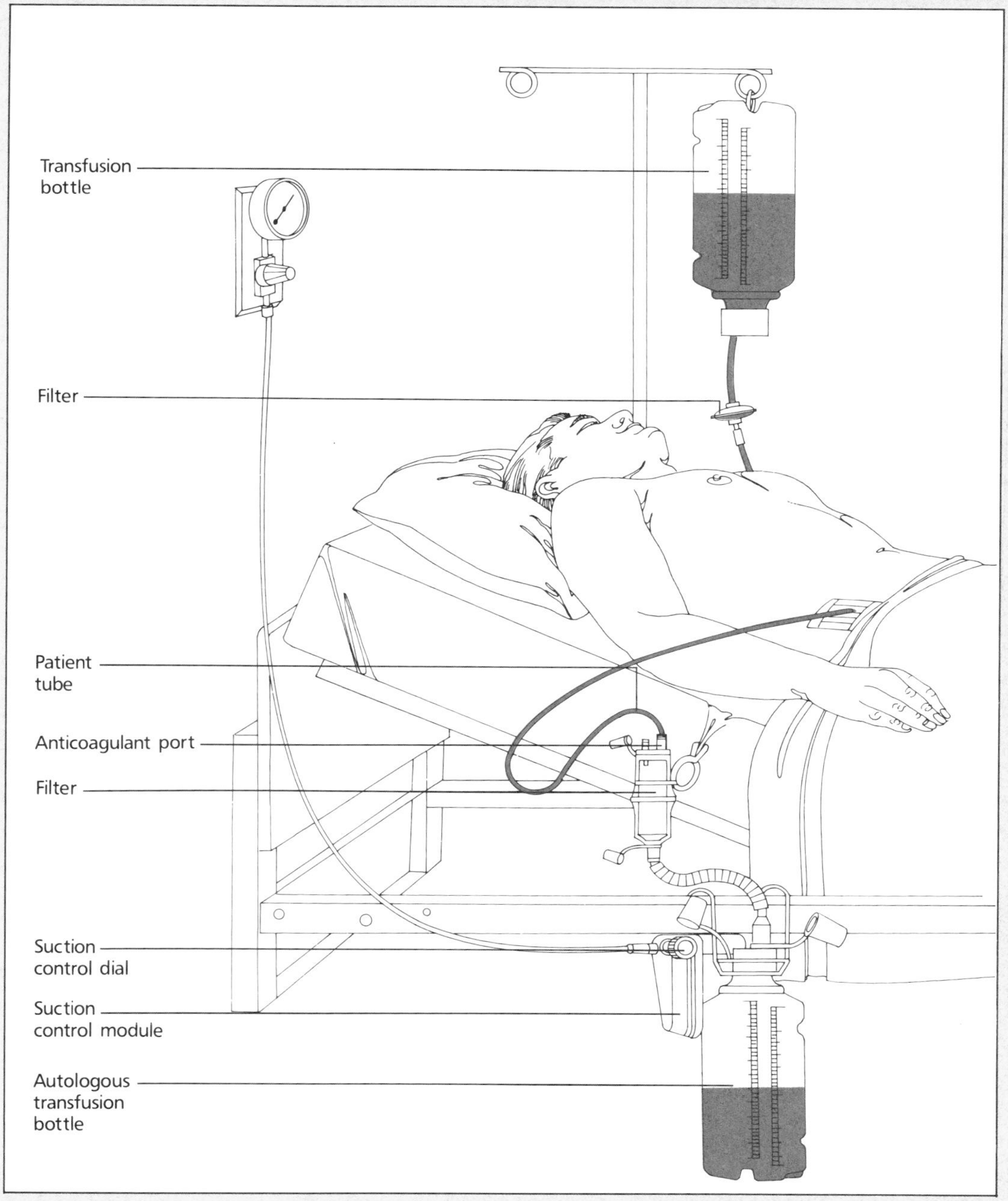

Transfusion bottle

Filter

Patient tube

Anticoagulant port

Filter

Suction control dial

Suction control module

Autologous transfusion bottle

• Insert the large-bore needle into the antecubital vein. Have the patient squeeze a rubber ball while you collect blood.
• Recheck vital signs after the collection.
• If ordered, provide replacement I.V. fluids immediately after the collection.
• Send a blood sample to the hospital laboratory to be tested.
• Before reinfusion, check vital signs again and make sure that the I.V. line is patent.
• Administer blood over 1½ to 4 hours, depending on the patient's cardiovascular status and hospital policy.

For perioperative blood donation using a Davol system
• Open the transfusion unit onto the sterile field. The doctor inserts the drain tube (from the patient) to the connecting tube of the unit.
• He injects 25 to 35 ml of ACD or CPD into the injection port on top of the filter and wets the filter with anticoagulant to keep the blood from clotting.
• Label the collection bag with the patient's name and the time the transfusion was started so that the reinfusion time is within guidelines.

After patient arrival in postanesthesia care unit or medical-surgical unit
• Note the amount of blood in the bag and on the postoperative sheet.
• Attach the tube from the suction source to the port on the suction control module.
• Adjust the suction source to between 80 and 100 mm Hg on the wall regulator. Pinch the suction tube. If the regulator exceeds 100 mm Hg, turn the suction down. Suction set at more than 100 mm Hg may cause the collection bag to collapse, resulting in lysing of blood cells. The potential for renal damage renders this blood unsafe. If the collection bag collapses, change the entire collection setup.
• If the doctor orders it, start reinfusing the blood when 500 ml has been collected or 4 hours have passed (whichever comes first). Blood reinfusion must be completed within 6 hours of initiating the collection in the operating room.
• If less than 200 ml is collected in 4 hours, record the amount on the intake and output sheet and the postoperative sheet. Discard the drainage appropriately because the proportion of anticoagulant (inserted in the operating room) to blood is too great to infuse. If this happens, switch from the container to a closed wound suction unit. First remove the suction tube from the suction control unit. Clamp the connecting tubing above the filter. Detach the connecting tubing from the patient's tube and cap the patient's tube. Connect a closed wound suction unit, such as a Hemovac, if you're not going to collect more blood for reinfusion. If more than 500 ml of blood is collected in the first 4 hours, connect a new autologous transfusion unit to the patient. Then reconnect the unit to suction. Monitor and record the drainage on the intake and output sheet.

To reinfuse the blood
• Prime the blood filter with 500 ml of 0.9% sodium chloride solution.
• Twist the suction control module to remove it.
• Remove the hanger assembly from the collection bag.
• Pull the clear cap from the top of the bag, and discard the cap and filter.
• Insert a spike adapter into the large port on top of the bottle.
• Remove the protective seal to expose the filtered vent.
• Attach the blood to the Y-connector of the blood filter.
• Invert the bag and hang it.
• Obtain vital signs and document them.
• Begin the infusion, following your hospital's instructions.
• Document the infusion on the patient's chart.
• Be sure to complete the infusion within 2 hours.

For perioperative blood donation using the Pleur-evac connected to a chest tube
• Establish underwater seal drainage. Following the steps printed on the Pleur-evac unit, connect the patient's chest tube. Inspect the blood collection bag and tubing, making sure

that all clamps are open and all connections are airtight.

• Before collection, add an anticoagulant such as heparin or CPD, if prescribed. With CPD, add one part to seven parts blood. Using an 18G (or smaller) needle, inject the anticoagulant through the red self-sealing port on the autologous transfusion connector. The system is now ready to use. You should see chest cavity blood begin to collect in the bag.

• To collect more than one bag of blood, open a replacement bag when the first one is nearly full. Close the clamps on top of the second bag. Before removing the first collection bag from the drainage unit, reduce excess negativity by using the high-negativity relief valve. Depress the button; then release it when negativity drops to the desired level (watch the water seal manometer).

• Close the white clamp on the patient tubing. Then close the two white clamps on top of the collection bag.

• Disconnect all connectors on the first bag. Attach the red (female) and blue (male) connector sections on top of the autologous transfusion bag.

• Remove the protective cap from the collection tubing on the replacement bag. Connect the collection tubing to the patient's chest drainage tube, using the red connectors.

• Remove the protective cap from the replacement bag's suction tube and attach the suction tube to the Pleur-evac unit, using the blue connectors. Make sure all connections are tight. Open all clamps, and inspect the system for airtight connections.

• Spread the metal support arms and disconnect them. Remove the first bag from the drainage unit by disconnecting the foot hook.

• Use the foot hook and support arm to attach the replacement bag.

• To reinfuse blood from the original collection bag, slide the bag off the support frame; then invert it so that the spike points upward. Remember to reinfuse blood within 6 hours of the start of collection. Never store collected blood.

• Remove the protective cap from the spike port and insert a microaggregate filter into the port, using a twisting motion. Prime the filter by gently squeezing the inverted bag. A new filter should be used with each bag.

• Continue squeezing until the filter is saturated and the drip chamber is half full. Then close the clamp on the reinfusion line and remove residual air from the bag. Invert the bag and suspend it from an I.V. pole. After carefully flushing the I.V. line to remove all air, infuse blood according to your hospital's policy.

Cautions

Monitor the patient closely during and after donation and autologous transfusion. Although vasovagal reactions are usually mild and easy to treat, they can quickly progress to severe reactions, such as loss of consciousness and seizures. Also, make sure that the patient isn't bacteremic when he donates blood. Bacteria can proliferate in the collection bag and cause sepsis when reinfused. Clearly label the collection bag: AUTOLOGOUS USE ONLY. This way, the blood won't be subjected to rigorous blood bank testing or be accidentally given to another patient. Before reinfusion, identify the patient and make sure that the collection bag is clearly marked with his name, hospital identification number, and an autologous blood label. If signs of a hemolytic reaction occur, the patient may have received the wrong unit of blood.

Monitoring and aftercare

For preoperative blood donation

• Caution the patient to remain supine for at least 10 minutes after donating blood.

• Encourage him to drink more fluids than usual for a few hours after blood donation and to eat heartily at his next meal.

• Tell him to keep an eye on the needle wound in his arm for a few hours after blood donation. If some bleeding occurs, he should apply firm pressure for 5 to 10 minutes. If the bleeding doesn't stop, he should notify the blood bank or his doctor.

• If the patient feels light-headed or dizzy, advise him to sit down immediately and to lower his head between his knees. Or he can lie down with his head lower than the rest of his body until the feeling subsides.

• Tell him that he can resume normal activities after resting 15 minutes.

For all donation methods
• Check the patient's laboratory data (coagulation profile and hemoglobin, hematocrit, and calcium levels) after he donates blood and again after reinfusion.
• Be alert for signs and symptoms of a hemolytic reaction: pain at the I.V. site, fever, chills, back pain, hypotension, and anxiety. If these occur, stop the transfusion and call the blood bank and doctor.
• Document the amount of blood that the patient donated and had reinfused, and how he tolerated each procedure.

Pneumatic antishock garment

Also known as medical antishock trousers, a MAST suit, military antishock trousers, and a G suit, a pneumatic antishock garment is made of inflatable bladders sandwiched between double layers of fabric. Three compartments in the garment can be inflated individually to compress the legs and abdomen. This raises the patient's MAP by selectively increasing peripheral vascular resistance in the lower body. The result is direct tamponade of bleeding, causing improved hemostasis and decreased blood flow to torn vessels under the garment. Although some preload occurs from autotransfusion of blood from the legs and abdomen, this effect is minimal. The dominant hemodynamic effect is a direct increase in afterload from vascular compression.

Pneumatic antishock garments are used mainly by emergency department and critical care unit nurses and by personnel on fire-rescue units, who are familiar with treating traumatic injuries and other emergencies. If you're working with a pneumatic antishock garment, your responsibilities include operating the garment, monitoring the patient's status, and observing for complications.

Indications
• Hypovolemic shock from traumatic injury
• Abdominal and lower extremity hemorrhage
• Stabilization and splinting of pelvic and femoral fractures

Contraindications and complications
A pneumatic antishock garment is contraindicated during cardiac resuscitation because it increases central venous pressure and doesn't increase coronary blood flow. It's also contraindicated in patients with cardiogenic shock, congestive heart failure, pulmonary edema, tension pneumothorax, or increased intracranial pressure. The suit should be used extremely cautiously in pregnant women because of the possibility of decreased blood flow to the fetus. And it probably shouldn't be used in patients who have foreign bodies in their abdomens or who have abdominal evisceration.

Complications of the garment include compartment syndrome of the legs; metabolic acidosis after prolonged use because of decreased tissue perfusion in the legs; impaired renal function; decreased diaphragmatic excursion and reduced vital capacity caused by inflation of the abdominal section; vomiting from abdominal compression; and skin breakdown after prolonged use.

Equipment
Pneumatic antishock garment in appropriate size (either pediatric or adult) • foot pump • resuscitative equipment

Preparation
• Explain the procedure to the patient. Tell him that he'll feel his legs and abdomen being compressed during inflation.
• Take the patient's baseline vital signs.
• Assess his physical condition to ensure that the garment isn't contraindicated.

Essential steps
• On a smooth surface, open the garment with the Velcro fasteners down. (See *Using a pneumatic antishock garment,* page 66).
• Open all stopcock valves so that the suit will inflate uniformly.

Using a pneumatic antishock garment

Open the pneumatic antishock garment on a flat surface with the Velcro fasteners down, as shown below.

After moving the patient onto the garment, close it. Make sure that all valves are properly positioned, as shown below.

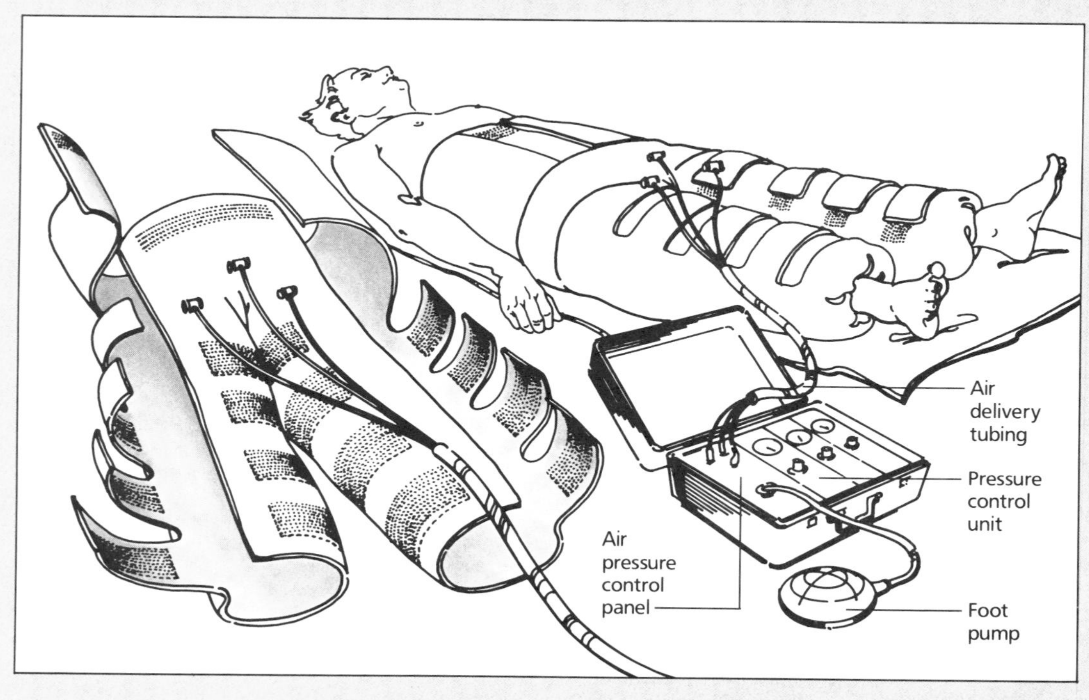

• Attach the foot pump tubing to the valve on the pressure control unit. If the patient can't be turned from side to side, slide the garment under him. If he can be turned, place the garment next to him and, with assistance, logroll him onto it.

• Before closing the garment, remove any sharp objects, such as pieces of glass, stones, keys, or a buckle, that could injure the patient or tear the garment. As appropriate, pad the pressure points and apply lanolin to protect the patient's skin from irritation.

• Double-check the stopcocks to ensure that they're all open.

• Place the upper edge of the garment just below the patient's lowest rib. Wrap the right leg compartment around the patient's right leg. Secure the compartment by fastening the Velcro straps from the ankle to the thigh.

• Repeat the above procedure for the left leg; then wrap the abdomen.

• Monitor the patient's vital signs while you inflate the garment slowly. Inflate the leg section of the garment first, then the abdominal section, to 20 to 30 mg Hg initially. Stop inflation when the patient's systolic blood pressure reaches 100 mm Hg or the desired level. Close all stopcocks to prevent accidental air loss.

Cautions

Before deflation, make sure that I.V. lines are patent, that a doctor is in attendance, and that emergency equipment is available.

Also, deflate each section of the garment slowly before removal. Deflating too quickly allows circulating blood to rush to the legs, causing potentially irreversible shock. Monitor blood pressure continuously during deflation, and don't remove the garment until the patient's blood volume is restored, his condition is stabilized, or he needs to be prepared for surgery. Keep fluids and blood available during deflation in case of hemodynamic instability.

Monitoring and aftercare

- To determine the patient's response to the pneumatic antishock garment, continue checking his vital signs every 5 minutes.
- Check the patient's pedal pulses and temperature periodically. If circulation is impaired, notify the doctor.
- If the garment is used for a long time, the patient may need a nasogastric tube because pressure on the abdomen can cause vomiting.
- Open the abdominal stopcock and begin to release small amounts of air while you closely monitor blood pressure. If the pressure of the antishock garment drops to 5 mm Hg, close the stopcock.
- If you need to stop deflation because the patient's blood pressure drops, increase the flow rate of the I.V. solution to help stabilize the blood pressure.
- If the blood pressure is stable, continue to deflate the garment slowly. After the abdominal section is deflated, deflate the legs simultaneously.
- When the garment is loose enough, gently pull it off.
- If necessary, clean the garment, but don't use solvents or autoclave it.
- Record the time of application and removal as well as the patient's vital signs before application, during treatment, and after removal.

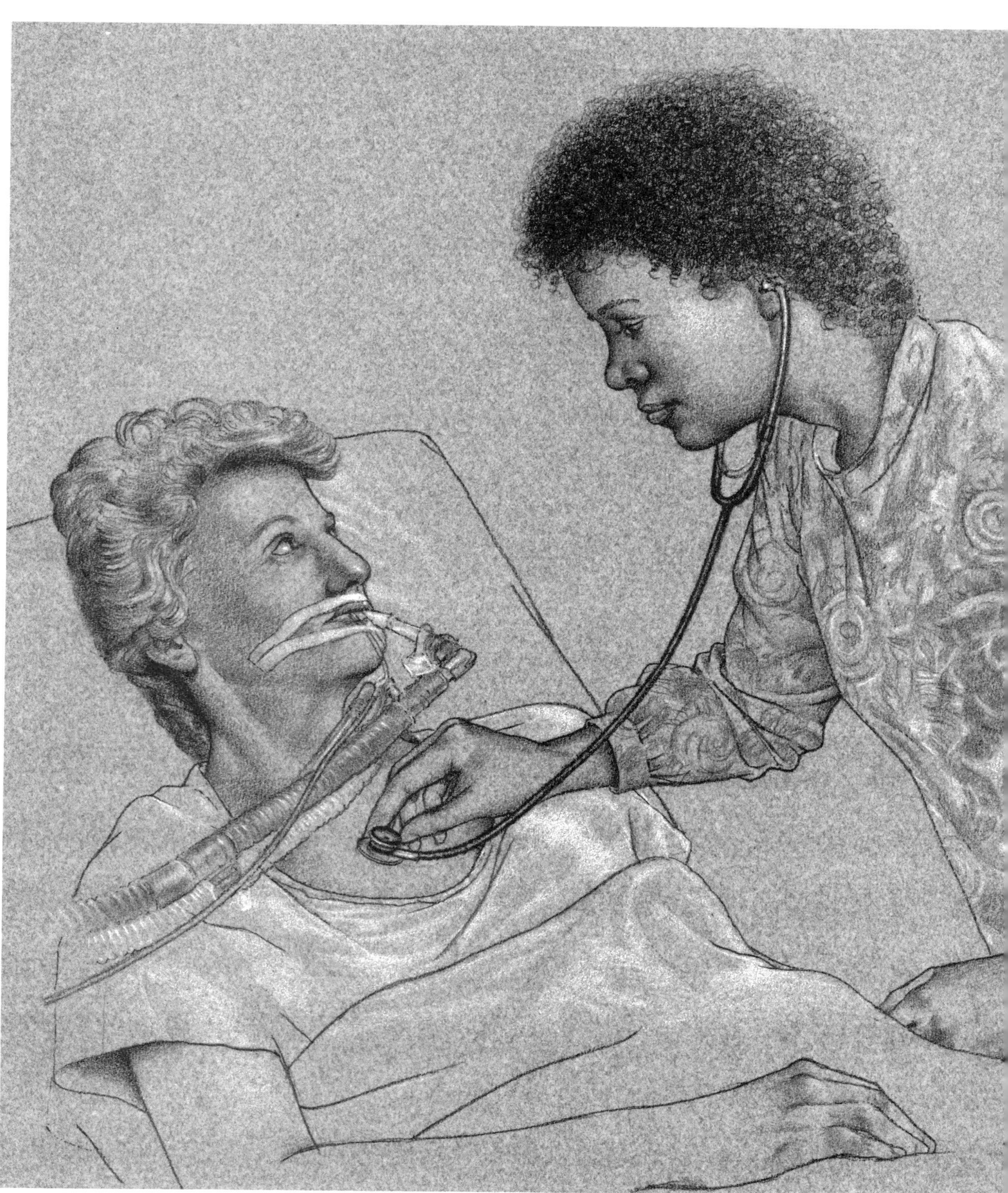

CHAPTER

Respiratory procedures

Impaired respiratory function can be a significant problem for any patient, but particularly for those with underlying pulmonary, musculoskeletal, neurologic, or cardiac disorders. Managing the respiratory care of patients like these will be one of your first priorities.

Whether your patient needs intermittent supplemental oxygen or complete ventilatory support, you'll need to be able to recognize and assess his condition—which can change quickly—and respond with appropriate care.

The number of respiratory procedures you're expected to perform or assist with has grown in recent years. And although many health care facilities have staff members who specialize in respiratory procedures, you must still know how to treat respiratory problems. To do this effectively, you need to keep current with advances in respiratory care.

This chapter presents the newest and most advanced respiratory procedures as well as established procedures. It includes entries on everything from extracorporeal membrane oxygenation to thoracic drainage, and from applying continuous positive airway pressure to performing thoracentesis. Each entry follows the same format, with an introduction, indications, contraindications and complications, equipment, preparation, essential steps, cautions, and monitoring and aftercare.

Extracorporeal membrane oxygenation

A highly technical procedure, extracorporeal membrane oxygenation (ECMO) helps treat patients with respiratory failure who don't respond to conventional therapy.

The procedure is used most commonly in neonates no more than 10 days old who have severe respiratory compromise. It's used less commonly in pediatric patients and in adults with adult respiratory distress syndrome (ARDS), pneumonia, pulmonary emboli, or inhalation injuries. ECMO results in a higher mortality in adults than neonates.

In an adaptation of cardiopulmonary bypass used during open-heart surgery, blood pumped by the heart is diverted from the lungs so that the lungs have a chance to rest and heal. A machine removes the blood from the body and oxygenates it, then returns it to the body. Blood removal and return takes place by one of two methods: venoarterial or venovenous. During oxygenation, the blood flows through a venous reservoir or bladder attached to a servoregulator that monitors reservoir filling. The blood passes through the oxygenator membrane and then through a heat exchanger before being returned to the patient. (See *Understanding the ECMO circuit.*)

Because ECMO is performed only for the acutely ill, the patient needs diligent nursing care. At many health care facilities, ECMO treatments are coordinated by a team, including a respiratory therapist, a perfusionist, and a nurse. You're responsible for the ongoing assessment and care of the patient, who requires hemodynamic monitoring and drug therapy to maintain a mean arterial pressure that's sufficient to perfuse vital organs and the extracorporeal membrane. You'll monitor his oxygenation continuously and provide psychological support to the patient and his family.

ECMO isn't performed unless the benefits outweigh the risks—after maximal ventilatory support has failed to improve oxygenation as indicated by a partial pressure of oxygen in arterial blood (PaO_2) level less than 40 mm Hg with an optimal positive end-expiratory pressure (PEEP) for at least 2 hours.

Indications

In neonates

- Meconium aspiration syndrome
- Respiratory distress syndrome
- Congenital diaphragmatic hernia with coexistent pulmonary hypoplasia
- Sepsis
- Persistent pulmonary hypertension
- Cardiac failure secondary to congenital or acquired problems
- Hyaline membrane disease
- Persistent fetal circulation

In adults

- ARDS
- Bacterial or viral pneumonia
- Pulmonary emboli
- Inhalation injuries
- Pulmonary hemorrhage
- Cardiogenic shock

Contraindications and complications

ECMO is contraindicated in any irreversible condition that hinders oxygenation, in profound neurologic impairment or intracranial hemorrhage, in incurable cancers, in uncontrollable bleeding disorders, in multisystem failure, and in neonates with a gestational age of less than 35 weeks whose birth weight is less than 2,000 g (because of an increased risk of intracranial hemorrhage). It's also contraindicated if the patient has been on mechanical ventilation for more than 10 days.

In some cases, ECMO may be contraindicated in a patient with significant congenital anomalies.

Understanding the ECMO circuit

An aggressive treatment that provides lung bypass, extracorporeal membrane oxygenation (ECMO) functions as a temporary artificial lung. ECMO diverts pulmonary blood flow, decompresses the pulmonary circuit, and supports systemic circulation. The process can minimize right-to-left shunt and correct hypoxia and hypercapnia.

The ECMO circuit can bypass the lungs venoarterially or venovenously. In the venoarterial (vein-to-artery) circuit, shown below, the patient's blood is removed through a venous access in the right internal jugular vein and advanced into the right atrium. A regulator monitors the blood volume. A pump moves the blood to the oxygenator through a warming device, then by the right carotid artery into the aortic arch.

The venovenous (vein-to-vein) method drains blood by gravity, usually from the right atrium, into the extracorporeal circuit. The blood is oxygenated and warmed, then returned by a catheter in the vena cava closer to the heart. An advantage of the venovenous system is the decreased incidence of embolism. Also, no major artery is cannulated. A disadvantage is that although the venovenous system provides respiratory support, it can't be used for cardiac support.

Pathway of venoarterial ECMO

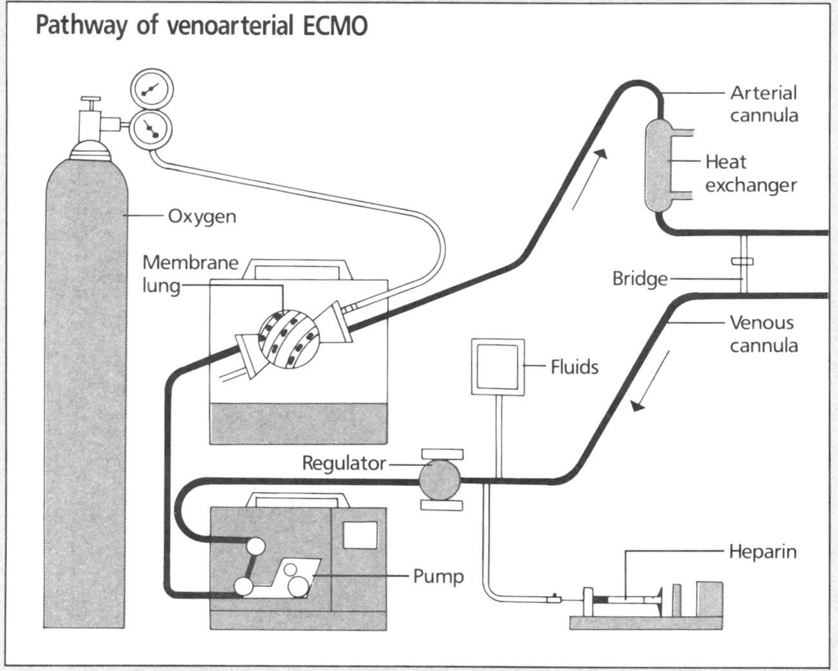

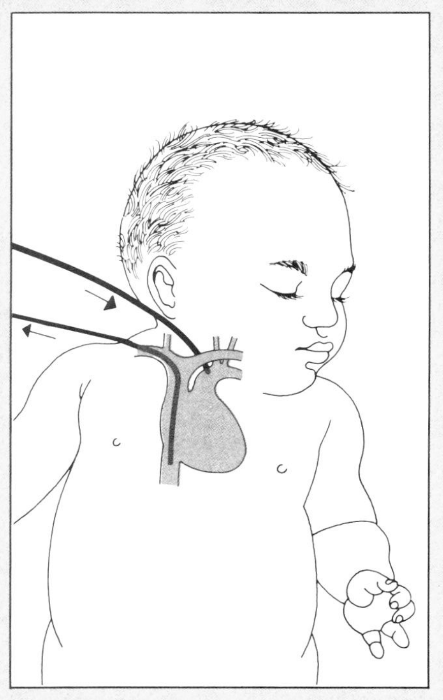

Of the mechanical complications associated with ECMO, the most common are hemorrhage and sepsis. The patient may suffer hemorrhage at the cannulation sites, or he may experience internal GI or intracranial hemorrhage as a result of the systemic heparin needed to prevent thrombus formation within the ECMO circuit. Sepsis may result from the patient's compromised state and the use of large, invasive cannulas.

Other mechanical complications include thrombus formation, cannula malposition, cannula dislodgment, patent ductus arteriosus, and perforation of the cannula outside the vein.

Equipment

Catheter • oxygenator (The main component of the oxygenator is a gas-permeable silicone polymer membrane that permits the diffusion of oxygen and carbon dioxide. Desaturated venous blood enters the oxygenator at one end and oxygen enters at the other, and these two phases are separated by the membrane. This process is similar to the action of the lungs diffusing oxygen into the blood while carbon monoxide is removed from the blood.) • ECMO circuit (The ECMO circuit will be assembled for use by a doctor or nurse specially trained to do so.) • sedation as ordered

Preparation

Help prepare the patient and his family for the emotional strain of the ECMO procedure. The parents of a neonate may need extra support, information, and reassurance as they adjust to the fact that their child was born with a serious health problem. With an older patient, you'll need to explain the procedure carefully and answer the patient's questions.

Prime the ECMO circuit. This is ordinarily done by the perfusionist or a respiratory therapist with specialized training in ECMO.

Essential steps

• Obtain a signed consent form from the patient or family.
• If time permits, arrange for testing before ECMO to rule out profound neurologic deficits. Tests usually include cranial ultrasound, EEG, a complete neurologic examination, and echocardiography.
• Make sure that all invasive procedures, such as arterial line placement, urinary catheter placement, and nasogastric tube placement, are performed before catheter cannulation, to prevent bleeding. Systemic anticoagulation is maintained after vessel cannulation.
• Ensure an adequate supply of blood products, including whole blood, packed cells, fresh frozen plasma, and platelets.
• Give medications—such as sedatives, muscle relaxants, or paralytic agents—as necessary for the cannulation process as well as analgesics for discomfort. Make sure that emergency medications are available and ready for administration.
• During the catheter insertion procedure (performed by a surgical team at the patient's bedside or in the operating room), monitor the patient's hemodynamic status. Give vasopressors as directed.
• After the vessels are exposed, give heparin at 30 to 100 units/kg to obtain systemic anticoagulation.
• Once the catheter is in place, the cannulas are connected to the ECMO circuit and the pump flow is gradually increased to approximately 80 to 120 ml/kg/minute.
• As flow to the ECMO circuit is increased, mechanical ventilator settings are decreased to allow the lungs a chance to rest. The settings vary, depending on the patient's age and condition.
• During ECMO, you may need to administer chest physiotherapy or arrange for daily chest X-rays. You'll monitor activated clotting times, give heparin, and continually assess the patient for volume overload or depletion. You'll also give diuretics or osmotic agents, sedatives, vasopressors, blood and blood products, and antibiotics, as necessary. All medications other than platelets may be given through the venous side of the circuit. Monitor arterial blood gas (ABG) levels (including arterial oxygen saturation [SaO_2]) and mixed venous oxygen saturation ($S\bar{v}O_2$) levels to determine the effectiveness of the therapy.
• Perform hygiene measures, such as mouth and skin care.
• Wean the patient from ECMO when the doctor is satisfied with his response to therapy. Decrease pump flow gradually, and take the patient off ECMO for 15 to 20 minutes at a time.
• Once adequate ABG levels are achieved, decannulation may take place. Monitor the patient carefully during this procedure because he may need increased ventilatory support.
• The operating staff clamps and removes the cannulas under sterile technique. (At many facilities, the cannulas are clamped but left in place for several hours to make sure they're no longer needed.) Infusions are switched from the circuit to the patient.

- Discontinue heparin and provide sedatives, anesthetics, or analgesics, as ordered. Dress the surgical site and check it for bleeding.
- Monitor platelet counts and anticoagulation studies.
- Continue mechanical ventilation. Extubation usually takes place in 3 to 5 days.
- Offer emotional support to the patient and his family.

Cautions

Because ECMO causes systemic anticoagulation, bleeding is the most common complication of the procedure; intracranial hemorrhage represents the most serious form of bleeding. Treat bleeding by carefully monitoring coagulation studies and by administering platelets. Although continual neurologic assessment may help prevent massive intracranial bleeding, neurologic deficits may be caused by asphyxia that occurred before the ECMO. Other areas at risk for bleeding include the cannula sites and the GI system. Monitor the surgical sites and the patient's abdominal girth to detect bleeding in these areas.

Fluid and electrolyte imbalances and renal failure may also result from ECMO. Treat fluid and electrolyte imbalances with diuretics or fluids. Detect early signs of renal failure by monitoring the patient's blood urea nitrogen level, serum creatinine level, and urine output.

Sepsis, another common complication, can develop because of the large cannulas in a main vascular tree and because the patient's physical state is compromised in general. Use strict sterile technique when changing dressings and monitoring the patient for signs of infection. You may need to monitor his white blood cell (WBC) count, his temperature, and any blood cultures taken. Antibiotics are commonly given prophylactically to prevent infection.

ECMO also may cause mechanical complications, some of which can be life-threatening. Monitor the ECMO circuit continuously for oxygenator failure, tubing rupture, perforation of the vessel, thrombus formation at the end of the cannula, and air emboli.

Monitoring and aftercare

- Make sure that the patient is getting enough oxygen by monitoring ABG and $S\bar{v}O_2$ levels throughout ECMO.
- Measure perfusion by mean arterial pressure, which should remain between 40 and 45 mm Hg in a neonate. (A child's mean arterial pressure varies according to his age; an adult's depends on his physical status, size, past medical history, and present condition.) Mean arterial pressure is used as a guide instead of systolic pressure because the ECMO circuit provides nonpulsatile blood flow. This causes damping of the arterial line waveform.
- When ECMO is discontinued, the patient may remain mechanically ventilated for 3 to 5 days before extubation. If he doesn't improve and extubation isn't possible, you'll need to provide extra support to the patient's parents or family as they decide whether to discontinue mechanical ventilation.
- When a patient has received ECMO, he'll need to be followed up closely throughout his life. Neurologic adverse effects may result from ECMO or from prolonged hypoxia, acidosis, or hypotension that occurred before ECMO. However, many patients experience no adverse effects from the procedure.
- Monitor for complications that may result from the ligation of a carotid artery after decannulation.
- As with any serious illness, the patient and his family may need follow-up psychological care, which you may want to recommend. If a patient dies or becomes permanently impaired, the family will need help adjusting to these events.
- Document the patient's tolerance; the date, time, and outcome; and your interventions during the procedure.

Transtracheal oxygen therapy

A simple outpatient procedure, transtracheal oxygen therapy is the administration of oxygen through a catheter inserted into the base of the neck and held in place with a chain necklace. A patient who finds oxygen therapy by nasal cannula uncomfortable or too restrictive may be better suited to transtracheal oxygen administration. It doesn't interfere with eating or talking, and it doesn't dry mucous membranes. The transtracheal catheter can easily be concealed by a shirt or scarf.

Compared with delivering oxygen through a nasal cannula, transtracheal oxygen therapy allows better oxygenation with lower oxygen flow. Transtracheal oxygen therapy uses half the oxygen that's required with a nasal cannula, so the cost of oxygen to the patient is cut in half. (See *Using a transtracheal catheter.*)

Indications

Transtracheal oxygen therapy can be used by patients who have spontaneous respirations but need a constant supply of supplemental oxygen, as in chronic obstructive pulmonary disease (COPD).

Contraindications and complications

Because this form of oxygen therapy requires a minor surgical procedure, it shouldn't be used in patients at risk for bleeding; patients with severe bronchospasm, uncompensated respiratory acidosis, or pleural herniation into the base of the neck; or patients receiving high corticosteroid dosages.

Transtracheal oxygen therapy also is contraindicated in patients with severe anxiety and in patients who aren't alert, who are unaware of their surroundings, and who show a low level of compliance. Additionally, it's contraindicated in patients unable to sustain interest in intensive patient education.

Complications include hematoma, pneumothorax, infection, and airway obstruction due to mucus plug accumulation.

Equipment

Lidocaine • syringe • 25G 3″ needle • scalpel • guide wire and needle • transtracheal oxygen therapy catheter, Johnson-Cary catheter, or Heimlich Micro-Trach catheter • povidone-iodine solution • 4″ × 4″ gauze sponges • tracheal catheter, such as the Spofford-Christian Oxygen Optimizing Prosthesis (SCOOP)

Commercially prepared trays with all of the required equipment for SCOOP insertion are available.

Preparation

• Before the procedure is performed, make sure that the patient is fully informed about the procedure and obtain a signed consent form.
• Administer a sedative and an antibiotic 1 hour before the procedure, if ordered.
• Drape the chain necklace—which comes with the catheter and is used to secure its position—around the patient's neck. Mark the spot where it crosses in front of the trachea to determine the location for catheter insertion. Remove the necklace.
• Help the patient into a sitting position in a chair with a head rest or into a lying position with a pillow under his shoulders.
• Clean the neck area with antimicrobial soap or povidone-iodine solution.

Essential steps

• Using the 25G needle, the doctor first numbs the skin around the puncture site with lidocaine.
• The doctor makes a vertical ½″ (1-cm) incision at the puncture site and inserts a needle into the trachea to confirm that air can be aspirated.
• The doctor then inserts a guide wire through the needle and removes the needle.
• Next, he passes a dilator over the guide wire. The dilator is left in place for 1 minute so the ligament can relax.
• Then, depending on the system used, the doctor inserts either a thin plastic stent or the catheter over the guide wire. You'll assist the doctor as he sutures the catheter or stent into place.
• If the patient will be using a SCOOP catheter, a stent is inserted first. After a week, the doctor replaces the stent with the SCOOP 1 catheter, which remains in place for the first 6 to 8 weeks while the tract is maturing. If the patient requires flow rates greater than 2 liters/minute, the SCOOP 1 catheter may be exchanged for a SCOOP 2 catheter, which has

HOME CARE

Using a transtracheal catheter

Before a patient is sent home with a transtracheal catheter, he'll need to learn how to care for the catheter as well as the skin surrounding it. In addition to teaching your patient to care for his catheter, tell him to call his doctor if he has a cough that's unrelieved by medication, increased shortness of breath or dyspnea, a fever, severe pain or bleeding at the catheter site, or blood in the sputum.

If the patient has a Heimlich Micro-Trach or a transtracheal oxygen therapy catheter, tell him to clean around the catheter twice a day using a soapy cotton-tipped applicator and water. He also needs to irrigate the catheter two to three times a day while it's in place, using 0.9% sodium chloride solution. Tell him that this loosens secretions and stimulates coughing. Instruct the patient to change the catheter once a month.

The Johnson-Cary catheter does not need cleaning at the tracheal insertion site because the catheter is tunneled subcutaneously. However, the insertion site on the chest wall should be kept clean with mild soap and water.

SCOOP catheter

If the patient has a SCOOP catheter, tell him to clean it two or three times a day to keep it free of mucus. Before he begins cleaning, he should put on a nasal cannula, disconnect the oxygen tubing from the catheter, and then connect it to the cannula. Instruct the patient to irrigate the catheter by instilling 1.5 ml of 0.9% sodium chloride solution into the catheter. Warn him that this may make him cough. Next, tell him to insert a cleaning rod (which he has cleaned beforehand) through the catheter as far as possible and then to pull it back.

After he has inserted and removed the rod three times, tell him to instill 1.5 ml of 0.9% sodium chloride solution into the catheter and then reconnect the oxygen tubing to the catheter. As a final step, instruct him to clean the rod with antimicrobial soap and to store it in a dry place.

In addition to cleaning the catheter while it remains in place, the patient with a SCOOP 2 catheter will remove the catheter at least once daily for a more thorough cleaning. After the catheter is removed, tell the patient to use antimicrobial soap, a cleaning rod, and lukewarm tap water to clean the catheter.

Next, he should insert a second SCOOP catheter coated with a water-soluble lubricant. Once the second catheter is secured, he can resume oxygen delivery through the catheter.

Irrigating a SCOOP catheter

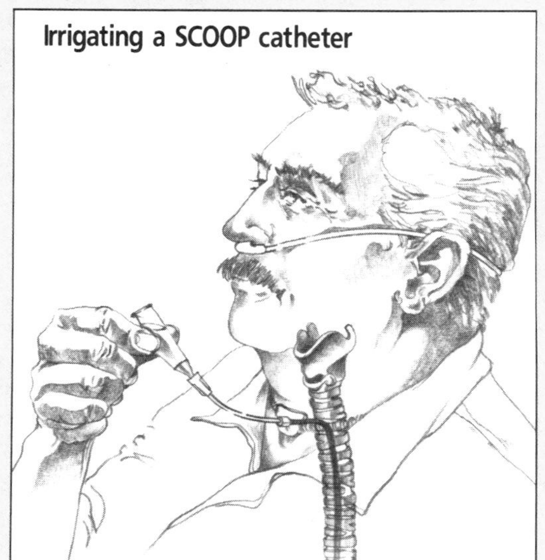

Inserting a cleaning rod in a SCOOP catheter

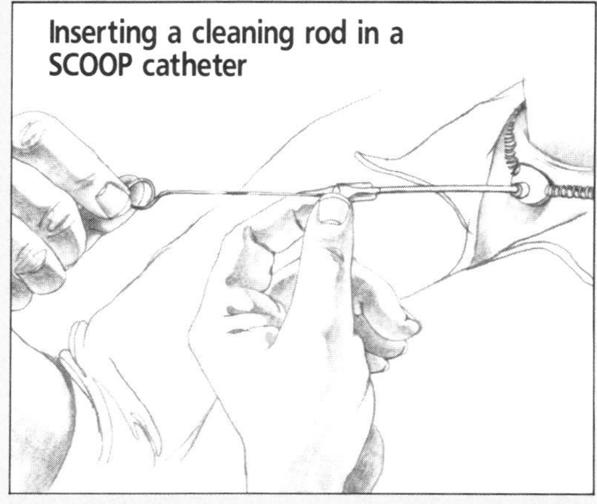

extra side holes to facilitate oxygen distribution.

• If a Johnson-Cary catheter is used, the tubing is tunneled subcutaneously from the trachea to the costophrenic margin, where it is brought out through the chest wall.

Cautions

Remind the patient never to remove or insert a SCOOP catheter while oxygen is flowing through it. Instead, he should put on a nasal cannula, disconnect the catheter from the oxygen source, and then remove the catheter. The SCOOP catheter should never be out of the tract for more than a few minutes or the tract may close.

If the patient is in respiratory distress and you suspect that the catheter isn't working, give him oxygen with a nasal cannula.

Monitoring and aftercare

• After insertion of the catheter, obtain a chest X-ray to confirm placement.

• The catheter must be cleaned regularly to prevent mucus plugs from blocking the catheter and causing irritation.

• Don't use the SCOOP stent for oxygen delivery. Some doctors allow the other tracheal catheters to be used immediately for oxygen delivery. Others wait 1 week for the stoma to heal and to lessen the risk of subcutaneous emphysema.

• Monitor the patient for bleeding, respiratory distress, pneumothorax, pain, coughing, hoarseness, or bleeding.

• Coughing is a normal response to a foreign object in the airway. Administer a cough suppressant or instill 0.5 ml of 1% lidocaine into the trachea.

Esophageal airways

Esophageal airways, such as the esophageal gastric tube airway (EGTA) and the esophageal obturator airway (EOA), are used to maintain ventilation temporarily (for up to 2 hours) in a comatose patient during cardiac or respiratory arrest. These devices avoid tongue obstruction, prevent air from entering the stomach, and keep stomach contents from entering the trachea. They can be inserted only after a patent airway is established.

Although endotracheal intubation is preferred in patients who are receiving advanced cardiac life support, esophageal airways can be used if endotracheal intubation isn't possible.

Nurses must have special training to insert an EGTA or EOA; however, insertion of these airways is much simpler than endotracheal intubation. One reason is that these devices don't require visualization of the trachea or hyperextension of the neck. This makes them useful for treating patients with suspected spinal cord injuries.

Esophageal airways are used most commonly by emergency medical technicians in the field.

Indications

The use of esophageal airways is indicated when loss of airway patency occurs with loss of consciousness resulting from cardiac or respiratory arrest.

Contraindications and complications

Because conscious and semiconscious patients will reject esophageal airways, these airways shouldn't be used unless the patient is unconscious and not breathing. They're also contraindicated if facial trauma prevents a snug mask fit or if the patient has an absent or weak gag reflex, has recently ingested toxic chemicals, has esophageal disease, or has taken an overdose of narcotics that can be reversed by naloxone. In addition, because pediatric sizes aren't currently available, these airways shouldn't be used in patients under age 16.

EOAs may be inferior to endotracheal intubation in providing adequate oxygenation and ventilation. Esophageal airways may cause esophageal injuries, including rupture; in semiconscious patients, they may cause laryngospasm, vomiting, and aspiration. The EOA doesn't prevent aspiration of foreign material from the mouth and pharynx into the trachea and bronchi.

Equipment
Esophageal tube • face mask • #16 or #18 French nasogastric (NG) tube (for EGTA) • 35-cc syringe • intermittent gastric suction equipment • oral suction equipment • optional: hand-held resuscitation bag, water-soluble lubricant

Preparation
• Explain the procedure to the patient, and gather the equipment you'll need.
• Fill the face mask with air to check for leaks.
• Inflate the esophageal tube's cuff with 35 cc of air to check for leaks; then deflate the cuff.
• Connect the esophageal tube to the face mask (the lower opening on an EGTA), and listen for the tube to click to determine proper placement.

Essential steps
• Lubricate the first inch (2.5 cm) of the tube's distal tip with a water-soluble lubricant, I.V. fluid, the patient's saliva, or tap water. With an EGTA, also lubricate the first inch of the NG tube's distal tip.

To insert the airway
• Assess the patient's condition to make sure that he's a candidate for an esophageal airway.
• If the patient's condition permits, place him in a supine position with his neck in a neutral or semiflexed position. Hyperextension of the neck may cause the tube to enter the trachea instead of the esophagus. Remove his dentures, if applicable.
• Insert your thumb deep into the patient's mouth behind the base of his tongue. Place your index and middle fingers of the same hand under the patient's chin, and lift his jaw straight up.
• With your other hand, grasp the esophageal tube just below the mask in the same way that you'd grasp a pencil. This promotes gentle maneuvering of the tube and reduces the risk of pharyngeal trauma.
• Still elevating the patient's jaw with one hand, insert the tip of the esophageal tube into the patient's mouth. Gently guide the airway over the tongue into the pharynx and then into the esophagus, following the natural pharyngeal curve. The tube should seat itself easily; you shouldn't need to use force. If you encounter resistance, withdraw the tube slightly and readvance it. When the tube is fully advanced, the mask should fit snugly over the patient's mouth and nose. When this is accomplished, the cuff will lie below the level of the carina. If the cuff is above the carina, it may, when inflated, compress the posterior membranous portion of the trachea and cause tracheal obstruction.
• Because the tube may enter the trachea, deliver positive-pressure ventilation before inflating the cuff. Watch for the chest to rise to confirm that the tube is in the esophagus.
• Once the tube is properly in place in the esophagus, draw 35 cc of air into the syringe, connect the syringe to the tube's cuff-inflation valve, and inflate the cuff. Avoid overinflation because this can cause esophageal trauma.
• If you've inserted an EGTA, insert the NG tube through the lower port on the face mask and into the esophageal tube, and advance it to the second marking so that it reaches 6" (15 cm) beyond the distal end of the esophageal tube. Suction stomach contents using intermittent gastric suction to decompress the stomach. This is particularly necessary after mouth-to-mouth resuscitation, which introduces air to the stomach. Leave the tube in place during resuscitation. (See *Esophageal gastric tube airway,* page 78.)
• With either type of airway, attach a hand-held resuscitation bag or a mechanical ventilator to the face mask port (upper port) on the EGTA. Up to 100% of the fraction of inspired oxygen (FIO_2) can be delivered this way.
• Monitor the patient to ensure adequate ventilation. Watch for chest movement, and suction the patient if mucus blocks the EOA tube perforations or in any way interrupts respiration.

To remove the airway
• Assess the patient's condition to determine if he's ready to have the airway removed. The airway may be removed if respirations are spontaneous and number 16 to 20 breaths/minute. If 2 hours have elapsed since airway insertion and respirations aren't spontaneous and at the normal rate, the patient must be

ADVANCED EQUIPMENT

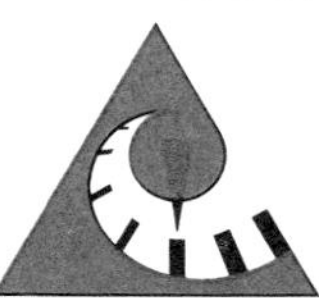

Esophageal gastric tube airway

A newer, modified version of the esophageal obturator airway, the esophageal gastric tube airway is an open tube that permits passage of a Salem sump or a nasogastric tube into the gastric area below the esophageal cuff.

Ventilating devices are attached to the mask rather than to the tube because the tube has no holes for the airflow. Ventilating gas is pushed into the lungs through the mask and prohibited from entering the gastric area by the esophageal cuff. (See the illustration at right.)

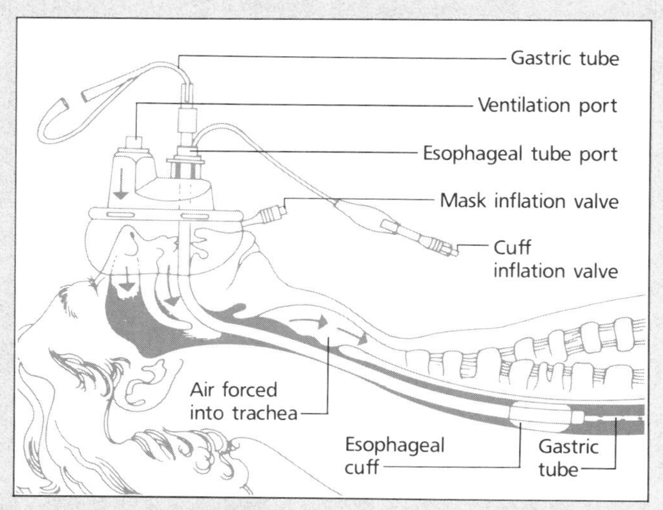

switched to an artificial airway that can be used for long-term ventilation, such as an endotracheal tube.
• Detach the mask from the esophageal tube.
• If the patient is conscious, place him on his left side, if possible, to avoid aspiration during removal of the esophageal tube. If he's unconscious and needs an endotracheal tube, insert it (or assist with its insertion) and inflate the cuff of the endotracheal tube before removing the esophageal tube. With the esophageal tube in place, the endotracheal tube can be guided easily into the trachea, and stomach contents are less likely to be aspirated when the esophageal tube is removed.
• Deflate the cuff on the esophageal tube by removing air from the inflation valve with a syringe. Don't try to remove the tube with the cuff inflated because it may perforate the esophagus.
• Turn the patient's head to the side, if possible, to avoid aspiration.
• Remove the EGTA or EOA in one swift, smooth motion, following the natural pharyngeal curve to avoid esophageal trauma.
• Perform oropharyngeal suctioning to remove any residual secretions.
• Assist the doctor as necessary in monitoring for and maintaining adequate ventilation for the patient.

Cautions

Store EGTAs and EOAs in the manufacturer's package until you're ready to use them. This preserves their natural curve.

To ease insertion, you may prefer to direct the airway along the right side of the patient's mouth because the esophagus is located to the right of and behind the trachea. Or you may advance the tube tip upward toward the hard palate, then invert the tip and glide it along the tongue surface and into the pharynx. This keeps the tube centered, avoids snagging it on the sides of the throat, and eases insertion in a patient with clenched jaws.

If the patient starts retching, remove the airway immediately because the accumulation of vomitus blocked by the airway cuff may perforate the esophagus. To help prevent complications, don't leave the EOA in place for more than 2 hours.

Monitoring and aftercare

• Watch the unconscious patient for signs that he's regaining consciousness.
• If the patient tries to remove the airway, restrain his hands. To reduce his apprehension, explain the procedure to him if possible.
• Record the date and time of the procedure, the type of airway inserted, the patient's vital signs and level of consciousness, and the time that you removed the airway. If another airway is inserted after extubation, document this too. Also record any complications that arose and subsequent interventions.

Endotracheal intubation

In endotracheal intubation, a flexible tube is inserted orally (orotracheal intubation) or nasally (nasotracheal intubation) through the larynx into the trachea to control the airway and mechanically ventilate the patient. Performed by a doctor, an anesthetist, a respiratory therapist, or a specially trained nurse, this procedure is usually done in emergency situations.

Endotracheal intubation establishes and maintains a patent airway, protects against aspiration by sealing off the trachea from the digestive tract, permits removal of tracheobronchial secretions in patients who can't cough effectively, and provides a route for mechanical ventilation. Its disadvantages are that it bypasses normal respiratory tract defenses against infection, reduces cough effectiveness, and prevents oral communication.

Some health care professionals prefer orotracheal intubation to nasotracheal intubation because oral insertion is easier and faster. However, maintaining exact tube placement is more difficult with oral insertion, and the tube must be well secured to avoid kinking and to prevent bronchial obstruction or accidental extubation. Orotracheal intubation is also poorly tolerated by conscious patients because it stimulates salivation, coughing, and retching.

Nasotracheal intubation is preferred for elective insertion when the patient is capable of spontaneous ventilation for a short period. It's typically used in conscious patients who risk imminent respiratory arrest or who have cervical spinal injury.

Although nasotracheal intubation is more comfortable than oral intubation, it's also more difficult to perform. Because the tube passes blindly through the nasal cavity, the procedure (sometimes called blind intubation) causes greater tissue trauma, increases the risk of infection by nasal bacteria introduced into the trachea, and risks pressure necrosis of the nasal mucosa. However, maintaining exact tube placement is easier and the risk of dislodgment is lower than with orotracheal intubation. The cuff on the endotracheal tube maintains a closed system that permits positive-pressure ventilation and protects the airway from aspiration of secretions and gastric contents.

Indications

• Cardiopulmonary arrest
• Airway compromise such as epiglottitis
• Deteriorating respiratory function due to pneumonia or other respiratory disorders
• Inability to maintain ventilation because of neuromuscular disorders

Contraindications and complications

Orotracheal intubation is contraindicated in patients with acute cervical spinal injury or degenerative spinal disorders; nasotracheal intubation is contraindicated in patients with apnea, bleeding disorders, chronic sinusitis, or nasal obstructions.

Endotracheal intubation can result in bronchospasm; aspiration of blood, secretions, or gastric contents; tooth damage or loss; injury to the lips, mouth, pharynx, or vocal cords; and apnea caused by reflex breath-holding or interruption of oxygen delivery. It can also result in laryngeal edema and erosion, and tracheal stenosis, erosion, and necrosis. Nasotracheal intubation can result in nasal bleeding, laceration, sinusitis, and otitis media.

Equipment

Two endotracheal tubes (one spare) in the appropriate size • 10-cc syringe • stethoscope • sterile gloves • lighted laryngoscope with a handle and blades of various sizes, both curved and straight • sedative • local anesthetic spray such as lidocaine (for conscious patients) • mucosal vasoconstricting agent (for nasal intubation) • overbed or other table • water-soluble lubricant • adhesive or other strong tape or Velcro tube holder • compound benzoin tincture • transparent adhesive dressing, if necessary • oral airway or bite block (for oral intubation) • suction equipment • hand-held resuscitation bag with sterile swivel adapter • humidified oxygen source • optional: prepackaged intubation tray, sterile gauze pad, stylet, Magill forceps, sterile water, and sterile basin

Preparation

• Explain the procedure to the patient as you quickly gather the individual supplies or use a prepackaged intubation tray. Select an endotracheal tube in the right size. Typically, tubes for adults range in size from 6 to 10 mm and are cuffed; those for children range from 2.5 to 5.5 mm and are uncuffed. The typical size of a tube used for oral intubation in women is 7.5 mm; in men, 9 mm. Select a sightly smaller tube for nasal intubation.

• Check the light in the laryngoscope by snapping the appropriate-sized blade into place. If the bulb doesn't light, replace the batteries or the laryngoscope (whichever will be quicker).

• Using sterile technique, open the package containing the endotracheal tube on an overbed table. Other sterile supplies can be opened at this time, as well. Pour the sterile water into the basin.

• To ease insertion, lubricate the first inch (2.5 cm) of the distal end of the endotracheal tube with the water-soluble lubricant, using aseptic technique. Do this by either placing some of the lubricant on the gauze pad and wiping it on the tube or by squeezing the lubricant directly onto the tube. Use only water-soluble lubricant because it can be absorbed by mucous membranes.

• Attach the syringe to the port on the tube's exterior pilot cuff. Slowly inflate the cuff, observing for uniform inflation. If you suspect a leak, you may submerge the tube in the sterile water and watch for air bubbles, which would indicate a leak. Then use the syringe to deflate the cuff.

• A stylet may be used in oral intubation to stiffen the tube. Lubricate the entire stylet so that it can be removed easily after intubation. Insert the stylet into the tube so that its distal tip lies about ½" (1 cm) inside the distal end of the tube. Make sure that the stylet doesn't protrude from the tube to avoid vocal cord trauma.

• Prepare the humidified oxygen source and the suction equipment for immediate use. If the patient is in bed, remove the headboard to provide easier access.

Essential steps

• Administer medication, as ordered, to decrease respiratory secretions, induce amnesia or analgesia, and help calm and relax the conscious patient. Remove dentures and bridgework, if necessary.

• To prevent hypoxia, administer oxygen until the tube is inserted.

• Place the supine patient in the sniffing position so that his mouth, pharynx, and trachea are extended. For a nasotracheal intubation, place the patient's head and neck in a neutral position.

• Put on gloves.

• For oral intubation, spray a local anesthetic (such as lidocaine) deep into the patient's posterior pharynx to diminish the gag reflex and reduce patient discomfort.

• For nasal intubation, spray a local anesthetic and a mucosal vasoconstricting agent into the patient's nasal passages to anesthetize and shrink the nasal turbinates and reduce the chance of bleeding.

• If necessary, suction the patient's pharynx just before tube insertion to improve visualization of the patient's pharynx and vocal cords.

• Time each intubation attempt, limiting attempts to less than 30 seconds to prevent hypoxia.

Intubation with direct visualization

• Stand at the head of the patient's bed. Using your right hand, hold the patient's mouth open by crossing your index finger over your thumb, placing your thumb on the patient's upper teeth and your index finger on his lower teeth. This technique provides greater leverage.
• Grasp the laryngoscope handle in your left hand, and gently slide the blade into the right side of the patient's mouth. Center the blade and push the patient's tongue to the left. Hold the patient's lower lip away from his teeth to prevent the lip from being traumatized.
• Advance the blade to expose the epiglottis. When using a straight blade, insert the tip under the epiglottis; when using a curved blade, insert the tip between the base of the tongue and the epiglottis.
• Lift the laryngoscope handle upward and away from your body at a 45-degree angle to reveal the vocal cords. Avoid pivoting the laryngoscope against the patient's teeth to prevent damaging them.
• If necessary, have an assistant apply pressure to the cricoid cartilage to occlude the esophagus and minimize gastric regurgitation.
• When performing an oral intubation, insert the endotracheal tube into the right side of the patient's mouth. When performing a nasotracheal intubation, insert the endotracheal tube through the nostril and into the pharynx. Then use Magill forceps to guide the tube through the vocal cords.
• Guide the tube into the vertical openings of the larynx between the vocal cords, being careful not to mistake the horizontal opening of the esophagus for the larynx. If the vocal cords are closed because of a spasm, wait a few seconds for them to relax and then gently guide the tube past them to avoid traumatic injury.
• Advance the tube until the cuff disappears beyond the vocal cords. Don't advance the tube farther to avoid occluding one of the mainstem bronchi and precipitating lung collapse.
• Holding the endotracheal tube in place, quickly remove the stylet, if present. Remove the laryngoscope.

Nasotracheal intubation

• Pass the endotracheal tube along the floor of the nasal cavity. If necessary, use gentle force to pass the tube through the nasopharynx and into the pharynx.
• Listen and feel for air movement through the tube as it's advanced to ensure that the tube is properly placed in the airway.
• Slip the tube between the vocal cords when the patient inhales because the vocal cords separate on inhalation.
• Once the tube is past the vocal cords, the breath sounds should become louder. If breath sounds disappear at any time during tube advancement, withdraw the tube until they reappear.
• Inflate the tube's cuff with 5 to 10 cc of air until you feel resistance. Once the patient is mechanically ventilated, you'll use the minimal-leak technique or the minimal occlusive volume technique to establish correct cuff inflation.
• If the patient was intubated orally, insert an oral airway or a bite block to prevent the patient from obstructing airflow or puncturing the tube with his teeth.
• To ensure correct tube placement, observe for chest expansion and auscultate for bilateral breath sounds. If the patient is unconscious or uncooperative, use a hand-held resuscitation bag while observing for upper chest movement and auscultating for breath sounds. Feel the tube's tip for warm exhalations and listen for air movement. Observe for condensation forming inside the tube.
• If you don't hear any breath sounds, auscultate over the stomach while ventilating the patient with the resuscitation bag. Stomach distention, belching, or a gurgling sound indicates esophageal intubation. If this occurs, immediately deflate the cuff and remove the tube. After reoxygenating the patient to prevent hypoxia, repeat insertion using a sterile tube to prevent contamination of the trachea.
• Auscultate lung fields bilaterally to rule out the possibility of endobronchial intubation. If you fail to hear breath sounds on both sides of the chest, you may have inserted the tube into one of the mainstem bronchi (usually the right one because of its wider angle at the bifurcation). This would occlude the other mainstem

SKILL TIP

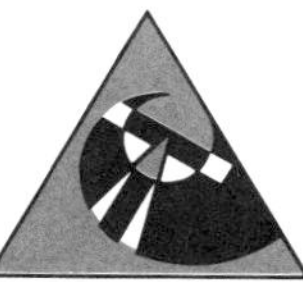

Taping an endotracheal tube

After tape has been in place for 24 hours or more and is saturated with sweat and secretions, finding its ends can be difficult. Tugging at tape ends causes shearing and possible skin avulsion.

When taping an endotracheal tube, you can avoid later problems by making tabs at the ends of each piece of tape you use. Fold ¼" (0.5 cm) of the tape end back on itself to form a tab as shown below.

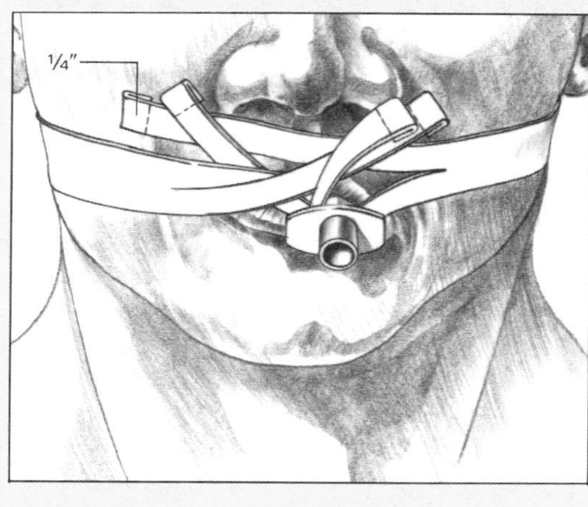

bronchus and lung and would result in atelectasis on the obstructed side. Or the tube may be resting on the carina, resulting in dry secretions that obstruct both bronchi. (The patient's coughing and fighting the ventilator will alert you to this problem.) To correct these situations, deflate the cuff, withdraw the tube 1 to 2 mm, auscultate for bilateral breath sounds, and reinflate the cuff.

Cautions

Although low-pressure cuffs have significantly reduced the incidence of tracheal erosion and necrosis caused by cuff pressure on the tracheal wall, overinflation of a low-pressure cuff can negate this benefit. Use the minimal-leak technique to avoid these complications. Inflating the cuff a bit more to make a complete seal with the least amount of air is the next most desirable method.

Always record the volume of air needed to inflate the cuff. A gradual increase in this volume indicates tracheal dilatation or erosion. A sudden increase in volume indicates rupture of the cuff and requires immediate reintubation if the patient is being ventilated or if he requires continuous cuff inflation to maintain a high concentration of delivered oxygen. Once the cuff has been inflated, measure its pressure every 8 hours or according to your hospital's policy to avoid overinflation. Normal cuff pressure is about 18 mm Hg.

Monitoring and aftercare

- Once you've confirmed correct tube placement, administer oxygen or initiate mechanical ventilation, and suction if indicated.
- To secure tube position, apply compound benzoin tincture to each cheek and let it dry for enhanced tape adhesion. Tape the tube firmly with adhesive tape or another strong tape, or use a Velcro tube holder. (See *Taping an endotracheal tube.*)
- Inflate the cuff with the minimal-leak technique or the minimal occlusive volume technique. For the *minimal-leak technique,* attach a 10-cc syringe to the port on the tube's exterior pilot cuff, and place a stethoscope on the side of the patient's neck. Inject small amounts of air with each breath until you hear no leaking around the cuff. Then aspirate 0.1 cc of air from the cuff to create a minimal air leak. Record the amount of air needed to inflate the cuff for subsequent monitoring of tracheal dilatation or erosion. For the *minimal occlusive volume technique,* follow the first two steps of the minimal-leak technique, placing your stethoscope over the trachea instead of the side of the neck. Then aspirate until you hear a small leak on inspiration, and add just enough air to stop the leak. Record the amount of air needed to inflate the cuff for subsequent monitoring of tracheal dilatation or erosion.
- Clearly mark the tube's exit point from the mouth or nose with a pen or tape. If you can't mark the tube, note the centimeter marking on the tube where the tube exits the

mouth or nose. Monitor this mark periodically, checking for tube displacement.
• Make sure that a chest X-ray is taken to verify tube position.
• Place a swivel adapter between the tube and the humidified oxygen source to allow intermittent suctioning and reduce tube tension.
• Place the patient on his side with his head in a comfortable position to avoid tube kinking and airway obstruction.
• Auscultate both sides of the chest and watch chest movement, as needed, to ensure correct tube placement and full lung ventilation.
• Provide frequent oral care to the orally intubated patient, and position the endotracheal tube to prevent formation of pressure ulcers and to avoid excessive pressure on the sides of the mouth. Give frequent nasal and oral care to the nasally intubated patient to prevent formation of pressure ulcers and drying of oral mucous membranes.
• Suction secretions through the endotracheal tube, as needed, to clear secretions and prevent mucus plugs from obstructing the tube.
• Record the date and time of the procedure; its indication and success or failure; the tube type and size; the cuff size, amount of inflation, and inflation technique; each administration of medication, supplemental oxygen, or ventilation therapy; results of chest auscultation and the chest X-ray; and any complications and subsequent interventions. Also document the patient's reaction to the procedure.

Endotracheal tube care

The intubated patient requires meticulous care to ensure airway patency and prevent complications until he can breathe on his own. This care includes frequent assessment of the patient's airway, maintenance of proper cuff pressure to prevent tissue ischemia and necrosis, careful repositioning of the tube to avoid traumatic manipulation, and constant monitoring for complications. The endotracheal tube is repositioned for patient comfort or if a chest X-ray shows improper placement. Once every 24 hours, move the tube from one side of the mouth to the other in the orally intubated patient to prevent pressure ulcers.

Indications

You'll provide care to patients with oral or nasotracheal intubation needing the tube pulled out slightly or inserted further, as indicated by clinical assessment or chest X-ray.

Contraindications and complications

No contraindications exist. Traumatic injury to the larynx or trachea may result from manipulation of the tube, accidental extubation, or slippage of the tube into the right mainstem bronchus. Aspiration of upper airway secretions, underventilation, or coughing spasms may occur if a leak is created during cuff pressure measurement. Ventilatory failure and airway obstruction, caused by laryngospasm or marked tracheal edema, are the most serious complications of extubation.

Equipment

For maintaining the airway

Stethoscope • suction equipment • gloves

For repositioning the endotracheal tube

10-cc syringe • compound benzoin tincture • stethoscope • adhesive or nonallergenic tape or Velcro tube holder • suction equipment • handheld resuscitation bag with mask (in case of accidental extubation)

For measuring cuff pressure

10-cc syringe • three-way stopcock • cuff pressure manometer or blood pressure manometer with tubing • stethoscope • suction equipment • gloves

For removing the endotracheal tube

10-cc syringe • suction equipment • supplemental oxygen source with mask • cool-mist, large-volume nebulizer • gloves • equipment for reintubation

Preparation

For repositioning the endotracheal tube

• Assemble all equipment at the patient's bedside.

For measuring cuff pressure

• Assemble all equipment at the patient's bedside. If you're measuring with a blood pressure manometer, attach the syringe to one stopcock port; then attach the tubing from the manometer to another stopcock port.
• Turn off the stopcock port where you'll be connecting the pilot balloon cuff so that air can't escape from the cuff. Use the syringe to instill air into the manometer tubing until the pressure reading reaches 10 mm Hg. This will prevent sudden cuff deflation when you open the stopcock to the cuff and the manometer.

For removing the endotracheal tube

• Assemble all equipment at the patient's bedside. Set up the suction and supplemental oxygen equipment.

Essential steps

• Explain the procedure to the patient even if he doesn't appear to be alert. Provide privacy, wash your hands, and put on gloves.

To maintain airway patency

• Auscultate the patient's lungs at any sign of respiratory distress. If you detect an obstructed airway, determine the cause and treat it appropriately. If secretions are obstructing the tube's lumen, suction them from the tube.
• If the tube has slipped from the trachea into the right or left mainstem bronchus, breath sounds will be absent over one lung. As ordered, obtain a chest X-ray to verify tube placement. If necessary, reposition the tube.

To reposition the endotracheal tube

• Get help from a respiratory therapist or another nurse to prevent accidental extubation during the procedure if the patient coughs.
• Suction the patient's trachea through the endotracheal tube to remove any secretions, which can irritate the bronchi and cause the patient to cough. (Coughing increases the risk of traumatic injury to the vocal cords and the likelihood of dislodging the tube.) Then suction the patient's pharynx to remove any secretions that may have accumulated above the tube cuff. This helps to prevent aspiration of secretions during cuff deflation.
• To prevent traumatic manipulation of the tube, instruct the assisting nurse to hold it as you carefully untape the tube or unfasten the Velcro tube holder. When freeing the tube, be sure to locate any identifying landmark, such as a number on the tube, or measure the distance from the patient's mouth to the top of the tube so that you have a reference point when moving the tube.
• Deflate the cuff by attaching a 10-cc syringe to the pilot balloon port and aspirating air until you meet resistance and the pilot balloon deflates. Deflate the cuff before moving the tube because the cuff forms a seal within the trachea and movement of an inflated cuff can damage the tracheal wall and vocal cords.
• Reposition the tube as necessary, noting new landmarks or measuring the length. Then immediately reinflate the cuff. To do this, instruct the patient to inhale, and slowly inflate the cuff using a 10-cc syringe attached to the pilot balloon port. As you do this, use your stethoscope to listen to the patient's neck to determine whether an air leak exists. Once air leakage ceases, stop cuff inflation and, while still listening to the patient's neck with your stethoscope, aspirate a small amount of air until you detect a slight leak. This creates a minimal air leak, which indicates that the cuff is inflated at the lowest pressure possible to create an adequate seal. If the patient is being mechanically ventilated, aspirate to create a minimal air leak during the inspiratory phase of respiration because the positive pressure of the ventilator during inspiration will create a larger leak around the cuff. Note the number of cubic centimeters of air required to inflate the cuff to achieve a minimal air leak.
• Measure cuff pressure (as described below) and compare the reading with previous pressure readings to prevent overinflation. Then use benzoin and tape to secure the tube in place, or refasten the Velcro tube holder.

To measure cuff pressure

• Once the cuff is inflated, measure its pressure every 8 hours or according to your hospital's policy to avoid overinflation. (See *Measuring tracheal cuff pressure.*)

Measuring tracheal cuff pressure

An endotracheal or tracheostomy cuff provides a closed system for mechanical ventilation that allows the desired tidal volume to be delivered to the patient's lungs. It also protects the patient's lower respiratory tract from secretions or gastric contents that may accumulate in the pharynx.

To function properly, the cuff must exert enough pressure on the tracheal wall to seal the airway. Excessive pressure, however, can compromise blood flow to the tracheal mucosa. The ideal pressure is the lowest amount needed to seal the airway, known as minimal occlusive volume. Many experts recommend maintaining a cuff pressure lower than the venous perfusion pressure. The target range is 16 to 24 cm H_20. (More than 24 cm H_20 may exceed venous perfusion pressure.) Actual cuff pressure will vary with each patient; to keep it within safe limits, measure minimal occlusive volume at least once each shift or as directed at your hospital.

To measure cuff pressure, attach a cuff pressure manometer to the external balloon, as shown in the photograph at right. The reading you get will tell you how much the cuff is inflated.

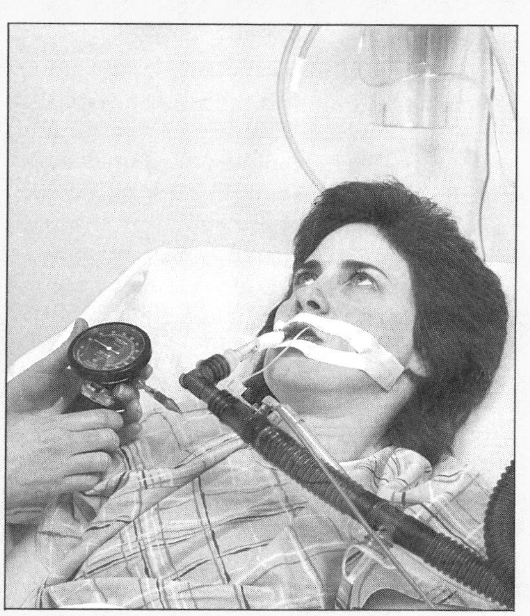

Special considerations

A patient with high airway pressure or positive end-expiratory pressure may need an extremely high cuff pressure to seal the airway. Ask the doctor if the patient can tolerate such a high cuff pressure or a minimal leak in the cuff, or if he should be reintubated. Then document the decision.

If the tube is too small, you may not be able to seal the airway without overinflating the cuff. Report this to the doctor because the tube may need to be replaced with a larger one.

Record the amount of air needed for reinflation. A gradual increase in the amount needed to reach minimal occlusive volume may indicate tracheal malacia (an abnormal softening of the tracheal tissue). Maintaining cuff pressure at the lowest possible level and inflating it to minimal occlusive volume will keep cuff-related complications to a minimum.

To remove the endotracheal tube

• When you're authorized to remove the tube, get another nurse's assistance to prevent traumatic manipulation of the tube when it's untaped or unfastened.

• Elevate the head of the patient's bed to approximately 90 degrees.

• Suction the patient's oropharynx and nasopharynx to remove any secretions that may have accumulated above the cuff and to help prevent aspiration of secretions when the cuff is deflated.

• Using a hand-held resuscitation bag or the mechanical ventilator, give the patient several deep breaths through the endotracheal tube to hyperinflate his lungs and increase his oxygen reserve.

• Attach a 10-cc syringe to the pilot balloon port and aspirate air until you meet resistance and the pilot balloon deflates. If you fail to de-

tect an air leak around the deflated cuff, notify the doctor immediately and don't proceed with extubation. Absence of an air leak may indicate marked tracheal edema and can result in total airway obstruction if the endotracheal tube is removed.
• If you detect the proper air leak, untape or unfasten the endotracheal tube while the assisting nurse stabilizes the tube.
• Insert a sterile suction catheter through the endotracheal tube. Then apply suction and ask the patient to take a deep breath and to open his mouth fully and pretend to cry out. This causes abduction of the vocal cords and reduces the risk of laryngeal trauma during withdrawal of the tube.
• Simultaneously remove the endotracheal tube and the suction catheter in one smooth outward and downward motion, following the natural curve of the patient's mouth. Suctioning during extubation removes secretions retained at the end of the tube and helps prevent aspiration.
• Give the patient supplemental oxygen. For highest humidity, use a cool-mist, large-volume nebulizer to help decrease airway irritation, patient discomfort, and laryngeal edema.
• Encourage the patient to cough and to breathe deeply. Remind him that a sore throat and hoarseness are to be expected and will gradually subside.
• After extubation, auscultate the patient's lungs frequently and watch for signs of respiratory distress. Be especially alert for stridor or other evidence of upper airway obstruction. If ordered, draw an arterial sample for blood gas analysis.

Cautions

When repositioning a tube, be especially careful in patients with highly sensitive airways. Sedation or direct instillation of 2% lidocaine to numb the airway may be indicated in such patients. Because the lidocaine is absorbed systemically, you must have a doctor's order to use it.

Never extubate a patient unless someone skilled at intubation is readily available. After extubation of a patient who has been intubated for an extended time, keep reintubation supplies readily available for at least 12 hours or until you're sure that the patient can tolerate extubation.

When measuring cuff pressure, keep the connection between the measuring device and the pilot balloon port tight to avoid an air leak that could compromise cuff pressure. Note the volume of air needed to inflate the cuff. A gradual increase in this volume indicates tracheal dilatation or erosion. A sudden increase in volume indicates rupture of the cuff and requires immediate reintubation if the patient is being ventilated or if he requires continuous cuff inflation to maintain a high concentration of delivered oxygen.

If you inadvertently cut the pilot balloon on the cuff, immediately call the person responsible for intubation in your health care facility, who will remove the damaged endotracheal tube and replace it with one that's intact. Don't remove the tube yourself before assistance arrives because a tube with an air leak is better than no airway.

Monitoring and aftercare

• Make sure that the patient is comfortable and the airway is patent. Clean or dispose of equipment properly.
• After tube repositioning, record the date and time of the procedure, the reason for repositioning (such as malposition shown by chest X-ray or prevention of pressure ulcers around the mouth), the new tube position, the total amount of air in the cuff after the procedure, any complications and subsequent interventions, and the patient's tolerance of the procedure.
• After cuff pressure measurement, record the date and time of the procedure, cuff pressure, the total amount of air in the cuff after the procedure, any complications and subsequent interventions, and the patient's tolerance of the procedure.
• After extubation, record the date and time of extubation, the presence or absence of stridor or other signs of upper airway edema, the type of supplemental oxygen administered, any complications and subsequent interventions, and the patient's tolerance of the procedure.

Tracheotomy

If all other attempts to establish an airway have failed, a doctor may perform a tracheotomy at a patient's bedside. In this procedure, an external opening in the trachea—called a tracheostomy—is surgically created and an indwelling tube is inserted to maintain the airway's patency.

A cuffed tracheostomy tube provides and maintains a patent airway, prevents the unconscious or paralyzed patient from aspirating food or secretions, allows removal of tracheobronchial secretions from the patient unable to cough, replaces an endotracheal tube, and permits the use of positive-pressure ventilation.

When laryngectomy accompanies a tracheotomy, the doctor may insert a laryngectomy tube (a shorter version of a tracheostomy tube). In addition, the patient's trachea is sutured to the skin surface. Consequently, with a laryngectomy, accidental tube expulsion doesn't lead to immediate closure of the tracheal opening. Once healed, the patient has a permanent neck stoma through which respiration takes place.

Indications

- Laryngeal edema
- Foreign body or tumor obstruction of airway
- Prolonged endotracheal intubation

Contraindications and complications

Contraindications to tracheotomy include patient refusal and bleeding tendencies. The procedure can cause airway obstruction, which may occur any time after tube placement. The obstruction may result from improper tube placement or from dry mucus secretions in the inner lumen of the tracheostomy tube. (See *Obstructed tracheostomy tube,* page 88.) Aspiration of secretions and tracheal necrosis (from cuff pressure) also may occur.

Potential complications from surgery include hemorrhage, edema, a perforated esophagus, subcutaneous or mediastinal emphysema, infection, and lacerations of arteries, veins, or nerves.

Equipment

Plastic or metal tracheostomy tube of the proper size (usually #13 to #38 French or #00 to #9 Jackson) with obturator • tracheostomy tape • sterile tracheal dilator • vein retractor • sutures and needles • sterile 4″ × 4″ gauze pads • sterile drapes, gloves, mask, and gown • sterile bowls • stethoscope • sterile tracheostomy dressing • pillow • tracheostomy ties • suction apparatus • alcohol sponge • povidone-iodine solution • sterile water • 5-ml syringe with 22G needle • local anesthetic such as lidocaine • oxygen therapy device and oxygen source • emergency equipment, including suctioning equipment, sterile obturator, sterile tracheostomy tube, sterile inner cannula, sterile tracheostomy tube and inner cannula one size smaller than tubes in use, sterile tracheal dilator or sterile hemostats

Preparation

- Make sure that one person stays with the patient while another obtains the necessary equipment.
- Wash your hands and then, maintaining sterile technique, open the tray and the packages containing the solution containers.
- Take the tracheostomy tube from its container, and place it on the sterile field. If necessary, set up the suction equipment and make sure that it works.
- Before the doctor begins, place a pillow under the patient's shoulders and neck and hyperextend his neck.
- Once the doctor opens the sterile bowls, pour in the appropriate solution.

Essential steps

- Explain the procedure to the patient.
- Assess the patient's condition and provide privacy. Maintain ventilation until the doctor performs the tracheotomy.
- The doctor will clean the area from the chin to the nipples with povidone-iodine solution. Next, he'll place sterile drapes on the patient and locate the area for the incision—usually ½″ to 1″ (1 to 2.5 cm) below the cricoid cartilage. Then he'll inject a local anesthetic.
- Wipe the top of the local anesthetic vial with an alcohol sponge. Invert the vial so that the

COMPLICATIONS

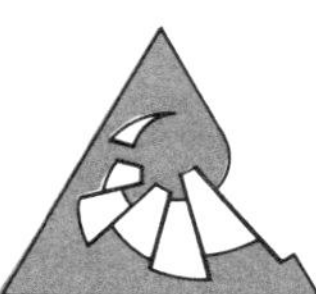

Obstructed tracheostomy tube

Suspect tube obstruction by a mucus plug if the patient appears pale and diaphoretic and if you hear a whistle sound with each breath. His labored respirations will be rapid and shallow, and you'll feel minimal airflow at the stoma. He may look cyanotic. If you hear a whistling sound and feel minimal airflow, you know he's receiving some air, but you must act quickly to remove the plug before he develops further respiratory distress.

Intervention

Call for assistance as you help the patient sit upright. Remove the tube's inner cannula and have him try to cough out the plug. (This may be difficult because he won't be able to perform Valsalva's maneuver or cough with an effective force.)

If this doesn't work, quickly attach a hand-held resuscitation bag with supplemental oxygen to his tracheostomy tube and deliver several vigorous hyperinflations. If they don't dislodge the plug or you feel resistance to inflation, you'll need to suction. Prepare a syringe of 2 ml sterile isotonic saline solution (without preservatives). Instill the solution and vigorously suction for no longer than 10 seconds at a time. Hyperinflate with the supplemental oxygen between each suctioning attempt.

If you still haven't been able to establish an effective airway, call the doctor immediately, cut the tracheostomy ties, and gently remove the entire tube. Keep the stoma open with a Kelly clamp and try to insert a new tube. If you can't get the tube in, insert a suction catheter instead, and thread the tube over the catheter.

If you still can't establish an effective airway and you no longer detect a pulse, call a code. Then either ventilate with a face mask and a resuscitation bag, or remove the Kelly clamp to close the stoma and perform mouth-to-mouth resuscitation until the doctor arrives. If air leaks from the stoma, cover the stoma with an occlusive dressing. (Remember, don't leave this patient alone until you're certain that he has an effective airway and can breathe comfortably.)

Once the patient has a new tracheostomy tube in place and can breathe more easily, provide supplemental humidified oxygen until he receives a full evaluation. Monitor his vital signs, skin color, and level of consciousness and, unless contraindicated, elevate the head of his bed.

Prevention

Help prevent future obstruction episodes by monitoring the patient for tenacious, blood-tinged tracheal mucus, the telltale whistling sound, and decreased airflow at the stoma during respirations.

Keep his secretions liquefied by ensuring that he's well hydrated and that any oxygen received is humidified. If he's not receiving oxygen, use an ultrasonic humidifier.

Have the patient routinely perform coughing and deep-breathing exercises to mobilize secretions and facilitate expectoration. If the exercises don't mobilize secretions, you can try routine chest physiotherapy.

doctor can withdraw the anesthetic, using the 22G needle attached to the 5-ml syringe.
• The doctor will make a horizontal or vertical incision into the skin. (A vertical incision helps avoid arteries, veins, and nerves on the lateral borders of the trachea.) Then he'll dissect subcutaneous fat and muscle and move the muscle aside with vein retractors to locate the tracheal rings.
• The doctor will make an incision between the second and third tracheal rings, using hemostats to control bleeding.
• He'll inject a local anesthetic into the tracheal lumen to suppress the cough reflex and then create a stoma in the trachea.
• Carefully apply suction to remove blood and secretions that may obstruct the airway or be aspirated into the lungs.
• The doctor will insert the tracheostomy tube and obturator into the stoma. After inserting the tube, he'll remove the obturator.

• Apply a sterile tracheostomy dressing, and anchor the tube with tracheostomy ties. Check for air movement through the tube, and auscultate the lungs to ensure proper tube placement.
• When the tube is in position, attach it to the appropriate oxygen therapy device.
• Inject air into the distal cuff port to inflate the cuff.
• The doctor will suture the corners of the incision.
• Put on sterile gloves and apply the sterile tracheostomy dressing under the tracheostomy tube flange. Place the tracheostomy ties through the openings of the tube flanges, and tie them on the side of the patient's neck. This allows easy access and prevents pressure necrosis at the back of the neck.
• Clean or dispose of the used equipment according to your facility's policy. Replenish all supplies as needed.
• Make sure that a chest X-ray is ordered to confirm tube placement.

Cautions

Make sure certain equipment is always at the patient's bedside so that you can handle emergency situations. Suctioning equipment is necessary because the patient may need his airway cleared at any time. The sterile obturator used to insert the tracheostomy tube should be available in case the tube is expelled. Have on hand a spare sterile tracheostomy tube and obturator the same size as the one used, in case the tube must be replaced quickly. Also have available a tube and an obturator one size smaller than those you used, in case the tube is expelled and the trachea begins to close.

Finally, make sure you have a spare sterile inner cannula that can be used if the cannula is expelled as well as a sterile tracheal dilator or sterile hemostats to maintain an open airway before inserting a new tracheostomy tube.

Review emergency first-aid measures, and always follow your facility's policy concerning an expelled or blocked tracheostomy tube.

Don't remove a partially expelled tracheostomy tube entirely; doing so may close the airway completely. Use extreme caution if you try to reinsert an expelled tracheostomy tube because of the risks of tracheal trauma, perforation, compression, and asphyxiation. Reassure the patient until the doctor arrives.

Monitoring and aftercare

• Assess the patient's vital signs and respiratory status every 15 minutes for 1 hour, then every 30 minutes for 2 hours, then every 2 hours until his condition is stable.
• Monitor the patient carefully for signs of infection. Ideally, the tracheotomy should be performed using sterile technique, as described. But in an emergency, this may not be possible.
• Record the reason for the procedure, the date and time it took place, and the patient's respiratory status before and after the procedure. Include any complications that occurred during the procedure, the amount of cuff pressure, the respiratory therapy initiated after the procedure, and the patient's response to the respiratory therapy.

Tracheostomy care

The goals of tracheostomy care are to ensure airway patency by keeping the tube free of mucus buildup, to maintain mucous membrane and skin integrity, to prevent infection, and to promote comfort and provide psychological support.

The patient may have a metal, plastic, or rubber tracheostomy tube. The metal tube, used mainly for long-term therapy, has three parts: an outer cannula, an inner cannula, and an obturator that guides insertion of the outer cannula. Some plastic tubes have the same three parts. Most, however, consist of an obturator, a cuff, and one single-walled tube that doesn't require removal for cleaning (because encrustations are less likely to form on nonmetal materials). The red rubber James tube, which doesn't have an inner cannula, is used infrequently because its surface may become roughened with use, making sterility difficult to guarantee. (See *Types of tracheostomy tubes,* page 90.)

Types of tracheostomy tubes

Various types of tracheostomy tubes are available, including plastic and metal. Plastic tubes are commonly used in emergencies because they have a universal adapter for respiratory support equipment, such as a mechanical ventilator, and a cuff to allow positive-pressure ventilation.

One type of plastic tracheostomy tube is the Bivonakaamen-Wilkinson Fome cuff. This tube has a cuff made of expandable foam that causes the least tracheal trauma since it doesn't need to be inflated. Instead, before inserting the tube, you withdraw air from the cuff to deflate the foam. The foam then expands by itself after insertion.

Metal tubes, which aren't cuffed, are used for laryngectomies and home care. They can't be used for mechanical ventilation.

Some tracheostomy tubes have an inner cannula that makes cleaning easy and allows for attachment to a mechanical ventilator. Tracheostomy tubes without inner cannulas must be changed regularly.

Fenestrated tracheostomy tubes, which are also plastic and are available cuffed or uncuffed, have a hole cut into the outer cannula to allow the patient to breathe around the tracheostomy tube. A fenestrated tube may be used to wean the patient from a mechanical ventilator. If the tube has a cuff and the cuff is inflated, an inner cannula seals off the fenestration and forms a sealed tracheal airway. The outer cannula plug can seal off the tracheostomy and allow for a patent upper airway if the cuff is deflated.

Cuffed tracheostomy tube with inner cannula

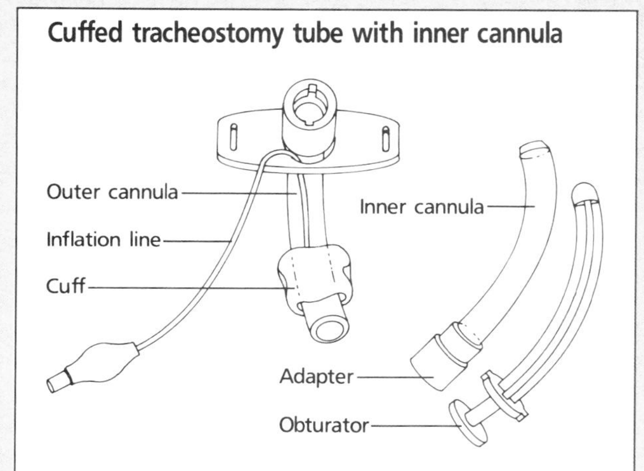

Fenestrated tracheostomy tube

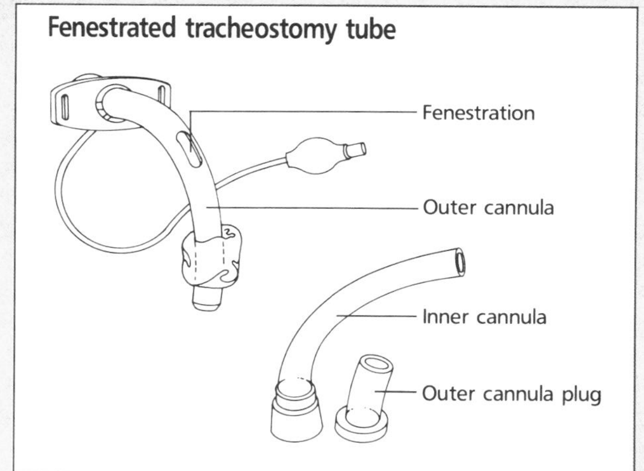

Whichever tube is used, tracheostomy care should be performed using aseptic technique until the stoma has healed. For recently performed tracheotomies, use sterile gloves for all manipulations at the tracheostomy site. Once the stoma has healed, substitute clean gloves for sterile ones.

Indications

All patients with tracheostomy tubes need care. Not all tubes, however, require inner cannula care.

Contraindications and complications

Tracheostomy care has no contraindications.

Secretions may collect under dressings, and twill tape can promote skin excoriation and infection. Hardened mucus or a slipped cuff can occlude the cannula opening and obstruct the airway. Tube displacement may stimulate the cough reflex if the tip rests on the carina, or it can cause blood vessel erosion and hemorrhage. Just the presence of the tube or cuff pressure can produce tracheal erosion and necrosis.

Equipment

For aseptic stoma and outer-cannula care

Waterproof trash bag • two sterile solution containers • 0.9% sodium chloride solution • hydrogen peroxide • sterile cotton-tipped applicators • sterile 4″ × 4″ gauze pads (or prepackaged sterile tracheostomy dressing) • sterile gloves • equipment and supplies for suctioning and for mouth care • water-soluble lubricant or topical antibiotic cream • materials as needed for cuff procedures and for changing tracheostomy ties (see below)

For aseptic inner-cannula care

All of the above equipment plus a prepackaged commercial tracheostomy care set and sterile forceps • sterile nylon brush • sterile 6″ (15-cm) pipe cleaners • clean gloves • a third sterile solution container • disposable temporary inner cannula (for a patient on a ventilator)

For changing tracheostomy ties

30″ (76-cm) length of tracheostomy twill tape • bandage scissors • sterile gloves • hemostat

For cuff procedures

5- or 10-cc syringe • padded hemostat • stethoscope

Preparation

• Assess the patient's condition to determine his needs. Provide privacy.
• Explain the procedure to the patient, even if he's unresponsive.
• Wash your hands and assemble all equipment and supplies in the patient's room. Check the expiration date on each sterile package and inspect for tears.
• Open the waterproof trash bag and place it next to you so that you can avoid reaching across the sterile field or the patient's stoma when discarding soiled items. Form a cuff by turning down the top of the trash bag to ensure a wide opening and to prevent contamination of instruments or gloves on the bag's edge.
• Establish a sterile field near the patient's bed (usually on the overbed table), and place equipment and supplies on it.
• Pour 0.9% sodium chloride solution, hydrogen peroxide, or a mixture of equal parts of both solutions into one of the sterile solution containers; then pour 0.9% sodium chloride solution into the second sterile container for rinsing.
• For inner-cannula care, you may use a third sterile solution container to hold the gauze pads and cotton-tipped applicators saturated with cleaning solution.
• If you'll be replacing the disposable inner cannula, open the package containing the new inner cannula while maintaining sterile technique. Obtain or prepare new tracheostomy ties, if indicated.

Essential steps

• Place the patient in semi-Fowler's position (unless it's contraindicated) to decrease abdominal pressure on the diaphragm, thereby promoting lung expansion.
• Remove any humidification or ventilation device.
• Using sterile technique, suction the entire length of the tracheostomy tube to clear the airway of any secretions that may hinder oxygenation.
• Reconnect the patient to the humidifier or ventilator, if necessary.

To clean a stoma and outer cannula

• Put on sterile gloves if you're not already wearing them.
• With your dominant hand, saturate a sterile gauze pad with the cleaning solution.
• Squeeze out the excess liquid to prevent accidental aspiration. Then wipe the patient's neck under the tracheostomy tube flanges and twill tapes.
• Saturate a second pad and wipe until the skin surrounding the tracheostomy is cleaned. Use additional pads or cotton-tipped applicators to clean the stoma site and the tube's flanges. Wipe only once with each pad and then discard it to prevent contamination of a clean area with a soiled pad.
• Rinse debris and peroxide (if used) with one or more sterile 4″ × 4″ gauze pads dampened in 0.9% sodium chloride solution. Dry the area thoroughly with additional sterile gauze pads;

HOME CARE

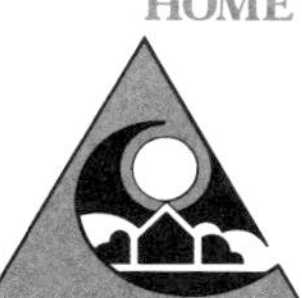

Applying a tracheostomy dressing

If you're caring for a patient in his home and a prepackaged gauze tracheostomy dressing is unavailable, refold a sterile 3" × 3" gauze pad to create a customized dressing, as shown below.

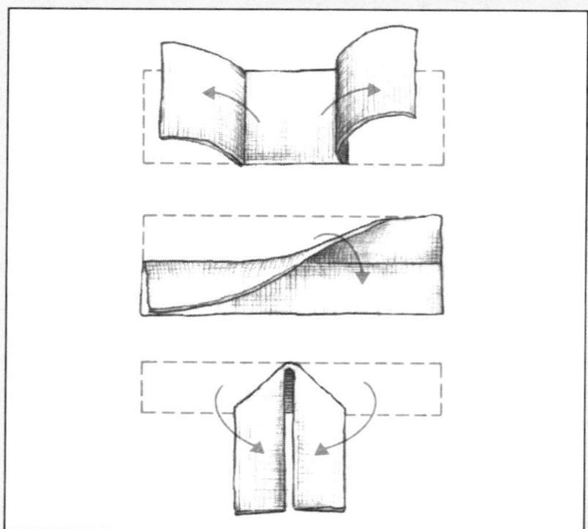

Never cut a gauze dressing to fit around the stoma; the patient could aspirate loose fibers through the tube, causing irritation deep within the airways.

Fasten the neck twill tapes to the openings in the neck plate of the tracheostomy tube. For the patient's comfort, tie the tape ends to the side of the neck rather than in back.

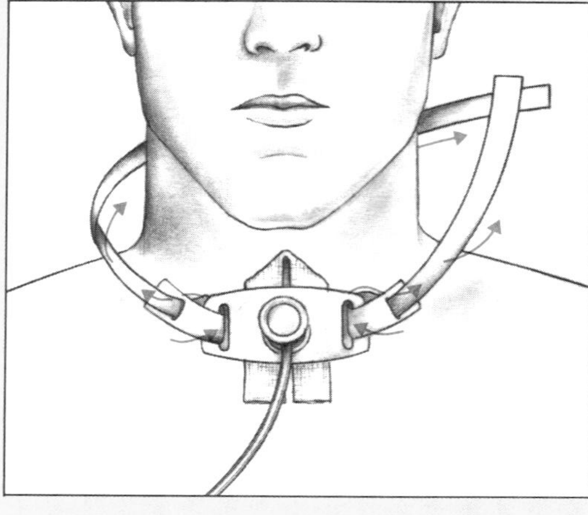

then apply a new sterile tracheostomy dressing. (See *Applying a tracheostomy dressing.*)
• Remove and discard your gloves.

To clean a nondisposable inner cannula
• Put on sterile gloves.
• Using your nondominant hand, remove and discard the patient's tracheostomy dressing. Then, with the same hand, disconnect the ventilator or humidification device and unlock the tracheostomy tube's inner cannula by rotating it counterclockwise. Place the inner cannula in the container of hydrogen peroxide.
• Working quickly, use your dominant hand to scrub the cannula with the sterile nylon brush. If the brush doesn't slide easily into the cannula, use a sterile pipe cleaner.
• Immerse the cannula in the container of 0.9% sodium chloride solution, and agitate it for about 10 seconds to rinse it thoroughly.
• Inspect the cannula for cleanliness, and repeat the cleaning process if necessary. If the cannula is clean, tap it gently against the inside edge of the sterile container to remove excess liquid and prevent aspiration. Don't dry the outer surface because a thin film of moisture acts as a lubricant during insertion.
• Reinsert the inner cannula into the patient's tracheostomy tube. Lock it in place and then gently pull on it to ensure that it's positioned securely. Reconnect the mechanical ventilator, and apply a new sterile tracheostomy dressing.
• If the patient can't tolerate being disconnected from the ventilator for the time it takes to clean the inner cannula, replace the existing inner cannula with a clean one and reattach the mechanical ventilator. Then clean the cannula just removed from the patient and store it in a sterile container until the next time tracheostomy care is performed.

To care for a disposable inner cannula
• Put on clean gloves.
• Using your dominant hand, remove the patient's inner cannula. After evaluating the secretions in the cannula, discard it properly.
• Pick up the new inner cannula, touching only the outer locking portion. Insert the cannula into the tracheostomy and, following the manufacturer's instructions, lock it securely.

To change tracheostomy ties

- Get help from another nurse or a respiratory therapist because of the risk of accidental tube expulsion during this procedure. Patient movement or coughing can dislodge the tube.
- Assist the patient into semi-Fowler's position, if possible.
- Wash your hands thoroughly and put on sterile gloves if you're not already wearing them.
- If you're not using commercially packaged tracheostomy ties, prepare new ties from a 30″ (76-cm) length of twill tape by folding one end back 1″ (2.5 cm) on itself. Then, with the bandage scissors, cut a ½″ (1-cm) slit down the center of the tape from the folded edge.
- Prepare the other end of the tape in the same way.
- Hold both ends together and, using scissors, cut the resulting circle of tape so that one piece is approximately 10″ (25 cm) long, and the other is about 20″ (51 cm) long.
- After your assistant puts on gloves, instruct her to hold the tracheostomy tube in place to prevent its expulsion during tie replacement. However, if you must perform the procedure without assistance, fasten the clean ties in place before removing the old ties to prevent tube expulsion.
- With the assistant's gloved fingers holding the tracheostomy tube in place, cut the soiled tracheostomy ties with the bandage scissors or untie them and discard the ties. Be careful not to cut the tube of the pilot balloon.
- Thread the slit end of one new tie a short distance through the eye of one tracheostomy tube flange from the underside; use the hemostat, if necessary, to pull the tie through. Then thread the other end of the tie completely through the slit end, and pull it taut so that it loops firmly through the tube's flange. This avoids knots that can cause discomfort, tissue irritation, pressure, and necrosis at the patient's throat.
- Fasten the second tie to the opposite flange in the same manner.
- Instruct the patient to flex his neck while you bring the ties around to the side and tie them together with a square knot. Flexion produces the same neck circumference as coughing and helps prevent a tie that's too tight. Instruct your assistant to place one finger under the tapes as you tie them to ensure that they're tight enough to avoid slippage but loose enough to prevent choking or jugular vein constriction. Placing the closure on the side allows easy access and prevents pressure necrosis at the back of the neck when the patient is prone.
- After securing the ties, cut off the excess tape with the scissors and instruct your assistant to release the tracheostomy tube.

To deflate and inflate a tracheostomy cuff

- Read the cuff manufacturer's instructions because cuff types and procedures vary widely.
- Assess the patient's condition, explain the procedure to him, and reassure him. Wash your hands thoroughly.
- Help the patient into semi-Fowler's position, if possible, or place him in a supine position so that secretions above the cuff site will be pushed up into the mouth if he's receiving positive-pressure ventilation.
- Suction the oropharyngeal cavity to prevent any pooled secretions from descending into the trachea after cuff deflation.
- Release the padded hemostat clamping the cuff inflation tubing (if a hemostat is present).
- Insert a 5- or 10-cc syringe into the cuff pilot balloon, and very slowly withdraw all air from the cuff. Leave the syringe attached to the tubing for later cuff reinflation. Slow deflation allows positive lung pressure to push secretions upward from the bronchi. Cuff deflation may also stimulate the patient's cough reflex, producing additional secretions.
- Remove any ventilation device. Suction the lower airway through any existing tube to remove all secretions. Then return the patient to the ventilation device.
- Maintain cuff deflation for the prescribed period of time. Observe the patient for adequate ventilation, and suction as necessary. If the patient has difficulty breathing, reinflate the cuff immediately by depressing the syringe plunger very slowly. Inject the least amount of air necessary to achieve an adequate tracheal seal.
- When inflating the cuff, you may use the minimal-leak technique or the minimal occlu-

sive volume technique to help gauge the proper inflation point.

• If you're inflating the cuff using cuff pressure measurement, don't exceed 25 mm Hg. If the pressure exceeds 25 mm Hg, notify the doctor because you may need to change to a larger size tube, use higher inflation pressures, or permit a larger air leak. A cuff pressure of about 18 mm Hg is usually recommended.

• Cuff pressure can be measured by the same procedure as endotracheal cuff pressure.

• After you've inflated the cuff, if the tubing doesn't have a one-way valve at the end, clamp the inflation line with a padded hemostat (to protect the tubing) and remove the syringe.

• Check for a leak-free cuff seal. Even with minimal cuff inflation, you should feel no air coming from the patient's mouth, nose, or tracheostomy site, and a conscious patient shouldn't be able to speak.

• Be alert for air leaks from the cuff itself. Suspect a leak if injection of air fails to inflate the cuff or increase cuff pressure, if you can't inject the amount of air you withdrew, if the patient can speak, if ventilation fails to maintain adequate respiratory movement with pressures or volumes previously considered adequate, or if air escapes during the ventilator's inspiratory cycle.

• Note the exact amount of air used to inflate the cuff to detect tracheal malacia if more air is consistently needed.

Cautions

Keep all necessary equipment at the patient's bedside for immediate use in an emergency. Consult the doctor about first-aid measures that you can use for your tracheostomy patient if an emergency occurs.

Don't change tracheostomy ties unnecessarily during the immediate postoperative period before the stoma track is well formed (usually 4 days) to avoid accidental dislodgment and expulsion of the tube. Unless secretions or drainage is a problem, you can change ties once a day.

Refrain from changing a single-cannula tracheostomy tube or the outer cannula of a double-cannula tube. Because of the risk of tracheal complications, the doctor usually changes the cannula as often as the patient's condition warrants.

Monitoring and aftercare

• Reconnect the patient to the humidification device, if necessary.

• Observe soiled dressings and any suctioned secretions for amount, color, consistency, and odor.

• Properly clean or dispose of all equipment, supplies, solutions, and trash, according to your hospital's policy.

• Make sure that the patient is comfortable and that he can easily reach the call button.

• Provide oral care, as needed, because the oral cavity can become dry and malodorous or develop sores from encrusted secretions.

• For the patient with a traumatic injury, radical neck dissection, or cardiac failure, check tracheostomy-tie tension frequently because neck diameter can increase from swelling and cause constriction; also check a neonate or restless patient frequently because ties can loosen, possibly leading to tube dislodgment.

• Tracheostomy care may be given at various intervals, depending on the patient's need. It may be necessary as often as every 30 minutes just after tube insertion; it should never be suspended for more than 8 hours. If the patient will be discharged with a tracheostomy, care measures include teaching him home care using clean technique.

• Change the dressing as often as necessary, whether or not you also perform the entire cleaning procedure. A dressing wet with exudate or secretions predisposes the patient to skin excoriation, breakdown, and infection.

• If the patient's neck or stoma is excoriated or infected, apply a water-soluble lubricant or topical antibiotic cream, as ordered. Remember not to use a powder or an oil-based substance on or around a stoma because aspiration can cause infection and abscess.

• Replenish any used supplies, including solutions, regularly according to facility policy to reduce the risk of nosocomial infections.

• Record the date and time of the procedure; the type of procedure; the amount, consistency, color, and odor of secretions; stoma and

skin condition; the patient's respiratory status; tracheostomy tube changes by the doctor; the duration of any cuff deflation; the amount of any cuff inflation; and cuff pressure readings and specific body position. Note any complications and subsequent interventions; any patient or family teaching and their comprehension and progress; and the patient's tolerance of the treatment.
• If the patient is being discharged with a tracheostomy, start self-care teaching as soon as he's receptive. Teach the patient how to change and clean the tube. If he's being discharged with suction equipment (a few patients are), make sure that he and his family feel knowledgeable and comfortable about using this equipment.

Manual ventilation

In this procedure, oxygen or room air is manually delivered to the lungs of a patient who can't breathe by himself. The procedure uses a hand-held resuscitation bag—an inflatable device that can be attached to a face mask or directly to an endotracheal or tracheostomy tube.

Usually performed in an emergency, manual ventilation is also used while a patient is temporarily disconnected from a mechanical ventilator—for example, during a tubing change, during transport, or before suctioning. Using the hand-held resuscitation bag maintains ventilation. Oxygen administration with a resuscitation bag improves oxygenation.

Indications
Manual ventilation is indicated for patients who can't breathe independently.

Contraindications and complications
Manual ventilation has no contraindications.

Gastric distention may result from air forced into the patient's stomach; this can cause vomiting, aspiration, and pneumonia.

Equipment
Hand-held resuscitation bag • mask • oxygen source (wall unit or tank) • oxygen tubing • nipple adapter attached to oxygen flowmeter • optional: PEEP valve, oxygen accumulator, suction equipment

Preparation
• Select a mask that fits snugly over the mouth and nose, unless the patient is intubated or has had a tracheotomy. Attach the mask to the resuscitation bag.
• If oxygen is readily available, connect the hand-held resuscitation bag to the oxygen. Attach one end of the tubing to the bottom of the bag and the other end to the nipple adapter on the flowmeter of the oxygen source.
• Turn on the oxygen and adjust the flow rate according to the patient's condition. For example, if the patient has a low PaO_2, he'll need a higher FIO_2. To increase the concentration of inspired oxygen, you can add an oxygen accumulator (also called an oxygen reservoir). This device, which attaches to an adapter on the bottom of the bag, permits an FIO_2 of up to 100%. Then, if time allows, set up the suction equipment.

Essential steps
• Before using the hand-held resuscitation bag, check the patient's upper airway for foreign objects. If you find any, remove them because this alone may restore spontaneous respirations in some instances. Also, foreign matter or secretions can obstruct the airway and impede resuscitation efforts. Suction the patient to remove any secretions that may obstruct the airway. If necessary, insert an oropharyngeal or nasopharyngeal airway to maintain airway patency. If the patient has a tracheostomy or endotracheal tube in place, suction the tube.
• If appropriate, remove the bed's headboard and stand at the head of the bed to help keep the patient's neck extended and to free space at the side of the bed for other activities, such as cardiac compressions.
• Tilt the patient's head backward, if not contraindicated, and pull his jaw forward to move the tongue away from the base of the pharynx

and prevent potential airway obstruction. (See *Applying a hand-held resuscitation bag and mask.*)

• Keeping your nondominant hand on the patient's mask, exert downward pressure to seal the mask against his face. For the adult patient, use your dominant hand to compress the bag every 5 seconds to deliver about 1 liter of air. For a child, deliver 15 breaths/minute, or one compression of the bag every 4 seconds; for the infant, 20 breaths/minute, or one compression every 3 seconds. Infants and children should receive 250 to 500 cc of air with each bag compression.

• Deliver breaths with the patient's own inspiratory effort, if present. Don't attempt to deliver a breath as the patient exhales.

• Observe the patient's chest to ensure that it rises and falls with each compression. If ventilation fails to occur, check the fit of the mask and the patency of the patient's airway. If necessary, reposition the patient's head and ensure patency with an oral airway.

Applying a hand-held resuscitation bag and mask

Place the mask over the patient's face so that the apex of the triangle covers the bridge of his nose and the base lies between his lower lip and chin.

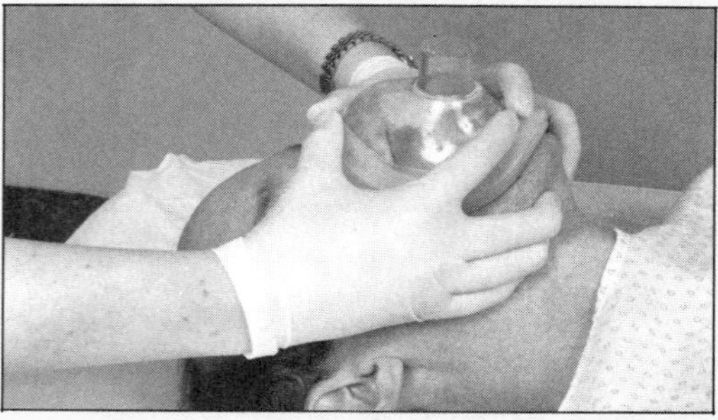

Make sure that the patient's mouth remains open underneath the mask. Attach the bag to the mask and to the tubing leading to the oxygen source.

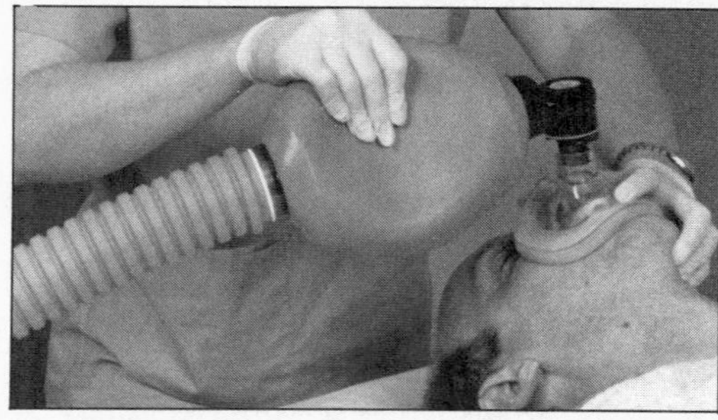

Or, if the patient has a tracheostomy or endotracheal tube in place, remove the mask from the bag and attach the hand-held resuscitation bag directly to the tube.

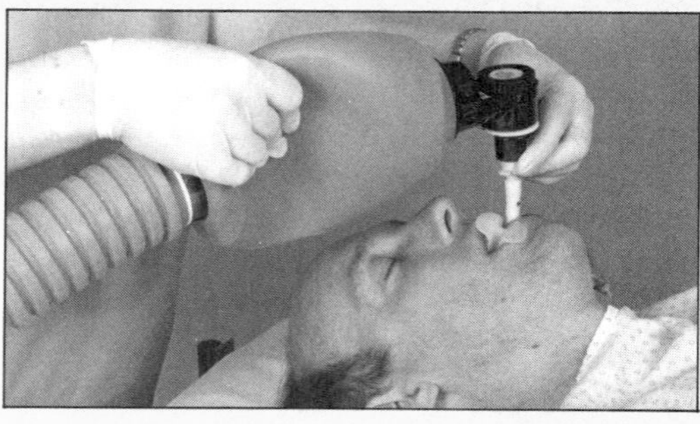

Cautions

Avoid neck hyperextension if the patient may have a cervical injury; instead, use the jaw-thrust technique to open the airway. If you need both hands to keep the patient's mask in place and maintain hyperextension, have another person compress the bag or, if necessary, use the lower part of your arm to compress the bag against your side.

Observe for vomiting through the clear part of the mask. If vomiting occurs, stop the procedure immediately, lift the mask, wipe and suction the vomitus, and resume resuscitation.

Underventilation commonly occurs because it's difficult to keep the hand-held resuscitation bag positioned tightly on the patient's face while ensuring an open airway. What's more, the volume of air delivered to the patient varies with the type of bag used and the hand size of the person compressing the bag. An adult with a small or medium-sized hand may not consistently deliver 1 liter of air. For these reasons, have someone assist with the procedure, if possible.

Monitoring and aftercare

• You can add a PEEP valve to most resuscitation bags to improve oxygenation if the patient hasn't responded to the increased FIO_2 levels. A PEEP valve is recommended for patients who have been receiving PEEP on a ventilator and are switching to manual ventilation.
• In an emergency, record the date and time of the procedure; manual ventilation efforts; any complications and subsequent interventions; and the patient's response to treatment.
• In a nonemergency situation, record the date and time of the procedure, the reason and length of time the patient was disconnected from mechanical ventilation and received manual ventilation, any complications and subsequent interventions, and the patient's tolerance of the procedure.

Tracheal suctioning

This procedure involves the removal of secretions from the trachea or bronchi by means of a catheter inserted through the mouth, nose, tracheal stoma, tracheostomy tube, or endotracheal tube. Besides removing secretions, tracheal suctioning also stimulates the cough reflex. The procedure helps maintain a patent airway to promote optimal exchange of oxygen and carbon dioxide and to prevent pneumonia that results from pooling of secretions. You should perform tracheal suctioning as frequently as the patient's condition warrants, always using strict aseptic technique.

Indications

• Impaired cough reflex
• Copious respiratory secretions
• Presence of tracheostomy, laryngectomy, or endotracheal tube

Contraindications and complications

Use extreme caution when you perform nasotracheal suctioning in patients with a history of nasopharyngeal bleeding or patients taking anticoagulants. You should also be cautious with patients who have had a tracheotomy recently, who have a blood dyscrasia, or who have increased intracranial pressure.

Because oxygen is removed along with secretions, the patient may experience hypoxia and dyspnea. Anxiety may alter respiratory patterns. Cardiac arrhythmias can result from hypoxia and stimulation of the vagus nerve in the tracheobronchial tree. Tracheal or bronchial trauma can result from traumatic or prolonged suctioning.

If the patient experiences laryngospasm or bronchospasm (rare complications) during suctioning, disconnect the suction catheter from the connecting tube and allow the catheter to act as an airway. Discuss with the patient's doctor whether bronchodilators or lidocaine can be used to reduce the risk of this complication.

Patients with compromised cardiovascular or pulmonary status are at risk for hypoxia, arrhythmias, hypertension, or hypotension.

Equipment

Wall or portable oxygen source (or a handheld resuscitation bag with a mask, 15-mm adapter, or PEEP valve, if indicated) • wall or portable suction apparatus • collection container • connecting tube • suction catheter kit (or sterile suction catheter, one sterile glove, one clean [nonsterile] glove, and a disposable sterile solution container) • 1-liter bottle of sterile water or 0.9% sodium chloride solution • sterile water-soluble lubricant (for nasal insertion) • syringe for deflating cuff of endotracheal or tracheostomy tube • waterproof trash bag • sterile towel (optional)

Preparation

• Get a doctor's order if required.
• Assess the patient's vital signs, breath sounds, and general appearance to establish a baseline for comparison after suctioning.
• Review the patient's ABG values and oxygen saturation levels if they're available.
• Evaluate the patient's ability to cough and breathe deeply because these actions will help move secretions up the tracheobronchial tree. If you'll be performing nasotracheal suctioning, check the patient's history for a deviated sep-

tum, nasal polyps, nasal obstruction, nasal trauma, epistaxis, or mucosal swelling.
• Choose a suction catheter of appropriate size. The diameter should be no larger than half the inside diameter of the tracheostomy or endotracheal tube to minimize the risk of hypoxia during suctioning. (A #12 or #14 French catheter may be used for an 8-mm or larger tube.) Place the suction apparatus on the patient's overbed table or bedside stand. Position the table or stand on your preferred side of the bed to facilitate suctioning.
• Attach the collection container to the suction unit and the connecting tube to the collection container. Label and date the bottle of 0.9% sodium chloride solution or sterile water.

Essential steps

• Wash your hands. Explain the procedure to the patient, even if he's unresponsive. Tell him that suctioning usually causes transient coughing or gagging but that coughing is helpful for removal of secretions. If the patient has been suctioned previously, summarize the reasons for suctioning. Continue to reassure him throughout the procedure to minimize anxiety, promote relaxation, and decrease oxygen demand.
• Unless contraindicated, place the patient in semi-Fowler's or high Fowler's position to promote lung expansion and productive coughing.
• Remove the top from the bottle of sterile water or 0.9% sodium chloride solution.
• Open the package containing the sterile solution container.
• Using strict aseptic technique, open the suction catheter kit and put on the gloves. If using individual supplies, open the suction catheter and the gloves, placing the sterile glove on your dominant hand and the nonsterile glove on your nondominant hand.
• Using your nondominant (nonsterile) hand, pour the 0.9% sodium chloride solution or sterile water into the solution container.
• Place a small amount of water-soluble lubricant on the sterile area of the packaging. The lubricant may be used to facilitate passage of the catheter during nasotracheal suctioning.
• Place a sterile towel over the patient's chest, if desired, to provide an additional sterile area.
• Using your dominant (sterile) hand, remove the catheter from its wrapper. Keep it coiled so that it can't touch a nonsterile object. Using your other hand to manipulate the connecting tubing, attach the catheter to the tubing.
• Occlude the suction port to assess suction pressure, which should be set according to facility policy. Typically, pressure may be set between 80 and 120 mm Hg. Higher pressures don't enhance secretion removal and may cause traumatic injury.
• Dip the catheter tip into the 0.9% sodium chloride solution to lubricate the outside of the catheter and reduce tissue trauma during insertion.
• With the catheter tip in the sterile solution, occlude the control valve with the thumb of your nondominant hand. Suction a small amount of solution through the catheter to lubricate the inside of the catheter. This will facilitate passage of secretions through it.
• For nasal insertion of the catheter, lubricate the tip of the catheter with the sterile, water-soluble lubricant to reduce tissue trauma during insertion.
• If the patient isn't intubated, or is intubated but not receiving supplemental oxygen or aerosol, instruct him to take three to six deep breaths to help minimize or prevent hypoxia during suctioning.
• If the patient isn't intubated but is receiving oxygen, evaluate his need for preoxygenation. If indicated, instruct the patient to take three to six deep breaths while using his supplemental oxygen. (If he needs it, the patient may continue to receive supplemental oxygen during suctioning by leaving his nasal cannula in one nostril or by keeping the oxygen mask over his mouth.)
• If the patient is being mechanically ventilated, preoxygenate him by using either a hand-held resuscitation bag or the sigh mode on the ventilator. To use the resuscitation bag, set the oxygen flowmeter at 15 liters/minute, disconnect the patient from the ventilator, and deliver three to six breaths with the resuscitation bag.
• If the patient is being maintained on PEEP, evaluate the need to use a resuscitation bag with a PEEP valve.
• To preoxygenate using the ventilator, first adjust the FIO_2 and tidal volume according to the

policy at your hospital and the patient's need. Then use the sigh mode or manually deliver three to six breaths. If you have an assistant for the procedure, the assistant can manage the patient's oxygen needs while you perform the suctioning.

Nasotracheal insertion in a nonintubated patient

• Remove the oxygen from the patient, if applicable.
• Using your nondominant hand, raise the tip of the patient's nose to straighten the passageway and facilitate insertion of the catheter.
• With your dominant hand, insert the catheter into the patient's nostril while gently rolling it between your fingers to help it advance through the turbinates.
• As the patient inhales, quickly advance the catheter as far as possible. Do not apply suction during insertion to avoid oxygen loss and tissue trauma.
• If the patient coughs as the catheter passes through the larynx, briefly hold the catheter still and then resume advancement when the patient inhales.

Nasotracheal insertion in an intubated patient

• Using your nondominant hand, disconnect the patient from the ventilator.
• Using your dominant hand, gently insert the suction catheter into the artificial airway. Advance the catheter, without applying suction, until you meet resistance. If the patient coughs, pause briefly and then resume advancement.

Suctioning the patient

• After inserting the catheter, apply suction intermittently by removing and replacing the thumb of your nondominant hand over the control valve. Simultaneously use your dominant hand to withdraw the catheter as you roll it between your thumb and forefinger. This rotating motion prevents the catheter from pulling tissue into the tube as it exits, thus avoiding tissue trauma. Never suction more than 10 seconds at a time to prevent hypoxia.
• If the patient is intubated, use your nondominant hand to stabilize the tip of the endotracheal tube as you withdraw the catheter. This prevents mucous membrane irritation or accidental extubation.
• If applicable, resume oxygen delivery by reconnecting the source of oxygen or ventilation and hyperoxygenating the patient's lungs before continuing, to prevent or relieve hypoxia.
• Observe the patient and allow him to rest for a few minutes before the next suctioning. The timing of each suctioning and the length of each rest period depend on his tolerance for the procedure and the absence of complications. To enhance secretion removal, encourage the patient to cough between suctioning attempts. (See *Suctioning thick secretions.*)
• If the patient's heart rate and rhythm are being monitored, observe for arrhythmias. If they occur, stop suctioning and ventilate the patient.

SKILL TIP

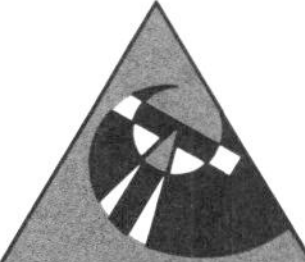

Suctioning thick secretions

Using a standard suction catheter may not be effective for thick and copious oral secretions. If not, try a Yankauer tonsil-tip catheter and frequently flush 0.9% sodium chloride solution or sterile water through the catheter and tubing to prevent clogging the suction apparatus. For neonates and infants, use a tuberculin syringe. Remove the plunger and needle, and cut off the wings at the plunger end. Now the syringe will fit into the suction tubing and will handle thick secretions.

After suctioning

• After the procedure, hyperoxygenate the ventilated patient with the hand-held resuscitation bag or by using the ventilator's sigh mode, as described earlier.
• Readjust the FIO_2 and, for ventilated patients, the tidal volume to the ordered settings.
• After suctioning the lower airway, assess the patient's need for upper airway suctioning. If the cuff of the endotracheal or tracheostomy tube will be deflated, suction the upper airway before deflating the cuff with a syringe. Al-

HOME CARE

Teaching tracheal suctioning

If a patient can't move secretions effectively by coughing, he may have to perform tracheal suctioning at home, using either clean or aseptic technique. Most patients use clean technique; they perform thorough hand washing and may wear a clean glove. But if a patient has poor hand-washing technique, recurrent respiratory infections, or a compromised immune system, or has recently had surgery, he may need to use aseptic technique.

Clean technique

Because the cost of disposable catheters can be prohibitive, many patients reuse disposable catheters, but the practice remains controversial. If the catheter has thick secretions adhering to it, the patient may clean it with a quaternary compound, such as Control III.

Nondisposable, red rubber catheters are an alternative to disposable catheters. Consult your hospital's policy regarding the care and cleaning of suction catheters in the home setting. Some protocols recommend soaking such catheters in soapy water, then placing them in boiling water for 10 minutes; or soaking them in 70% alcohol for 3 to 5 minutes, then rinsing them in 0.9% sodium chloride solution.

Supplies needed

Obviously, the supplies needed will vary with the technique used. If the patient will be using clean technique, he'll need suction catheter kits (or clean gloves, suction catheters, and a basin) and distilled water. If he'll be using aseptic technique, the suction catheters and gloves will need to be sterile, as will the basin and the water (or 0.9% sodium chloride solution).

The type of suction machine necessary will depend on the patient's needs. You'll need to evaluate the amount of suction the machine provides, how easy it is to clean, the volume of the collection bottles, how much the machine costs, and whether it has an overflow safety device to prevent secretions from entering the compressor. You'll also need to determine whether the patient needs a machine that operates on batteries and, if so, how long the batteries will last, and if and how they can be recharged.

Nursing goals

Before discharge, have the patient and his family demonstrate the suctioning procedure to you. Make sure that they know the indications for suctioning, the signs and symptoms of infection, the importance of adequate hydration, and when to use adjunct therapy, such as aerosol therapy, chest physiotherapy, oxygen therapy, or a hand-held resuscitation bag. At discharge, arrange for a home health care provider and a reliable medical equipment vendor to follow up with the patient.

ways change the catheter and sterile glove before resuctioning the lower airway to avoid introducing microorganisms into the lower airway.

• Discard the gloves and the catheter in the waterproof trash bag. Clear the connecting tubing by aspirating the remaining 0.9% sodium chloride solution or sterile water. Discard and replace suction equipment and supplies according to the policy at your hospital. Wash your hands.

Cautions

Because tracheal suctioning can cause complications and increased mucus production, perform it only when necessary. Do not allow the collection container to become more than three-quarters full to keep from damaging the machine.

Raising the patient's nose into the sniffing position helps align the larynx and pharynx and may facilitate passing the catheter during nasotracheal suctioning. If the patient's condition permits, have an assistant extend the patient's head and neck above his shoulders. The patient's lower jaw may need to be moved up and forward. If the patient is responsive, ask him to stick out his tongue so that he won't be able to swallow the catheter during insertion.

During suctioning, the catheter is usually advanced as far as the mainstem bronchi. The tracheobronchial structure causes the catheter to enter the right mainstem bronchus instead of the left. Using an angled catheter (such as a coudé or Bronchitrac L) may help you guide the catheter into the left mainstem bronchus, if needed. Rotating the patient's head to the right also seems to help.

In addition to the closed tracheal method, oxygen insufflation offers a new approach to suctioning. This type of suctioning uses a double-lumen catheter that allows oxygen insufflation during the suctioning procedure, preventing hypoxia.

Monitoring and aftercare

- If sputum is thick, clear the catheter periodically by dipping the tip in the 0.9% sodium chloride solution and applying suction. Normally, sputum is watery and tends to be sticky. Tenacious or thick sputum usually indicates dehydration. Also watch for color variations. A white or translucent color is normal; yellow indicates pus; green indicates retained secretions or *Pseudomonas* infection; brown usually indicates old blood; red indicates fresh blood; and a red jellylike consistency indicates *Klebsiella* infection.
- Auscultate the lungs bilaterally and take vital signs, if indicated, to assess the procedure's effectiveness.
- Inject 0.9% sodium chloride solution into the trachea before suctioning to stimulate the patient's cough. (Studies have shown that this doesn't liquefy the patient's secretions.) Keep the patient adequately hydrated, and use good bronchial hygiene techniques.
- Record the date and time of the procedure, the technique used, and the reason for suctioning; the amount, color, consistency, and odor (if any) of the secretions; any complications and subsequent interventions; and pertinent data regarding the patient's subjective response to the procedure. (See *Teaching tracheal suctioning.*)

Closed tracheal suctioning

The newest way to facilitate suctioning while reducing its complications, closed tracheal suctioning is used for patients on mechanical ventilation who require suctioning or who are being weaned with a T-piece. The procedure poses a lower risk of suction-induced hypoxemia because the patient can maintain the tidal volume, oxygen concentration, and PEEP delivered by the ventilator while being suctioned. And because the catheter remains in a protective sleeve, closed tracheal suctioning reduces the risk of infection, even when the same catheter is used many times. Gloves are not required for closed tracheal suctioning.

The procedure is safer for you than conventional suctioning because the patient can't cough secretions into your face and eyes. Also, closed tracheal suctioning can be performed more quickly than conventional suctioning because it involves fewer steps. And the costs are usually lower because fewer supplies are used.

Indications

Closed tracheal suctioning is indicated for patients on mechanical ventilation who require suctioning.

Contraindications and complications

Closed tracheal suctioning has the same contraindications as conventional tracheal suctioning. Use it with extreme caution in patients taking anticoagulants, patients who've had a tracheotomy recently, patients who have a blood dyscrasia, or patients who have increased intracranial pressure.

Possible complications during suctioning include arterial oxygen desaturation, bradycardia, hypotension, bronchoconstriction, tachyarrhythmias, premature ventricular contractions, and asystole.

Equipment

Closed suction control valve • T-piece (to connect the artificial airway to the ventilator breathing circuit) • catheter sleeve that encloses the catheter and has connections for the control valve and T-piece • 0.9% sodium chloride solution in a unit-dose container or a 6-cc syringe • clean gloves (optional)

Preparation

Wash your hands and explain the procedure to the patient.

Essential steps

• Attach the closed tracheal suction system to the ventilator tubing and wall suction.
• Suction the patient. (See *Performing closed tracheal suctioning.*)

Cautions

Hyperoxygenation may still be necessary before suctioning, especially for sensitive patients prone to arrhythmias or hypotension due to hypoxia. Allow 1 to 2 minutes of 100% oxygen flow before suctioning.

Depress the suction control valve when setting the vacuum to achieve adequate suction.

Don't use the tracheal suction setup for naso-oral suctioning. You'll need to use a separate suctioning setup. Use a Y-adapter at the suction canister to change the setup, and use a clean pair of gloves for the new setup.

If you use tracheal lavage to remove secretions, a technique whose efficacy remains controversial, the catheter should be inserted 6" (15 cm) into the airway before the 0.9% sodium chloride solution is instilled.

Make sure that you maintain the system's patency by rinsing secretions from the catheter after each use.

Monitoring and aftercare

• Auscultate the lungs bilaterally and take the patient's vital signs, if necessary, to assess the procedure's effectiveness.
• Dispose of and replace the suction equipment and supplies according to your facility's policy.
• Change the closed suction system every 24 hours to minimize the risk of infection.
• Record the date and time of the procedure; the technique used; the reason for suctioning; the amount, color, and consistency of secretions; any complications and subsequent interventions; and the patient's response to suctioning.

Mechanical ventilation

A mechanical ventilator moves air in and out of a patient's lungs. Although the equipment ventilates a patient, it doesn't ensure adequate gas exchange. For mechanical ventilation to be effective, you may have to administer a sedative or neuromuscular blocking agent to relax the patient and prevent spontaneous breathing efforts, which can interfere with the ventilator's action. Mechanical ventilators may use either positive or negative pressure to ventilate patients.

Positive-pressure ventilators exert a positive pressure on the airway, which causes inspiration and, at the same time, increases the patient's tidal volume. The inspiratory cycles of these ventilators may vary according to volume, pressure, or time. For example, a volume-cycled ventilator—the type used most commonly—delivers a preset volume of air to the patient each time, regardless of the amount of resistance by the patient's lungs. A pressure-cycled ventilator generates flow until the machine reaches a preset pressure, regardless of the volume delivered or the time required to achieve the pressure. A time-cycled ventilator generates flow for a preset amount of time.

High-frequency jet ventilation is the newest type of positive-pressure ventilation. This technique prevents fluctuation of pressure within the lungs and doesn't cause the detrimental effects on the cardiovascular system that other positive-pressure ventilators do. (See *High-frequency jet ventilation,* page 107.)

Negative-pressure ventilators create negative pressure, which pulls the patient's thorax outward and allows air to flow into his lungs. Examples of negative-pressure ventilators are the iron lung, the cuirass ventilator (turtle shell), and the body wrap (Pneumowrap or Pulmo-wrap).

(Text continues on page 107).

Performing closed tracheal suctioning

Closed tracheal suctioning allows you to provide suctioning during mechanical ventilation without disconnecting the patient from the ventilator.

To use a closed tracheal suction system, first remove the suction system from the package.

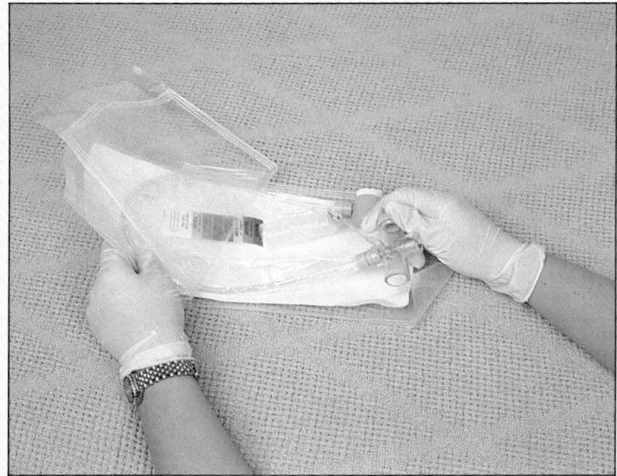

Attach the thumb control valve to the wall suction tubing.

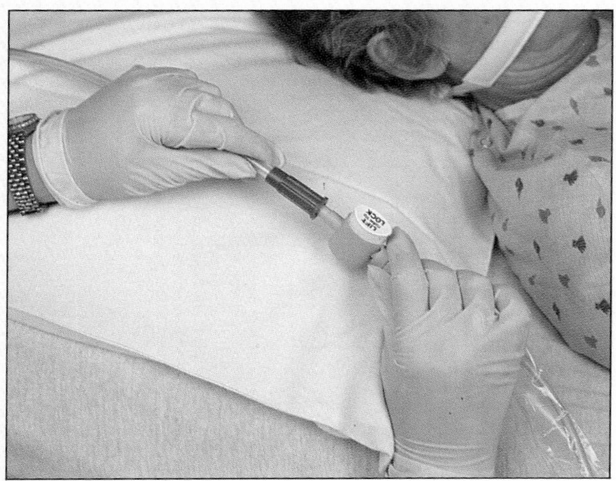

Now depress the thumb control valve.

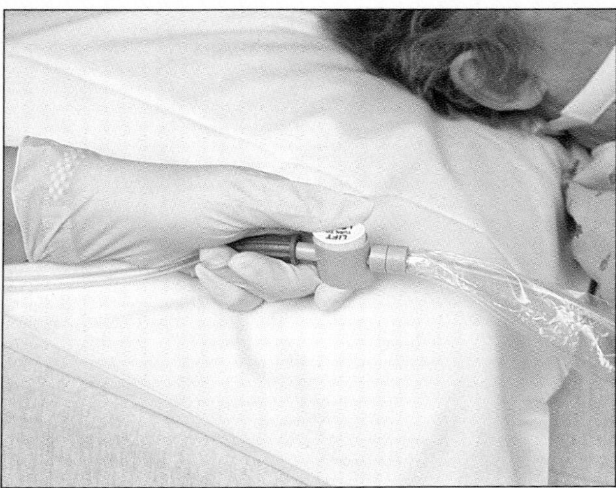

Keep the valve depressed while you set the suction to the desired level.

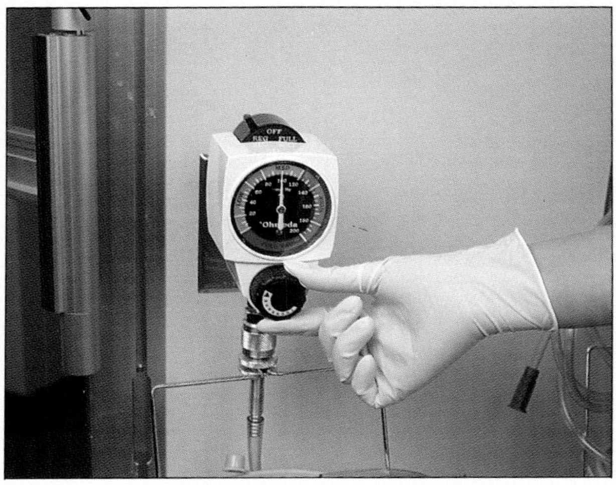

(continued)

Performing closed tracheal suctioning *(continued)*

Attach the T-piece to the ventilator circuit, using the flex tube between the circuit and the T-piece, if needed.

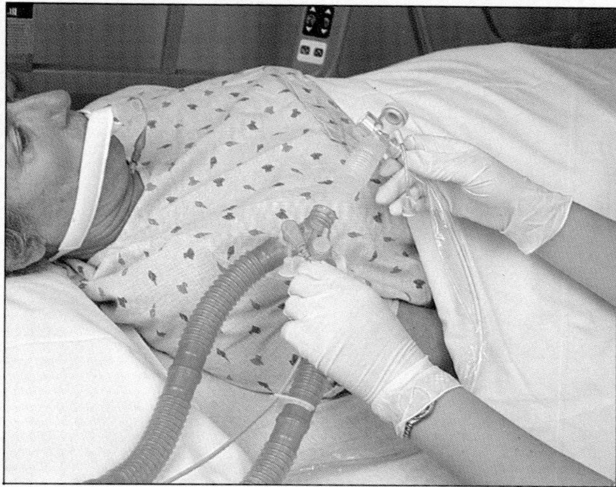

Make sure that the irrigation port is closed and in the up position.

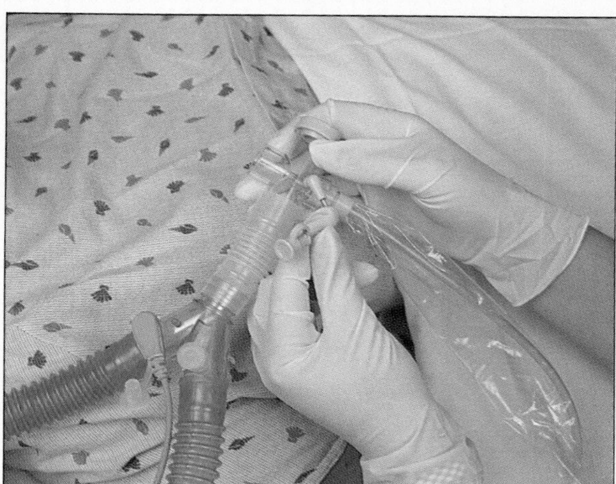

Attach the T-piece to the endotracheal tube, keeping a straight line between it and the suction catheter. The system is now ready for use.

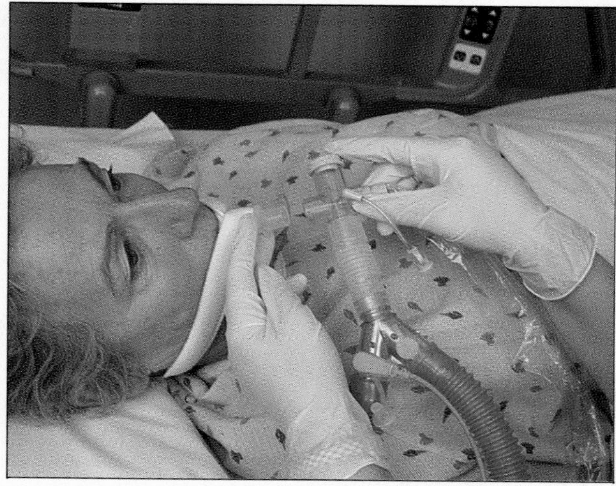

If the system has already been set up, attach the suction catheter to the suction tubing (if this was disconnected). Then turn the thumb piece on the control valve 180 degrees to the unlocked position.

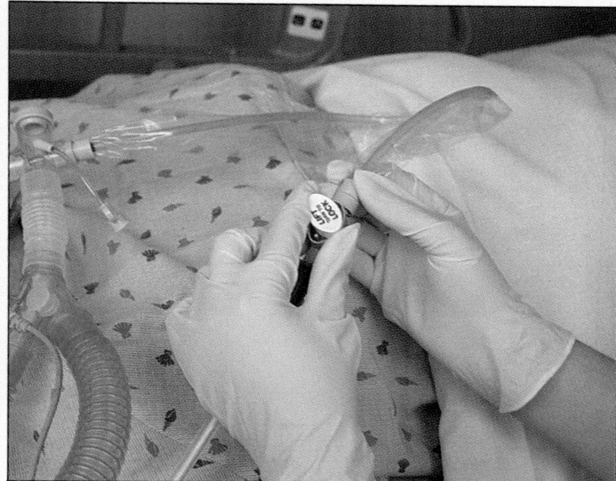

Performing closed tracheal suctioning *(continued)*

Because the patient will continue to receive oxygen during suctioning, you may not need to hyperoxygenate and hyperinflate his lungs. But if you need to do so, hyperoxygenate by either adjusting the FIO_2 to 100% or by pressing the 100% oxygen button. Allow 1 to 2 minutes for the oxygen to "wash" through the ventilator circuitry before you suction.

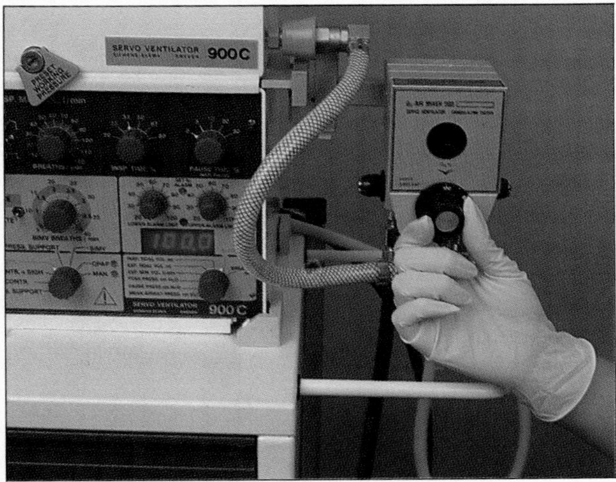

Holding the T-piece stable with one hand, advance the catheter 4" to 5" (10 to 13 cm) down the endotracheal tube with your other hand.

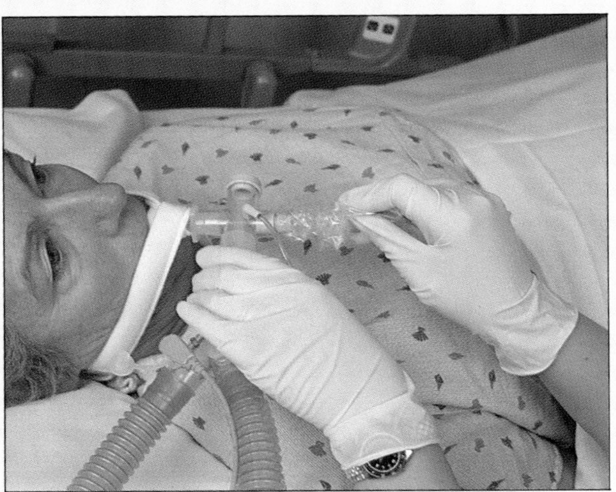

If you need to irrigate the tube, do so by instilling a few milliliters of preservative-free 0.9% sodium chloride solution through the irrigation port after the catheter has been advanced. Don't apply suction during this procedure.

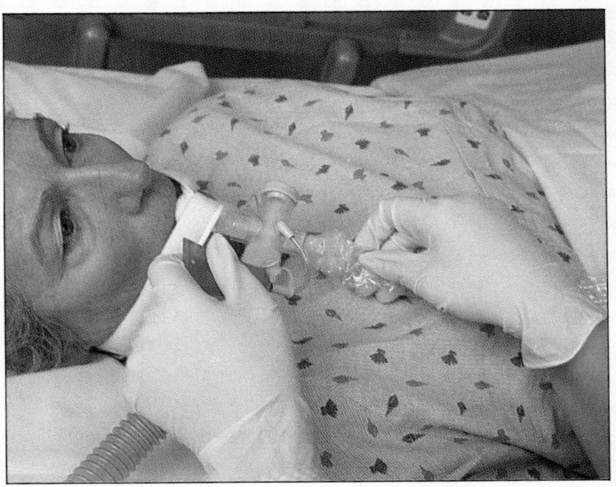

After advancing the catheter to the desired depth or when you feel resistance, withdraw it and apply suction by depressing the thumb control valve.

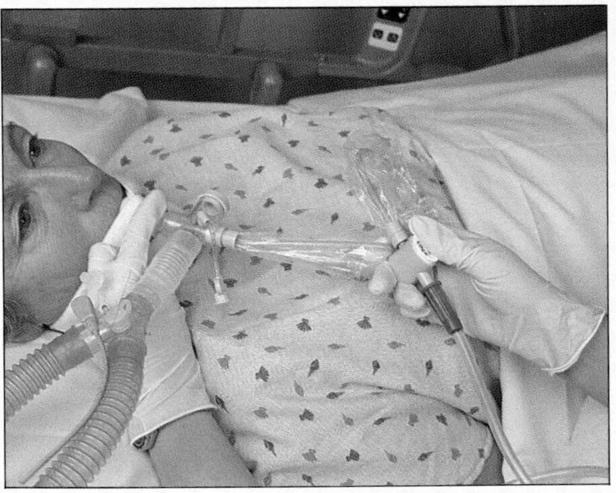

(continued)

Performing closed tracheal suctioning *(continued)*

Maintaining a grip on the T-piece, gently withdraw the catheter until the black mark on it is visible at the back of the T-piece. Never apply suction for more than 10 seconds.

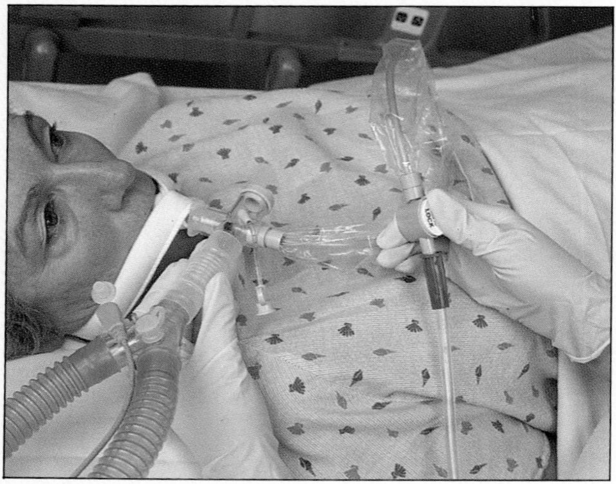

To clear the catheter after suctioning, depress the control valve. Then slowly instill the flush solution.

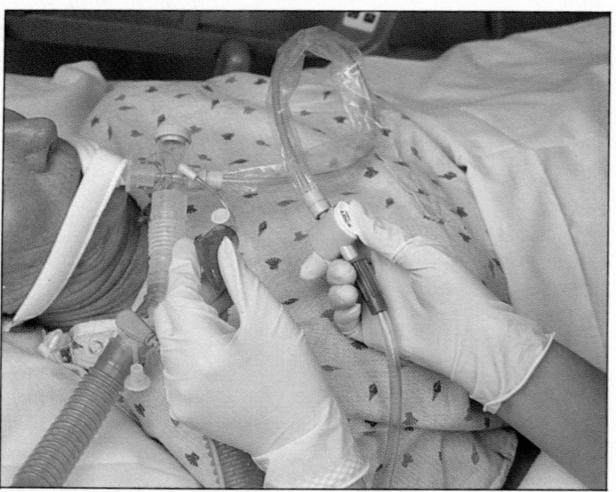

After clearing the catheter, lock it by lifting and turning the thumb piece on the control valve 180 degrees to the locked position.

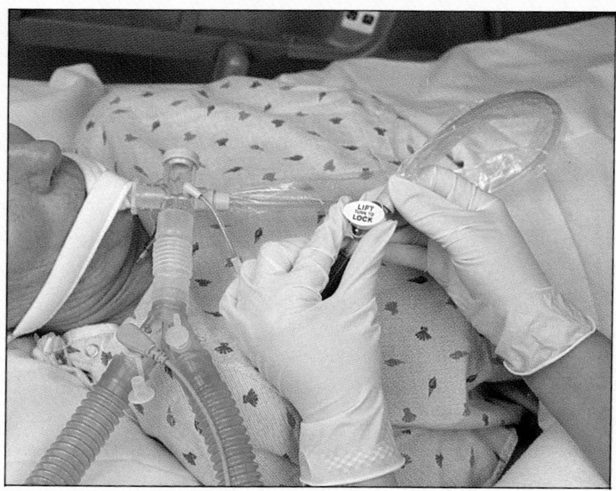

Finally, place the catheter and suction tubing alongside the ventilator tubing, or disconnect the catheter from the suction tubing.

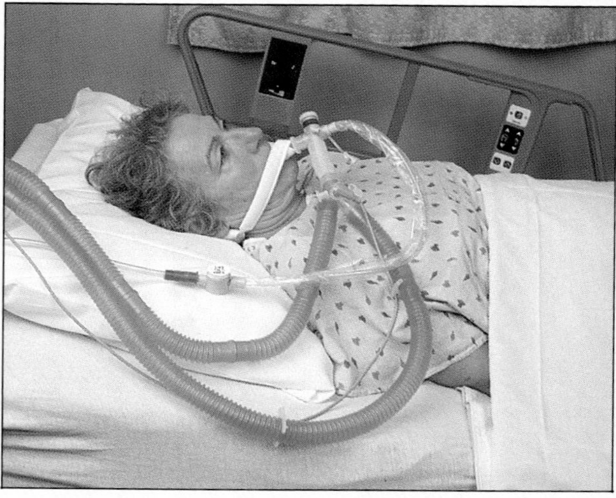

Indications

• Neuromuscular disorders, such as Guillain-Barré syndrome, myasthenia gravis, and poliomyelitis
• Central nervous system disorders or injuries, such as cerebral hemorrhage and spinal cord transection
• Respiratory disorders, such as ARDS, pulmonary edema, and COPD

Contraindications and complications

Mechanical ventilation has no contraindications.

Possible complications include tension pneumothorax, decreased cardiac output, oxygen toxicity, infection, fluid volume excess caused by humidification, and such GI complications as abdominal distention or bleeding from stress ulcers.

Equipment

Oxygen source • air source that can supply 50 psi • mechanical ventilator • humidifier • ventilator circuit tubing, connectors, and adapters • condensation collection trap • spirometer, respirometer, or electronic device to measure flow and volume • in-line thermometer • probe for gas sampling and measuring airway pressure • bacterial filter • gloves • hand-held resuscitation bag with reservoir • suction equipment • sterile distilled water • equipment for ABG analysis • soft restraints, if indicated • oximeter (optional)

Preparation

• Set up the ventilator, unless the respiratory therapist has already done so. If necessary, check the manufacturer's instructions for setting it up. In most cases, you'll need to add sterile distilled water to the humidifier and connect the ventilator to the appropriate gas source.
• Verify the doctor's order for ventilatory support. If the patient isn't already intubated, prepare him for intubation.
• Explain the procedure to the patient and his family to help reduce anxiety and fear. Assure them that staff members are nearby to provide care.

ADVANCED EQUIPMENT

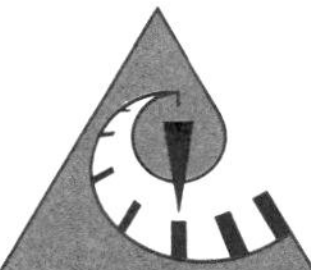

High-frequency jet ventilation

This technique was developed for use when high peak-airway pressures or large intrapleural air leaks preclude conventional mechanical ventilation. The high-frequency jet ventilation (HFJV) system employs a narrow injector cannula to deliver short, rapid bursts of oxygen to the airways under low pressure.

This combination of high rate, low tidal volumes, and low pressure enhances alveolar gas exchange without elevating peak inspiratory pressures and compromising cardiac output—the major drawback of conventional high-volume, high-pressure mechanical ventilation. Thus, HFJV is valuable for patients with hemodynamic instability and those at high risk for pulmonary barotrauma, such as young children. It's also useful for ventilating patients during bronchoscopy, laryngoscopy, and laryngeal surgery because its narrow cannula doesn't obstruct the operating field.

A potential new use of HFJV is in emergency respiratory situations. Because the cannula can be inserted directly into the trachea through a cricothyrotomy, HFJV may be used when upper airway trauma or obstruction precludes intubation. Use of HFJV in cardiopulmonary resuscitation allows continuous ventilation during chest compression. And its use in patients with chest trauma decreases chest wall movement and improves stability, enhancing ventilation.

• Perform a complete cardiopulmonary assessment, and draw blood for ABG analysis to establish a baseline.
• Suction the patient if necessary.

Essential steps

• Plug the ventilator into the electrical outlet and turn it on. Adjust the settings on the ventilator as ordered. Make sure that the ventilator's alarms are set as ordered and that the humidifier is filled with sterile distilled water.
• Put on gloves if you haven't already done so. Connect the endotracheal tube to the ventilator. Observe for chest expansion and auscultate

TROUBLESHOOTING

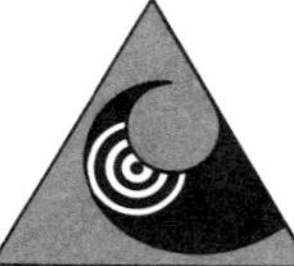

Responding to ventilator alarms

SIGNAL	POSSIBLE CAUSE	INTERVENTIONS
Low-pressure alarm	• Tube disconnected from ventilator	• Reconnect the tube to the ventilator.
	• Endotracheal tube displaced above vocal cords or tracheostomy tube extubated	• If displacement or extubation has occurred, ventilate the patient manually and call the doctor immediately.
	• Leaking tidal volume from low cuff pressure (from an underinflated or ruptured cuff or a leak in the cuff or one-way valve)	• Listen for a whooshing sound around the tube, indicating an air leak. If you hear one, check cuff pressure. If you can't maintain pressure, call the doctor; he may need to insert a new tube.
	• Ventilator malfunction	• Disconnect the patient from the ventilator, and ventilate him manually if necessary. Obtain another ventilator.
	• Leak in ventilator circuitry (from loose connection or hole in tubing, loss of temperature-sensitive device, or cracked humidification jar)	• Make sure that all connections are intact. Check for holes or leaks in the tubing and replace the tube if necessary. Check the humidification jar and replace it if it's cracked.
High-pressure alarm	• Increased airway pressure or decreased lung compliance caused by worsening disease	• Auscultate the lungs for evidence of increasing lung consolidation, barotrauma, or wheezing. Call the doctor if indicated.
	• Patient biting on oral endotracheal tube	• Insert a bite block if needed.
	• Secretions in airway	• Assess for secretions in the airway by auscultating for breath sounds. To remove secretions, suction the patient or have him cough.
	• Condensate in large-bore tubing	• Check tubing for condensate and remove any fluid.
	• Intubation of right mainstem bronchus	• Check tube position (by auscultating for bilateral breath sounds) and call the doctor if the tube has slipped; he may need to reposition it.
	• Patient coughing, gagging, or attempting to talk	• The doctor may order a sedative or a neuromuscular blocking agent if the patient fights the ventilator.
	• Chest wall resistance	• Reposition the patient if doing so improves chest expansion. If repositioning doesn't help, administer the prescribed analgesic.
	• Failure of high-pressure relief valve	• Have the faulty equipment replaced.
	• Bronchospasm	• Assess the patient for the cause. Report to the doctor and treat the patient as ordered.

for bilateral breath sounds to verify that the patient is being ventilated.

Cautions

Make sure that the ventilator alarms are on at all times. These alarms alert the nursing staff to potentially hazardous conditions and to changes in the patient's status. If an alarm sounds and the problem can't be identified easily, disconnect the patient from the ventilator and use a hand-held resuscitation bag to ventilate him. (See *Responding to ventilator alarms.*)

If the patient is receiving a neuromuscular blocking agent, make sure that he also receives a sedative. Neuromuscular blocking agents cause paralysis without altering the patient's level of consciousness. Reassure the patient and his family that the paralysis is temporary. Also make sure that emergency equipment is readily available in case the ventilator malfunctions or the patient is extubated accidentally. Continue to explain all procedures to the patient, and take extra steps to ensure the safety of a paralyzed patient, such as raising the bed rails during turning and covering and lubricating his eyes.

Monitoring and aftercare

• Monitor the patient's ABG values after the initial ventilator setup (usually 20 to 30 minutes), after any changes in ventilator settings, and as the patient's condition warrants, to determine whether the patient is being adequately ventilated and oxygenated. Be prepared to adjust the ventilator settings, depending on the results of the ABG analysis.
• Check the ventilator tubing frequently for condensation, which can cause resistance to airflow and which the patient could aspirate. Drain the condensate into a collection trap, or briefly disconnect the patient from the ventilator (ventilating him with a hand-held resuscitation bag if necessary) and empty the water into a receptacle. Don't drain the condensate into the humidifier because the condensate may be contaminated by the patient's secretions.
• Check the in-line thermometer to make sure that the temperature of the air delivered to the patient is close to body temperature.
• When monitoring the patient's vital signs, count spontaneous breaths as well as ventilator-delivered breaths.
• Change, clean, or dispose of the ventilator tubing and equipment according to the policy at your health care facility. Typically, ventilator tubing should be changed every 24 to 48 hours, sometimes more often.
• Provide emotional support to the patient during all phases of mechanical ventilation to reduce anxiety and promote successful treatment. Even if the patient is unresponsive, continue to explain all procedures and treatments to him, using a normal tone of voice. To lessen his anxiety, stop in frequently to see him and let him know when you'll return.
• Because intubation and mechanical ventilation impair the patient's ability to speak, you'll need to help him find another way of communicating, such as nodding his head, mouthing words, or writing.
• Unless contraindicated, turn the patient from side to side every 1 to 2 hours to facilitate lung expansion and removal of secretions. Perform active or passive range-of-motion (ROM) exercises for all extremities to reduce the hazards of immobility. If the patient's condition permits, position him upright at regular intervals to increase lung expansion.
• Assess the patient's peripheral circulation, and monitor his urine output for signs of decreased cardiac output. Watch for signs and symptoms of fluid volume excess or dehydration.
• Administer a sedative or neuromuscular blocking agent, as ordered, to relax the patient and prevent spontaneous breathing efforts, which can interfere with the ventilator's action. Remember that the patient receiving a neuromuscular blocking drug requires close observation because of his inability to breathe or communicate.
• Make sure that the patient gets adequate rest and sleep because fatigue can delay weaning from the ventilator. Provide subdued lighting, safely muffle equipment noises, and restrict staff access to the area to promote quiet during rest periods.
• Document the date and time that mechanical ventilation was begun. Note the type of ventilator used for the patient and its settings. Describe the patient's subjective and objective responses to mechanical ventilation (including vital signs, breath sounds, use of accessory muscles, intake and output, and weight). List any complications and subsequent interventions. Record all pertinent laboratory data, including ABG analysis results and oxygen saturation levels. If the patient was receiving pressure support ventilation or using a T-piece or tracheostomy collar, note the duration of spontaneous breathing and the patient's ability to maintain the weaning schedule. If the patient was receiving intermittent mandatory ventilation, with or without pressure support ventilation, record the control breath rate, the time of each breath reduction, and the rate of spontaneous respirations.
• If the patient will be discharged on a ventilator, evaluate the family's or caregiver's ability and motivation to provide the necessary home care. Well before discharge, develop a teaching

plan that will address the patient's needs. Teaching should include information about ventilator care and settings, artificial airway care, suctioning, respiratory therapy, communication, nutrition, therapeutic exercise, signs and symptoms of infection, and ways to troubleshoot minor equipment malfunctions.

• Evaluate the patient's need for adaptive equipment, such as a hospital bed, a wheelchair or walker with a ventilator tray, a patient lift, and a bedside commode. If the patient needs to travel, recommend appropriate portable equipment. At discharge, contact a durable medical equipment vendor and a home health nurse to follow up with the patient. Also, refer the patient to community resources, if available.

Weaning from the ventilator

To wean a patient from a mechanical ventilator, you'll first need to determine his readiness to breathe on his own. The patient's breathing must be sufficient to keep him ventilated, he must have a stable cardiovascular system, and he must have sufficient respiratory muscle strength and level of consciousness to sustain the breathing. You'll provide care to the patient and monitor his progress during the weaning period.

For the patient who has received mechanical ventilation for a long time, weaning can be accomplished by switching the ventilator to pressure support ventilation with or without intermittent mandatory ventilation. This way, each of the patient's spontaneous breaths is augmented by the ventilator. As the patient's own respirations improve, the intermittent mandatory ventilation and pressure support ventilation can be decreased.

For the patient who has received ventilation a short time, the T-piece method of weaning is used. The T-piece method weans the patient by progressively decreasing the frequency and tidal volume of the ventilated breaths.

Indications

• PaO_2 of at least 60 mm Hg (50 mm Hg or the ability to maintain baseline levels if the patient has chronic lung disease) or an FIO_2 at or below 40%
• Carbon dioxide (CO_2) of less than 40 mm Hg (or normal for the patient) or an FIO_2 of 40% or less if his partial pressure of carbon dioxide in arterial blood ($PaCO_2$) is 60 mm Hg or more
• Vital capacity of more than 10 ml/kg of body weight
• Maximum inspiratory pressure greater than −20 cm H_2O.
• Minute ventilation under 10 liters/minute with a respiratory frequency of less than 28 breaths/minute
• Forced expiratory volume in the first second of more than 10 ml/kg of body weight
• Ability to double spontaneous resting minute ventilation
• Adequate natural airway or a functioning tracheostomy that allows the patient to cough and mobilize secretions
• Successful withdrawal of any neuromuscular blocking agent, such as pancuronium
• Clear or clearing chest X-ray
• Absence of infection, acid-base or electrolyte imbalance, hyperglycemia, arrhythmias, renal failure, anemia, fever, or excessive fatigue

Contraindications and complications

Weaning is contraindicated in any patient who doesn't meet the three basic criteria for weaning: spontaneous respiratory effort, a stable cardiovascular system, and sufficient respiratory muscle strength and level of consciousness to sustain the breathing.

In addition, failed weaning attempts can result in psychological setbacks. Physical complications include respiratory muscle fatigue, respiratory alkalosis, and possibly respiratory arrest.

Equipment

Stethoscope • respirometer • maximum-inspiratory-pressure manometer for assessment • aerosol adapter with T-piece • pulse oximeter

Preparation

• Plan to start the weaning process in the morning when the patient is well rested.
• Explain the weaning procedure to the patient and his family.
• Assess the patient's breath sounds and suction if necessary. Obtain baseline pulse oximeter readings or a baseline ABG analysis.

Essential steps

• Disconnect the patient from the ventilator, and place him on heated aerosol via a T-piece or tracheal collar for 5 to 10 minutes.
• Watch the patient for signs of fatigue; monitor his pulse oximeter and cardiac monitor readings for arrhythmias.
• Place the patient back on the ventilator for the remainder of the hour.
• Repeat the procedure the next hour, gradually increasing the time off the ventilator, until the patient can tolerate being off of the ventilator totally.
• Be prepared to place him back on the ventilator if he shows signs of fatigue.
• Consider placing the patient back on the ventilator at night to conserve his energy and to ensure adequate rest.

Cautions

A decreased tidal volume, an increased respiratory rate, and some decrease in PaO_2 and increase in $PaCO_2$ are expected while weaning. But return the patient to mechanical ventilation if he displays signs or symptoms of distress or respiratory muscle fatigue. Help the patient avoid other activities that will cause fatigue during the weaning process. (See *When to stop weaning a patient.*)

Don't remove the ventilator from the immediate area until the patient's stability is established.

Monitoring and aftercare

• Take the patient's vital signs every 5 to 10 minutes for 30 minutes, every 30 minutes for 1 hour, and then every 1 to 2 hours during the weaning process and after extubation.
• Suction the patient as needed.
• Don't leave the patient unattended during the weaning process.

When to stop weaning a patient

Discontinue weaning and return the patient to the ventilator if you detect any of these signs:
• blood pressure increase of more than 20 mm Hg systolic or more than 10 mm Hg diastolic
• heart rate increase of more than 20 beats/minute or a rate above 120 beats/minute
• respiratory rate increase of more than 10 breaths/minute or a rate above 30 breaths/minute
• arrhythmias
• reduced tidal volume
• elevated $PaCO_2$
• anxiety
• dyspnea
• accessory muscle use or deteriorating breathing pattern.

• Help the patient avoid panicking during weaning by encouraging him to breathe in a regular pattern. Try using a metronome, which can be set at different rates. The regular ticking may calm the patient and allow him to focus on slower, fuller breathing.

Continuous positive airway pressure

A spontaneously breathing patient may receive continuous positive airway pressure (CPAP), during which he exhales against the positive pressure. With CPAP, the functional residual capacity in the lungs increases and collapsed alveoli are distended. CPAP can be administered with or without an artificial airway, but the patient must be able to breathe on his own.

In the past, a patient receiving CPAP needed to be intubated and placed on a mechanical ventilator with a CPAP mode. Now the patient wears a tightly fitting CPAP mask that delivers pressure to the airway. CPAP can also be delivered through a nasal mask or cannula. Widely used in critical care units, CPAP therapy is being used more often for patients in medical-surgical units also. And home care patients can use nasal CPAP to treat sleep apnea.

You'll need to monitor the patient on CPAP carefully, assessing his respiratory status regularly. If at any time he can't breathe spontaneously, he'll require intubation. He'll also need cardiac assessment. Because the positive airway pressure can cause an increase in intrathoracic pressure, the venous return to the heart decreases, as does cardiac output. If the patient can't compensate for this decrease in cardiac output, oxygenation will worsen.

Indications

- Pulmonary edema
- Pneumonia (viral and aspiration)
- Atelectasis
- Sleep apnea

Contraindications and complications

CPAP is contraindicated in patients who can't breathe on their own and in patients with hypotension due to hypovolemia, shock, or decreased cardiac output. The positive pressure may exacerbate the decrease in blood pressure.

CPAP is also contraindicated in patients with disorders affecting only one lung and in patients with chest trauma, such as pulmonary contusion, pneumothorax, or fractured ribs.

The tight fit of the mask may cause anxiety in some patients.

Other complications include barotrauma from the increased pressure and gastric distention. If the patient vomits while wearing a CPAP mask, he's at risk for aspirating the vomitus. The CPAP mask can also cause hypoventilation from overdistention of the lung.

Equipment

Delivery apparatus (mask or nasal cannula in the appropriate size for the patient) • oxygen source • flow generator to regulate oxygen flow • humidification system • straps to ensure a tight fit (straps come with the mask, but extra straps may be indicated)

Preparation

- Thoroughly explain CPAP to the patient before applying the mask. Make sure he understands that the mask fits very tightly and may be slightly uncomfortable. Tell the patient that anxiety and claustrophobia are common reactions. If he experiences these reactions, give him reassurances, such as telling him you'll stay with him, open the curtains, and turn on the light.
- Obtain a baseline respiratory assessment and ABG analysis so that you'll be able to assess the therapy's effectiveness.
- Make sure that you have the necessary equipment, and prepare it for setup (unless your facility's respiratory therapy department has already set it up).

Essential steps

- Attach the flow generator to the oxygen outlet and the air entrainment port to the flow generator. Set the dial to the desired pressure. Next, attach the humidification system to the flow generator and tubing.
- Turn on the generator and adjust the FIO_2 dial to provide the desired flow. If necessary, use an oxygen analyzer to determine the correct setting.
- Attach the oxygen tubing to the inlet valve of the mask or nasal cannula.
- If ordered, attach a PEEP valve and dial in the ordered amount of PEEP. (The addition of PEEP helps to increase the area of gas exchange at the end of expiration.)
- Apply the mask or nasal cannula. (See *Positioning a CPAP mask.*)

Cautions

Because a patient on CPAP may experience a decrease in cardiac output, you should regularly measure his heart rate and blood pressure during therapy. Make sure that he has an adequate intake and output. If his blood pressure drops, position him with his head below his heart, and contact the doctor if blood pressure continues to drop.

Because of the risk of tension pneumothorax, assess the patient's respiratory status regularly. If you note an increase in respiratory rate, asymmetrical chest expansion, and absent breath sounds on one side, let the doctor know immediately. Other signs include cyanosis, tachycardia, tachypnea, tracheal deviation away from the affected side, hypoxia, and distended neck veins.

Call the doctor if you suspect CO_2 retention. To monitor the patient for hypoventilation, continually assess his respiratory effort and ABG levels.

Monitoring and aftercare

• Check the mask or nasal cannula regularly for a tight seal. Any leak in the system can cause the system to lose positive pressure. Because the mask fits so snugly, providing frequent skin care to the patient is important. Assess the patient's face regularly for signs of redness or skin breakdown.
• Watch the patient for signs of gastric distention. To gauge distention, assess the patient's abdomen at the beginning of therapy and then every 2 to 4 hours during therapy. If the patient shows signs of gastric distention, he may need a nasogastric tube.
• Monitor the patient for any acute changes in heart rate and blood pressure that may be caused by the positive pressure.
• Monitor the patient's respiratory status, including respiratory rate, respiratory effort, oxygen saturation levels (by pulse oximetry), ABG levels, and breath sounds. If the patient's condition worsens, or if he becomes fatigued and has a decrease in respiratory drive, he may need intubation and mechanical ventilation.
• Monitor the CPAP circuit for adequate delivery of pressure. If you detect a decrease in positive pressure, check all connections and ensure a tight seal. If the drop in pressure continues, contact the respiratory care department or the doctor.
• Provide continual reassurance. If the patient becomes anxious, you may need to administer a mild sedative.
• Prepare the patient for CPAP therapy at home, if indicated.
• Once CPAP therapy is discontinued, continue to assess the patient for complications that may occur with positive-pressure ventilation. Continue to monitor the patient's respiratory status.

Positioning a CPAP mask

When applying a CPAP mask, position one strap behind the patient's head and the other strap over his head. The fit should be snug but not too tight.

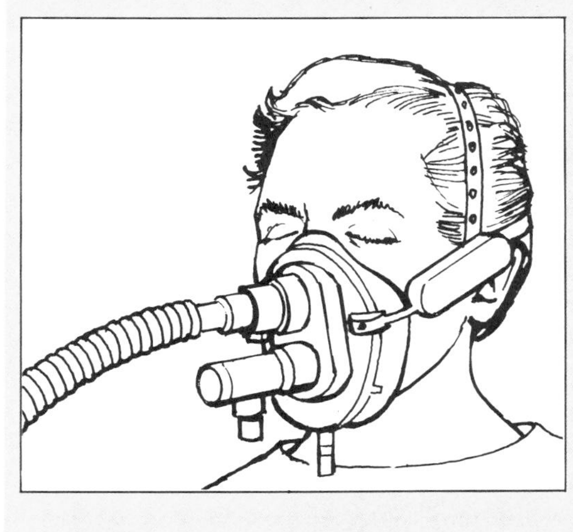

Thoracentesis

This procedure involves the aspiration of fluid or air from the pleural space. Thoracentesis relieves pulmonary compression and respiratory distress by removing accumulated air or fluid that results from injury or such conditions as tuberculosis or cancer. It also provides a specimen of pleural fluid or tissue for analysis and allows instillation of chemotherapeutic agents or other medications into the pleural space. Emergency thoracentesis may be necessary for life-threatening tension pneumothorax. (See *Performing needle thoracentesis,* page 114.)

Indications

• Pleural effusion (caused by malignancy, nephrotic syndrome, tuberculosis, tumor, or lymphatic disorders)
• Pneumothorax resulting from trauma or lung disease

Performing needle thoracentesis

For a patient with life-threatening tension pneumothorax, needle thoracentesis temporarily relieves pleural pressure until a doctor can insert a chest tube.

How needle thoracentesis works

A needle attached to a flutter valve is inserted into the affected pleural space (see inset). Trapped air escapes through the flutter valve when the patient exhales, instead of being retained under pressure. A flutter valve consists of a length of rubber tubing with one end flattened. This valve allows air and fluid to leave the pleural space but prevents them from reentering. A plastic cylinder encasing the valve protects it from compression or occlusion; if the cylinder breaks, the flutter valve will still work.

How to perform the procedure

Clean the skin around the second intercostal space at the midclavicular line with povidone-iodine solution. Use a circular motion, starting at the center and working outward.

Insert a sterile 16G (or larger) needle over the superior portion of the rib and through the tissue covering the pleural cavity. The vein, artery, and nerve lie behind the rib's inferior border. Listen for a hissing sound; this signals the needle's entry into the pleural cavity.

Attach the flutter valve securely to the needle. Make sure that the connection is airtight; then tape it to prevent dislodgment. The arrow on the valve indicates the direction of airflow.

You may leave the distal end open if only air is being evacuated. But this can compromise sterility, so you should connect the distal end to a drainage bag—especially when draining blood. A sterile glove works nicely as an emergency drainage bag. Just be sure to vent the glove (or bag) so that air leaving the chest doesn't become trapped.

Leave the needle in place until a chest tube can be inserted.

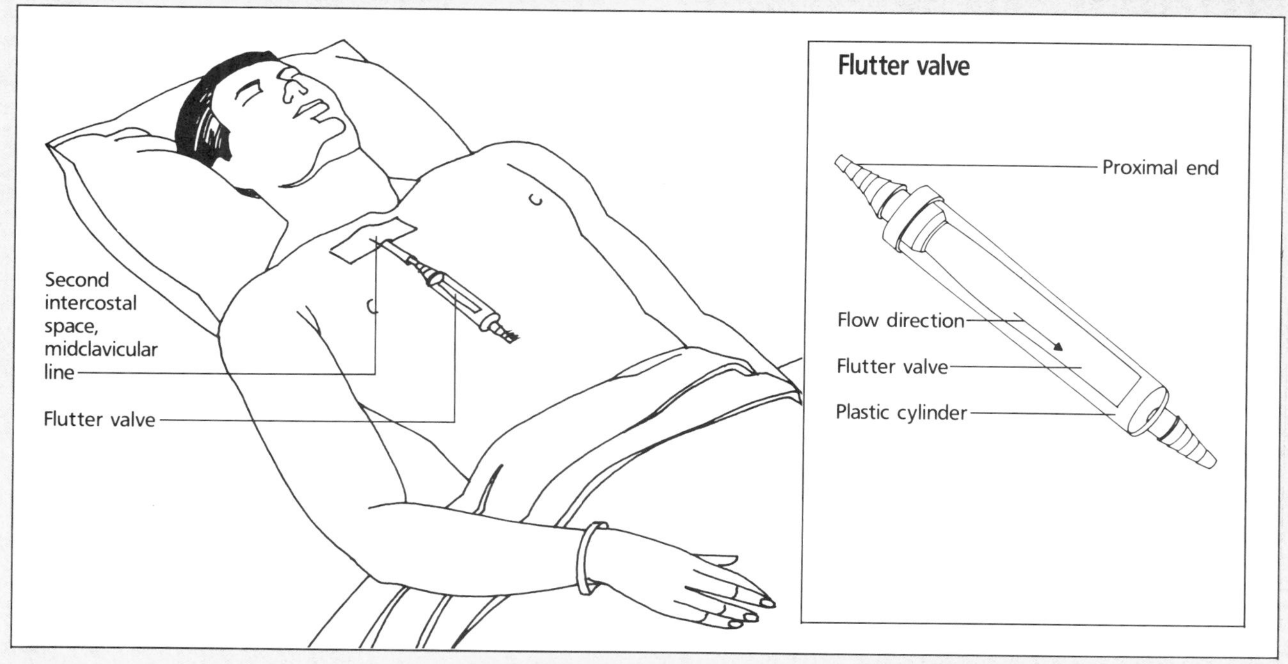

Contraindications and complications

Thoracentesis is contraindicated in patients with bleeding disorders.

Pneumothorax (possibly leading to mediastinal shift and requiring chest tube insertion) can occur if the needle punctures the lung and allows air to enter the pleural cavity. Pleuritic or shoulder pain may indicate pleural irritation by the needle point. Pyogenic infection can result from contamination during the procedure. Other potential complications include pain, coughing, anxiety, dry taps, and subcutaneous hematoma.

Equipment

Most hospitals use a prepackaged thoracentesis tray including sterile gloves • sterile drapes • 70% isopropyl alcohol or povidone-iodine solution • 1% or 2% lidocaine • 5-ml syringe with 21G and 25G needles for anesthetic injection • 17G thoracentesis needle for aspiration • 50-ml syringe • three-way stopcock and tubing • sterile specimen containers • sterile hemostat • sterile 4″ × 4″ gauze pads.

You'll also need the following: adhesive tape • sphygmomanometer • gloves • stethoscope • laboratory request slips • optional: drainage bottles (if the doctor expects a large amount of drainage), Teflon catheter, shaving supplies, biopsy needle, prescribed sedative with 3-ml syringe and 21G needle.

Preparation

- Assemble all equipment at the patient's bedside or in the treatment area. Check the expiration date on each sterile package and inspect it for tears.
- Prepare the necessary laboratory request form. Be sure to list current antibiotic therapy on the laboratory forms because this will be considered in analyzing the specimens.
- Make sure that the patient has signed an appropriate consent form. Note any drug allergies, especially to the local anesthetic. Have the patient's chest X-rays available.
- Explain the procedure to the patient. Tell him that he may feel some discomfort and a sensation of pressure during the needle insertion. Provide privacy and emotional support.
- Wash your hands.

Essential steps

- Administer the prescribed sedative, as ordered.
- Obtain baseline vital signs and assess respiratory function.
- Position the patient. Make sure that he's firmly supported and comfortable. Although the choice of position varies, you'll usually seat the patient on the edge of the bed with his legs supported and his head and folded arms resting on a pillow on the overbed table. Or you can have him straddle a chair backward and rest his head and folded arms on the back of the chair. If the patient can't sit, turn him on the unaffected side with the arm of the affected side raised above his head. Elevate the head of the bed 30 to 45 degrees if such elevation isn't contraindicated. Proper positioning stretches the chest or back and allows easier access to the intercostal spaces.
- Remind the patient not to cough, breathe deeply, or move suddenly during the procedure to avoid puncture of the visceral pleura or lung. If he coughs, the doctor will briefly stop the procedure and withdraw the needle slightly to prevent lung puncture.
- Expose the patient's entire chest or back.
- Shave the aspiration site if necessary.
- Wash your hands again before touching the sterile equipment. Then, using sterile technique, open the thoracentesis tray and assist the doctor as necessary in disinfecting the site.
- If an ampule of local anesthetic is not included in the sterile tray and a multidose vial of local anesthetic is to be used, wipe the rubber stopper with an alcohol sponge and hold the inverted vial while the doctor withdraws the anesthetic solution.
- After draping the patient and injecting the local anesthetic, the doctor attaches a three-way stopcock with tubing to the aspirating needle and turns the stopcock to prevent air from entering the pleural space through the needle.
- Attach the other end of the tubing to the drainage bottle.
- The doctor then inserts the needle into the pleural space and attaches a 50-ml syringe to the needle's stopcock.
- Check the patient's vital signs and the dressing for drainage every 15 minutes for 1 hour.

Then continue to assess his vital signs and respiratory status once every 2 hours.
• Put on gloves and assist the doctor as necessary in specimen collection, fluid drainage, and dressing the site.
• After the doctor withdraws the needle or catheter, apply pressure to the puncture site, using a sterile 4″ × 4″ gauze pad. Then apply a new sterile gauze pad, and secure it with tape.
• Label the specimens properly, and send them to the laboratory.

Cautions

To prevent postthoracentesis pulmonary edema and hypovolemic shock, fluid is removed slowly and no more than 1,000 ml of fluid is removed during the first 30 minutes. Removing the fluid increases the negative intrapleural pressure, which can lead to edema if the lung doesn't reexpand to fill the space.

Monitoring and aftercare

• Assess the patient's vital signs and respiratory status as warranted by his condition.
• Continually observe him for signs and symptoms of distress, such as pallor, vertigo, faintness, weak and rapid pulse, decreased blood pressure, dyspnea, tachypnea, diaphoresis, chest pain, blood-tinged mucus, and excessive coughing.
• Discard disposable equipment. Clean nondisposable items and return them for sterilization.
• A chest X-ray is usually ordered after the procedure to detect pneumothorax and evaluate the results of the procedure.
• Record the date and time of thoracentesis; location of the puncture site; volume and description (color, viscosity, odor) of the fluid withdrawn; specimens sent to the laboratory; vital signs and respiratory status before, during, and after the procedure; any postprocedural tests, such as chest X-ray; any complications and subsequent interventions; and the patient's reaction to the procedure.

Chest tube insertion

When a patient experiences a partial or total lung collapse, chest tube insertion allows the air or fluid to drain from the pleural space. This sterile procedure is usually performed by a doctor, with a nurse assisting him.

For pneumothorax, the second intercostal space is the most common site for chest tube insertion because air rises to the top of the intrapleural space. For hemothorax or pleural effusion, the sixth to eighth intercostal spaces are the most common sites because fluid settles at the lower levels of the intrapleural space. For removal of air and fluid, a chest tube is inserted into a high and a low site. After insertion, one or more chest tubes are connected to a thoracic drainage system that removes air, fluid, or both from the pleural space and prevents backflow, thus promoting lung reexpansion.

Indications

• Hemothorax (usually caused by trauma)
• Pneumothorax (spontaneous, or caused by trauma or lung disease)
• Pleural effusion (caused by malignancy or infection)

Contraindications and complications

Chest tube insertion has no contraindications.

The major complication is tension pneumothorax caused by an obstructed or dislodged tube.

Equipment

Two pairs of sterile gloves • sterile drape • povidone-iodine solution • vial of 1% lidocaine • 10-ml syringe • alcohol sponge • 22G 1″ needle • 25G ⅝″ needle • sterile scalpel (usually with #11 blade) • sterile forceps • two rubber-tipped clamps for each chest tube inserted • sterile 4″ × 4″ gauze pads • two sterile 4″ × 4″ drain dressings (gauze pads with slit) • 3″ or 4″ sturdy elastic tape • 1″ adhesive tape for connections • chest tube of appropriate size (#16 to #20 French catheter for air or serous fluid; #28 to #40 French catheter for blood, pus, or thick fluid), with or without a trocar • sterile Kelly clamp • suture material (usually 2-0 silk with cutting needle) • thoracic drainage system • sterile drainage tubing, 6′ (2 m) long, and connector • sterile Y-connector (for two chest tubes, same side)

Preparation

• Check the expiration date and integrity of the sterile packages. Make sure that the patient has signed the appropriate consent form. Then assemble all equipment in the patient's room, and set up the thoracic drainage system. Place it next to the patient's bed below chest level to facilitate drainage.

• Explain the procedure to the patient.

• After washing your hands, record baseline vital signs and respiratory status.

• Position the patient appropriately. (See *Positions for chest tube insertion,* page 118.)

Essential steps

• Place the chest tube tray on the overbed table. Open it, using sterile technique.

• The doctor puts on sterile gloves and prepares the insertion site by cleaning the area with povidone-iodine solution.

• Wipe the stopper of the lidocaine vial with an alcohol sponge. Invert the bottle and hold it for the doctor to withdraw the anesthetic.

• After the doctor anesthetizes the site, he makes a small incision and inserts the chest tube. Then he either immediately connects the chest tube to the thoracic drainage system or momentarily clamps the tube close to the patient's chest until he can connect it to the drainage system. He may then secure the tube to the skin with a suture.

• Open the packages containing the 4″ × 4″ drain dressings and gauze pads, and put on sterile gloves. If the doctor orders it, apply antimicrobial ointment to the insertion site. Then place two 4″ × 4″ drain dressings around the insertion site, one from the top and the other from the bottom. Place several 4″ × 4″ gauze pads on top of the drain dressings. Tape the dressings, covering them completely.

• Tape the chest tube to the patient's chest distal to the insertion site to help prevent accidental dislodgment of the tube.

• Tape the junction of the chest tube and the drainage tube to prevent their separation.

• Coil the drainage tube and secure it to the bed sheet with tape and a safety pin, providing enough slack for the patient to move; this measure also prevents accidental dislodgment of the chest tube.

• Immediately after the drainage system is connected, instruct the patient to take a deep breath, hold it momentarily, and slowly exhale to assist drainage of the pleural space and lung reexpansion.

• After the procedure, a chest X-ray is taken (by a portable unit) to check tube position.

Cautions

If the patient's chest tube comes out, immediately cover the site with petroleum gauze or 4″ × 4″ gauze pads and tape them in place. Stay with the patient and monitor his vital signs every 10 minutes. Watch for signs of tension pneumothorax (hypotension, distended neck veins, absent breath sounds, tracheal shift, hypoxemia, weak and rapid pulse, dyspnea, tachypnea, diaphoresis, and chest pain).

Place the rubber-tipped clamps at the bedside. If a drainage bottle breaks, a thoracic drainage system cracks, or a tube disconnects, clamp the chest tube momentarily as close to the insertion site as possible. Observe the patient closely for signs of tension pneumothorax while the clamp is in place.

Wrap a piece of petroleum gauze around the tube at the insertion site to make an airtight seal. Clamp the tube with large, smooth, rubber-tipped clamps for several hours before removal, and observe the patient for signs of respiratory distress.

Monitoring and aftercare

• Take the patient's vital signs every 15 minutes for 1 hour, then as often as his condition warrants. Auscultate his lungs at least every 4 hours after the procedure to assess air exchange in the affected lung. Diminished or absent breath sounds indicate that the lung hasn't reexpanded.

• Record the date and time of chest tube insertion, the insertion site, the drainage system used, the presence of drainage and bubbling, vital signs and auscultation findings, and any complications and subsequent interventions.

Positions for chest tube insertion

If the patient has a pneumothorax, place him in high Fowler's, semi-Fowler's, or the supine position. The doctor inserts the tube in the anterior chest at the midclavicular line in the second to third intercostal space.

Semi-Fowler's position

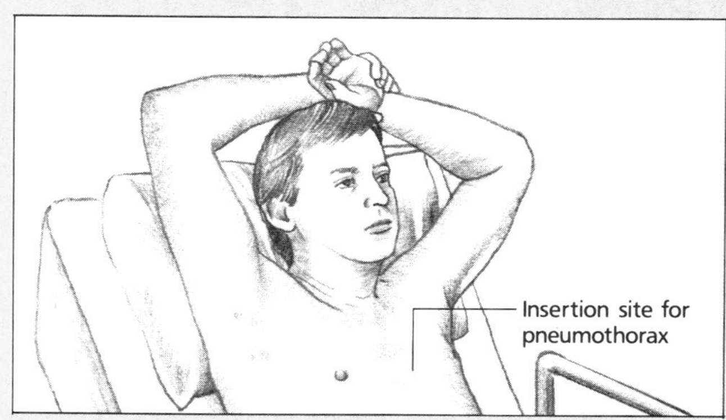

If the patient has a hemothorax, have him lean over the overbed table or straddle a chair with his arms dangling over the back. The tube is inserted in the fourth to sixth intercostal space at the midaxillary line.

Leaning forward

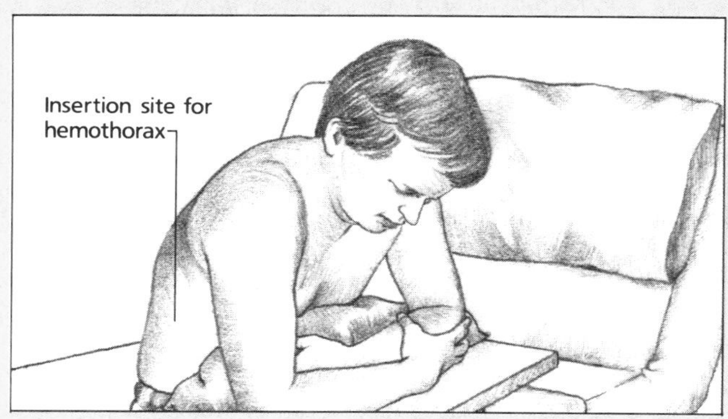

For either a pneumothorax or a hemothorax, the patient may lie on his unaffected side with his arms extended over his head.

If the patient has had a thoracotomy, the doctor usually will insert one or two chest tubes during surgery (typically a basilar tube and an apical tube). The patient will be positioned on his unaffected side with his arms elevated.

Lying on side

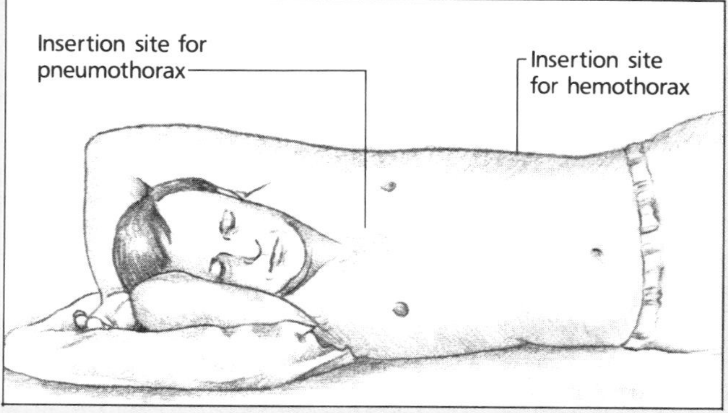

• Assist the doctor in chest tube removal. A chest tube is usually removed within 7 days of insertion to prevent infection.
• Administer an analgesic, as ordered, 30 minutes before the removal. The patient may feel a burning sensation, pain, pulling, or pressure.
• Place the patient in semi-Fowler's position or on his unaffected side. After putting a linen-saver pad under his affected side, put on clean gloves and remove the dressings. Don't dislodge the chest tube.
• The doctor holds the chest tube in place with sterile forceps and cuts the suture anchoring the tube. Make sure that the chest tube is clamped securely, and tell the patient to perform Valsalva's maneuver to increase intrathoracic pressure.
• Immediately after removing the tube, the doctor covers the insertion site with an airtight dressing. Cover the dressing completely with tape so that it's as airtight as possible.
• After properly disposing of the chest tube, soiled gloves, and other equipment, take the patient's vital signs. Assess the depth and quality of his respirations, and watch him carefully for signs and symptoms of pneumothorax, subcutaneous emphysema, or infection.

Thoracic drainage

Because negative pressure in the pleural cavity exerts a suction force that keeps the lungs expanded, any chest trauma that upsets this pressure may cause lung collapse. Consequently, one or more chest tubes may be surgically inserted and then connected to a thoracic drainage system. This system uses gravity and sometimes suction to restore negative pressure and remove any material that collects in the pleural cavity.

An underwater seal in the drainage system allows air and fluid to escape from the pleural cavity but doesn't allow air to reenter. The system may include one, two, or three bottles to collect drainage, create a water seal, and control suction, or it may be a self-contained, disposable system. The procedure here details use of a disposable system.

Thoracic drainage may be ordered to remove accumulated air, fluids (blood, pus, chyle, serous fluids, gastric juices), or solids (blood clots) from the pleural cavity; to restore negative pressure in the pleural cavity; or to reexpand a partially or totally collapsed lung.

Indications

• Pneumothorax
• Hemothorax
• Pleural effusion
• Empyema

Contraindications and complications

Thoracic drainage has no contraindications.

Tension pneumothorax may result from excessive accumulation of air or drainage, and eventually may exert pressure on the heart and aorta, causing a precipitous fall in cardiac output.

Equipment

Thoracic drainage system (Pleur-evac, Argyle, Ohio, or Thora-Klex system) • 1 liter sterile distilled water • adhesive tape • sterile clear plastic tubing • bottle or system rack • two rubber-tipped Kelly clamps • sterile 50-ml catheter-tip syringe • suction source (if ordered)

Preparation

• Explain the procedure to the patient, and wash your hands.
• Check the doctor's order for the type of drainage system and for specific procedural details. Collect the equipment, and take it to the patient's bedside.

Essential steps

• Open the packaged system, and place it on the floor in the manufacturer's rack. You may hang it from the side of the patient's bed.
• Remove the plastic connector from the short tube that's attached to the water-seal chamber. Using a 50-ml catheter-tip syringe, instill sterile distilled water into the water-seal chamber until it reaches the 2-cm mark or the mark specified by the manufacturer. Then replace the plastic connector.

• If suction is ordered, remove the cap (also called the *muffler* or *atmosphere vent cover*) on the suction-control chamber to open the vent. Next, instill sterile distilled water until it reaches the 20-cm mark or the ordered level, and recap the suction-control chamber. Using the long tube, connect the patient's chest tube to the closed drainage collection chamber. Secure the connection with tape.
• Connect the short tube on the drainage system to the suction source, and turn on the suction. Gentle bubbling should begin in the suction-control chamber, indicating that the correct suction level has been reached.

Cautions

Maintain sterile technique throughout the procedure and whenever you make changes in the system or alter any of the connections.

Be sure to keep two rubber-tipped clamps at the patient's bedside. You'll use these to clamp the chest tube if a bottle breaks, if the commercially prepared system cracks, or if you need to locate an air leak in the system.

When clots are visible, you may be able to strip (or milk) the tubing, depending on your hospital's policy. Stripping is a controversial procedure because it creates high negative pressure that could suck viable lung tissue into the drainage ports of the tube, resulting in ruptured alveoli and a pleural air leak. Strip the tubing only when clots are visible. Use an alcohol sponge or lotion as a lubricant on the tube, and pinch it between your thumb and index finger about 2″ (5 cm) from the insertion site. Using the other thumb and index finger, compress the tubing as you slide your fingers down the tube or use a mechanical stripper. Release the thumb and index finger, pinching near the insertion site.

If excessive continuous bubbling is present in the water-seal chamber, rule out a leak in the drainage system (especially if suction is being used). Try to locate the leak by clamping the tube briefly at various points. Work down toward the drainage system, paying special attention to the seal around the connections. If any connection is loose, push it back together and tape it securely. The bubbling will stop when a clamp is placed between the air leak and the water seal. If you clamp along the tube's entire length and the bubbling doesn't stop, the drainage unit may be cracked.

If the commercially prepared drainage collection chamber fills, replace it. To do this, double-clamp the tube close to the insertion site (using two clamps facing in opposite directions), exchange the system, remove the clamps, and retape the bottle connection. Never leave the tubes clamped for more than a minute or two to prevent a tension pneumothorax, which can occur when clamping stops air and fluid from escaping.

If the commercially prepared system cracks, clamp the chest tube momentarily with the two rubber-tipped clamps you placed at the bedside. Place the clamps close to each other near the insertion site; they should face in opposite directions to provide a more complete seal. Observe the patient for altered respirations while the tube is clamped. Then replace the damaged equipment. (Prepare the new unit before clamping the tube.)

Instead of clamping the tube, you can submerge the distal end of the tube in a container of 0.9% sodium chloride solution to create a temporary water seal while you replace the bottle. Check your hospital's policy.

Monitoring and aftercare

• Repeatedly note the character, consistency, and amount of drainage in the drainage collection chamber.
• Mark the drainage level in the drainage collection chamber by noting the time and date at the drainage level every 8 hours (or more often if there is a large amount of drainage).
• Check the water level in the water-seal chamber every 8 hours. If necessary, carefully add sterile distilled water until the level reaches the 2-cm mark indicated on the water-seal chamber of the commercial system.
• Check for fluctuation in the water-seal chamber as the patient breathes. Normal fluctuations of 2″ to 4″ (5 to 10 cm) reflect pressure changes in the pleural space during respiration. To check for fluctuation when a suction system is being used, momentarily disconnect the suction system so that the air vent is opened.

- Check for intermittent bubbling in the water-seal chamber. This occurs normally when the system is removing air from the pleural cavity. If bubbling isn't readily apparent during quiet breathing, have the patient take a deep breath or cough. The absence of bubbling indicates that the pleural space has sealed.
- Check the water level in the suction-control chamber. Detach the chamber or bottle from the suction source; when bubbling stops, observe the water level. If necessary, add sterile distilled water as ordered.
- Check for gentle bubbling in the suction-control chamber, which indicates that the proper suction level has been reached. Vigorous bubbling in this chamber increases the rate of water evaporation.
- Periodically check that the air vent in the system is working properly.
- Coil the system's tubing, and secure it to the edge of the bed with a rubber band or tape and a safety pin. Avoid creating dependent loops, kinks, or pressure on the tubing and lifting the drainage system above the patient's chest level because fluid may flow back into the pleural space.
- Encourage the patient to cough frequently and breathe deeply to help drain the pleural space and reexpand the lungs.
- Instruct him to sit upright for optimal lung expansion and to splint the insertion site while coughing to minimize pain.
- Check the rate and quality of the patient's respirations, and auscultate his lungs periodically to assess air exchange in the affected lung. Diminished or absent breath sounds may indicate that the lung hasn't reexpanded.
- Notify the doctor immediately if the patient develops cyanosis, rapid or shallow breathing, subcutaneous emphysema, chest pain, or excessive bleeding.
- Check the chest tube dressing at least every 8 hours. Palpate the area surrounding the dressing for crepitus or subcutaneous emphysema, which indicates that air is leaking into the subcutaneous tissue surrounding the insertion site. Change the dressing if necessary or according to your hospital's policy.
- Encourage active or passive ROM exercises for the patient's arm on the affected side if he has been splinting the arm. Usually, the thoracotomy patient will splint his arm to decrease his discomfort.
- Give ordered pain medication as needed for comfort and to help with deep breathing, coughing, and ROM exercises.
- Remind the ambulatory patient to keep the drainage system below chest level and to be careful not to disconnect the tubing, to maintain the water seal.
- Instruct staff members and visitors to avoid touching the equipment to prevent complications from separated connections.
- Record the date and time thoracic drainage began, the type of system used, the amount of suction applied to the pleural cavity, the presence or absence of bubbling or fluctuation in the water-seal chamber, the initial amount and type of drainage, and the patient's respiratory status. At the end of each shift, record the frequency of system inspection; how frequently chest tubes were milked or stripped; the amount, color, and consistency of drainage; the presence or absence of bubbling or fluctuation in the water-seal chamber; the patient's respiratory status; the condition of the chest dressings; any pain medication you gave; and any complications and subsequent interventions.

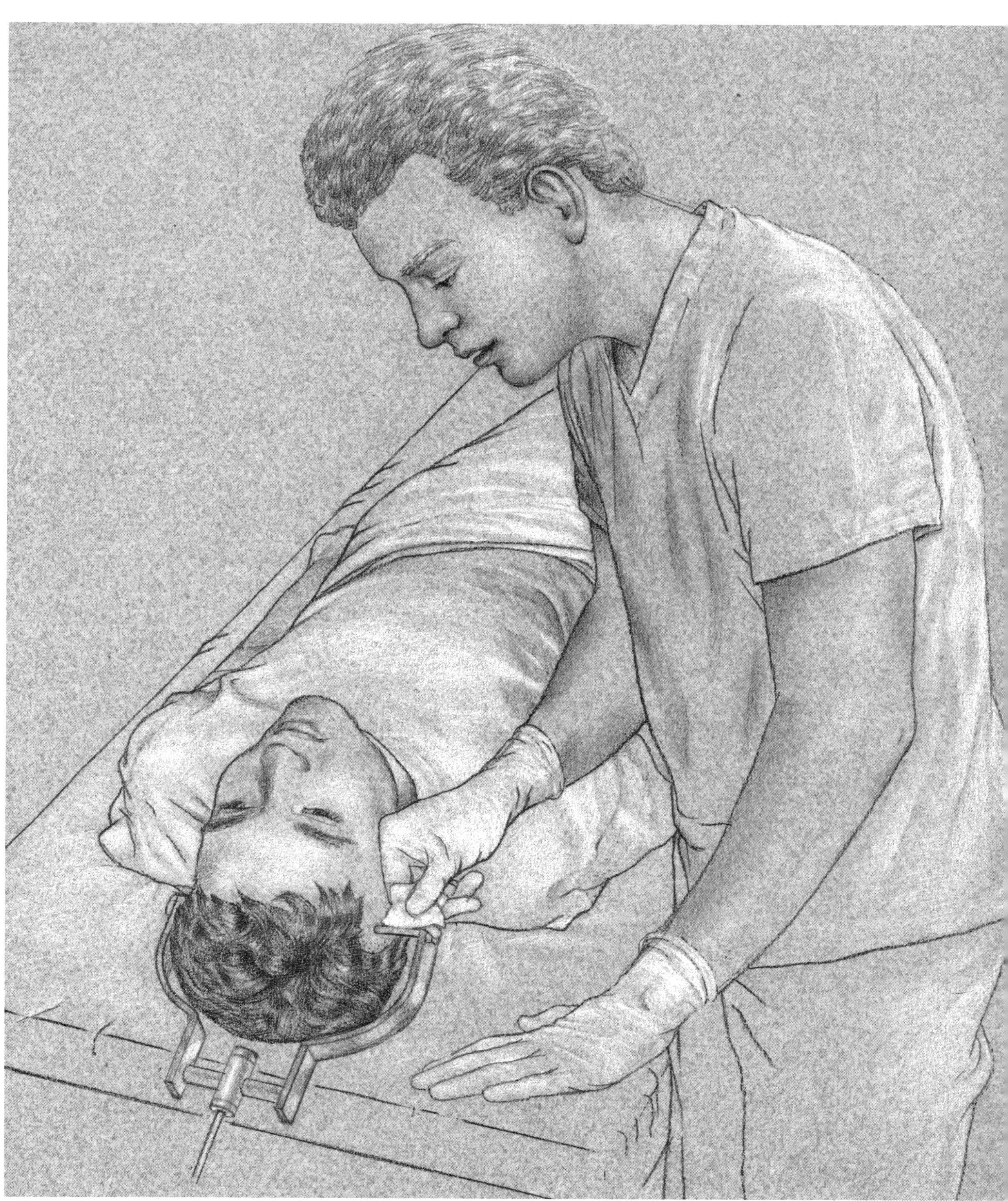

CHAPTER 4

Neurologic and musculoskeletal procedures

The neurologic and musculoskeletal systems control and coordinate the functions of all other body systems. When catastrophic illness or injury strikes them, restoration and preservation of function become the chief goals of nursing care. To achieve these goals, you'll need to master a plethora of sophisticated procedures, such as the latest techniques for intracranial pressure monitoring.

In this chapter, you'll find up-to-date instruction on such key procedures as cerebrospinal fluid drainage, care of skull tongs, mechanical traction, and continuous passive motion.

CSF drainage

Cerebrospinal fluid (CSF) drainage aims to manage increased intracranial pressure (ICP) and to promote spinal or cerebral dural healing after a traumatic injury or surgery. The drain may withdraw fluid from the lateral ventricle (ventriculostomy) or the lumbar subarachnoid space. Ventricular drainage is used to reduce increased ICP, whereas lumbar subarachnoid drainage aids healing of the dura mater.

In either case, a catheter or ventriculostomy tube drains CSF in a sterile, closed collection system. To place a ventricular drain, the doctor inserts a ventricular catheter through a burr hole in the patient's skull and dural lining. Usually, this procedure takes place in the operating room, with the patient under general anesthesia. In an emergency, however, it may be done at the patient's bedside. To place a lumbar subarachnoid drain, the doctor may administer a local spinal anesthetic at the bedside or in the operating room before suturing the drain in place or merely taping it externally. (See *CSF drainage techniques.*)

Your responsibilities include assessing the patency of the drain, regulating CSF output according to doctor's orders, and monitoring the patient's status and response to treatment. To manage a CSF drain, you must maintain strict sterile technique and be thoroughly familiar with the signs of increasing ICP.

Indications

- To monitor ICP
- To instill drugs or contrast media directly into the subarachnoid space
- To aspirate CSF for laboratory analysis

Contraindications and complications

There are no contraindications. However, CSF drainage may cause such complications as excessive drainage of CSF, clots in the catheter or ventriculostomy tube, increased ICP, and infection.

Signs and symptoms of excessive CSF drainage include headache, tachycardia, diaphoresis, and nausea. Acute overdrainage may result in collapsed ventricles, tonsillar herniation, and medullary compression. Cessation of drainage, in contrast, may indicate clot formation and occlusion of the catheter, and cause signs of increased ICP. If your patient has a lumbar drain to aid dural wound healing, blockage may cause CSF leakage in the wound area.

Infection may lead to meningitis. (See *Hazards of CSF drainage,* page 126.)

Equipment

Overbed table • sterile gloves • sterile cotton-tipped applicators • povidone-iodine solution • alcohol sponges • sterile fenestrated drape • 3-ml syringe for local anesthetic • 25G ¾" needle for injecting anesthetic • local anesthetic (usually 1% lidocaine) • 18G or 20G sterile spinal needle or Tuohy needle • #5 French whistle-tip catheter or ventriculostomy tube • external drainage set (includes drainage tubing and sterile collection bag) • suture material • 4" × 4" dressings • Kerlix or Kling gauze for head dressing • sterile towel to cover pillowcase • paper tape or a connector • lamp or other light source • I.V. pole • ventriculostomy tray with twist drill • pain medication • anti-infective agent

Preparation

- Explain the procedure to the patient and his family.
- Make sure the patient or a responsible family member has signed a consent form, and document this according to your hospital's guidelines.
- Open all equipment, using sterile technique. Check all packaging for breaks in seals and for expiration dates.
- Connect the catheter to the external drainage system tubing.
- Secure connection points with paper tape or a connector.
- Place the collection system, including drip chamber and collection bag, on an I.V. pole.

Essential steps

- Wash your hands thoroughly.
- Perform a baseline neurologic assessment, including vital signs, to help detect changes or signs of deterioration.

Insertion of a ventricular drain

- Place the patient in the supine position. Put a sterile towel over the pillowcase.

CSF drainage techniques

Cerebrospinal fluid (CSF) drainage aims to control intracranial pressure (ICP) during treatment for a traumatic injury or other conditions that cause ICP to rise. In the two procedures commonly used, a catheter is connected to the closed drainage system, as shown below.

Ventricular drain

The doctor inserts a catheter through a burr hole in the patient's skull and dural lining, into the ventricle. The distal end of the catheter is connected to a closed drainage system.

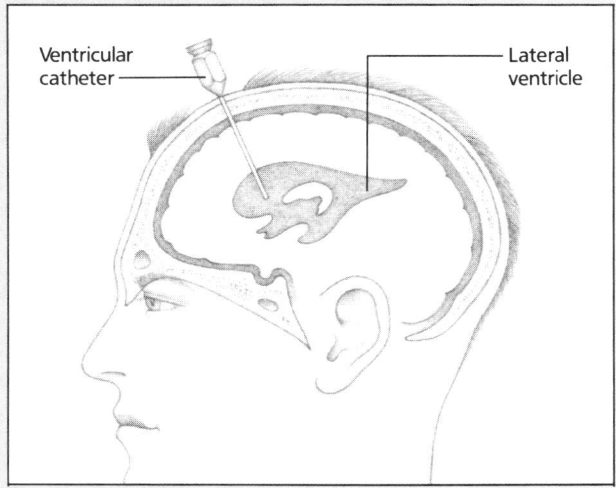

Lumbar subarachnoid drain

The doctor inserts a catheter beneath the dura into the L3-L4 interspace. The distal end of the catheter is connected to a closed drainage system.

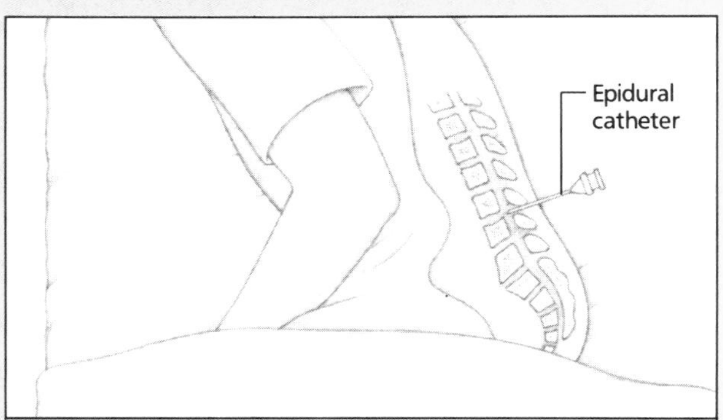

Closed drainage system

The catheter leads from the drain to a sterile, closed drainage system affixed securely to the bed or an I.V. pole. Make sure that you set the drip chamber at the level ordered by the doctor.

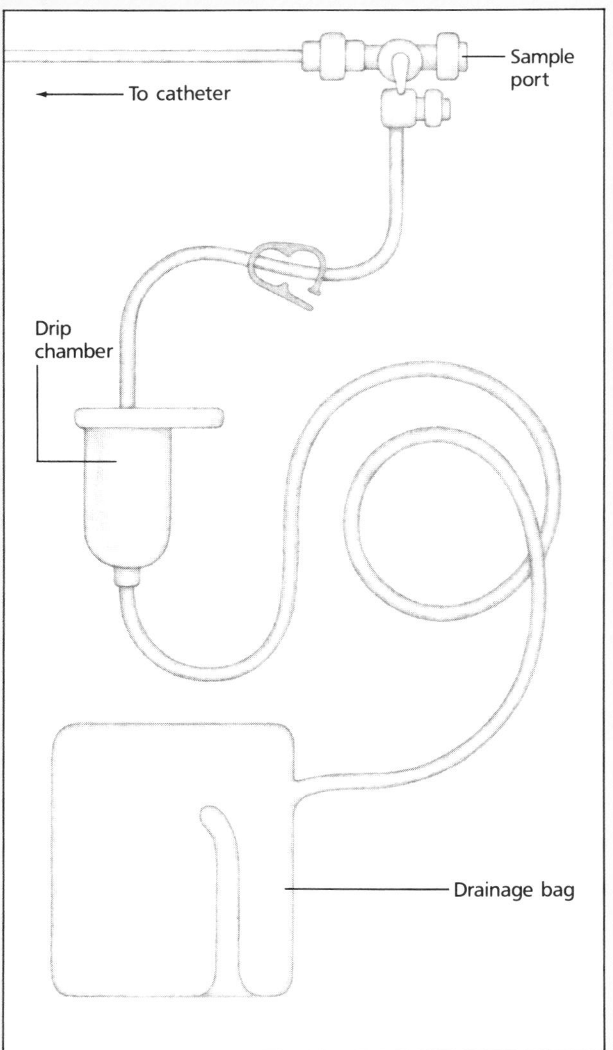

COMPLICATIONS

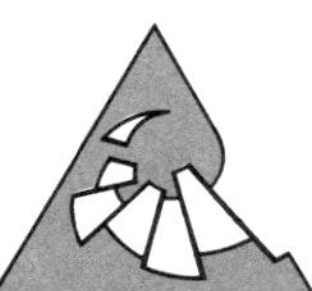

Hazards of CSF drainage

Supportive care for a patient undergoing cerebrospinal fluid (CSF) drainage involves careful monitoring for early signs of two life-threatening complications: infection and brain herniation. Here's what to look for, as well as ways to manage or help prevent these complications.

Infection

Both ventricular catheters and subarachnoid screws carry a high risk of infection, such as meningitis and ventriculitis. So stay alert for signs of infection – redness and warmth around the insertion site, fever, and drainage from the wound. Call the doctor if any of these signs occur. Also notify the doctor if your patient has an elevated white blood cell count, which also signals infection.

To help prevent infection, maintain strict asepsis around the equipment and insertion site. When changing dressings, use aseptic technique. Teach the patient that this area must remain clean at all times, and warn him never to touch or manipulate the equipment or insertion site.

Brain herniation

In brain herniation, brain structures are displaced. This leads to increased intracranial pressure (ICP) and eventually compresses the brain stem, causing death. Herniation typically results from improper positioning of the drain or from a sudden drop in ICP caused by excessive drainage.

Because increasing ICP may herald herniation, you must monitor your patient carefully for the often subtle early signs of increased ICP: altered level of consciousness, increased restlessness, personality changes, and disorganized motor behavior (such as repetitive pulling at the gown); headache; visual disturbances; and vital sign changes, such as widened pulse pressure and irregular or decreased respiratory rate.

• Set the equipment tray on the overbed table and unwrap it.
• Adjust the patient's bed height so the doctor can perform the procedure comfortably. Illuminate the site where the catheter will be inserted.
• Put on sterile gloves.
• The doctor then cleans the insertion site with povidine-iodine solution using sterile cotton-tipped applicators. He puts a sterile fenestrated drape in place, exposing only the insertion site. He then administers a local anesthetic. To insert the drain, he requests the ventriculostomy tray with a twist drill. After completing the ventriculostomy, he connects the drainage system.

Insertion of a lumbar subarachnoid drain
• Position the patient on his side, with his chin tucked into his chest and knees drawn up to his abdomen, as for a lumbar puncture.
• Instruct the patient to remain as still as possible during the procedure to minimize discomfort and traumatic injury.
• To insert the drain, the doctor attaches a Tuohy needle (or spinal needle) to the whistle-tip catheter. The needle guides the catheter into the subarachnoid space.
• After the doctor removes the needle, he connects the drainage system and sutures or tapes the catheter securely in place. The insertion site can be dressed using an anti-infective agent and 4″ × 4″ dressings or Kerlix or Kling gauze.

Cautions

If drainage accumulates rapidly, clamp the system and notify the doctor immediately. If drainage ceases and you can't quickly correct the cause of the obstruction, notify the doctor.

To prevent overdrainage or underdrainage, maintain a continuous hourly CSF output. Underdrainage or lack of CSF may result from kinked tubing, catheter displacement or occlusion, or a drip chamber placed higher than the catheter insertion site. Overdrainage can occur if the drip chamber is placed too far below the catheter insertion site. Raising or lowering the head of the bed can affect the CSF flow rate. When changing the patient's position, you must reposition the drip chamber as well.

During continuous CSF drainage, your patient may have a chronic headache. Reassure him that this isn't unusual, and administer analgesics as ordered.

Monitoring and aftercare

- To maintain CSF outflow, keep the drip chamber slightly below or at the level of the lumbar drain insertion site. In some cases, you may need to raise or lower the drip chamber carefully to increase or decrease CSF flow. If your patient has a ventricular drain to treat increased ICP, set the drip chamber higher than the foramen of Monro, approximately at the level of the canthus of the eye or 1" (2.5 cm) above the patient's ear.
- When measuring ICP, attach the transducer to an I.V. pole to allow a wide range of patient movement. Keep the transducer at a level 1" above the patient's ear. Be sure to recalibrate the system after repositioning the patient.
- Adjust the level of the drainage bag according to the doctor's orders.
- After draining and calibrating the system, check the position of the stopcocks.
- Observe your patient's ICP waveforms for possible damping, which may indicate that the system is losing patency.
- Assess the dressing frequently for drainage, which could indicate CSF leakage.
- Check the tubing for patency by watching CSF drops in the drip chamber.
- Observe CSF for color, clarity, amount, blood, and sediment. Obtain CSF specimens for laboratory analysis from the collection port attached to the tubing, not from the collection bag.
- Assess the tubing for kinks or areas of compression to ensure a flow of fluid.
- Change the collection bag when full or every 24 hours, according to your hospital's policy.
- Document the time and date of the drain insertion and your patient's response. Record vital signs and neurologic assessment findings every 4 hours.
- Document the color, clarity, and amount of CSF at least every 8 hours. Record hourly and 24-hour CSF outputs. Also describe the appearance of the dressing.

Care of skull tongs

Used to apply skeletal traction, skull tongs immobilize the cervical spine after injury or an invasive procedure. Three types of skull tongs are commonly used: Crutchfield, Gardner-Wells, and Vinke. (See *Types of skull tongs,* page 128.)

The doctor applies Crutchfield tongs by incising the skin with a scalpel, drilling holes in the exposed skull, and inserting the pins on the tongs into the holes. He applies Gardner-Wells and Vinke tongs less invasively. With Gardner-Wells tongs, for instance, he gently advances spring-loaded pins attached to the tongs into the patient's skull. After tightening the tongs to secure the apparatus, he creates traction by extending a rope from the center of the tongs over a pulley and attaching weights to it.

When caring for a patient with skull tongs, you must provide meticulous care of the pin sites and observe the traction apparatus frequently to make sure it's working properly. Be aware that home care and patient teaching can prove crucial to your patient's adjustment to the apparatus and the accompanying restrictions.

Indications

Skull tongs are used to stabilize the cervical spine after a fracture or dislocation, invasion by tumor or infection, or surgery.

Contraindications and complications

There are no contraindications. However, infection, excessive tractive force, or osteoporosis can cause skull pins to slip or pull out.

Equipment

Three medicine cups • one bottle each of ordered cleaning solution, 0.9% sodium chloride solution, and povidone-iodine solution • sterile cotton-tipped applicators • sandbags or hard cervical collar • fine-mesh gauze strips • 4" × 4" gauze pads • sterile gloves • sterile basin • sterile scissors • hair clippers • optional: turning frame, antibacterial ointment

ADVANCED EQUIPMENT

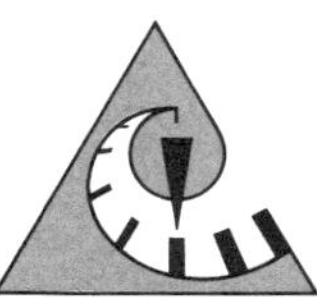

Types of skull tongs

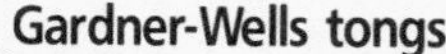

Skull (or cervical) tongs consist of a stainless steel body with a pin at the end of each arm. Each pin is about 1⁄8″ (0.3 cm) in diameter, with a sharp tip.

Crutchfield tongs
Pins are placed about 5″ (13 cm) apart, in line with the long axis of the cervical spine.

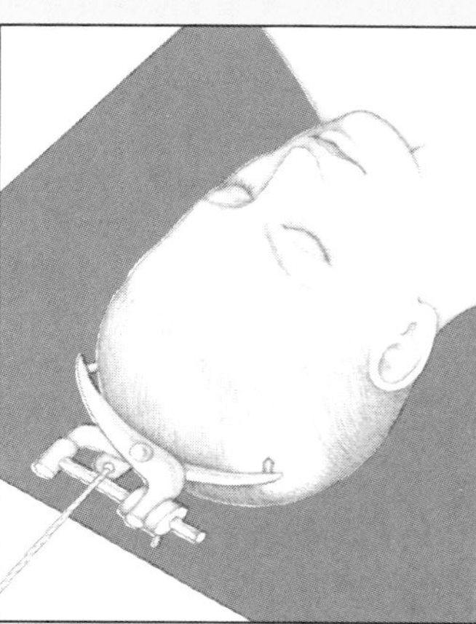

Gardner-Wells tongs
Pins are farther apart. They're inserted slightly above the patient's ears.

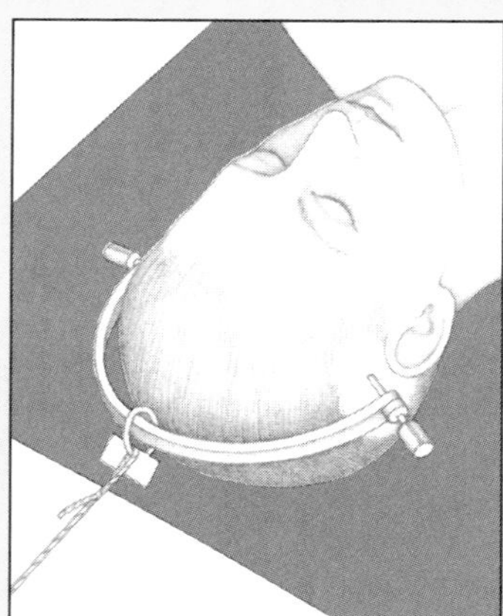

Vinke tongs
Pins are placed at the parietal bones, near the widest transverse diameter of the skull, about 1″ (2.5 cm) above the helix.

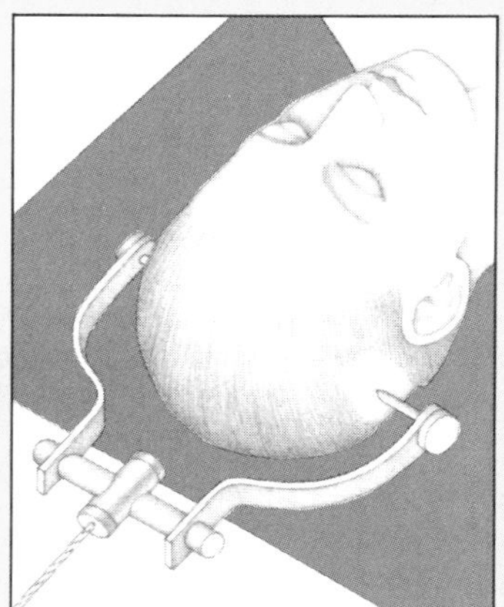

Preparation

- Explain the procedure to the patient, allowing time for him to ask questions.
- Bring the equipment to the room. Wash your hands.
- Place the medicine cups on the bedside stand. Fill one cup with 0.9% sodium chloride solution and another with povidone-iodine solution.
- Unwrap the sterile cotton-tipped applicators.
- Keep the sandbags or hard cervical collar on hand in case of emergency.

Essential steps

- Tell the patient that the pin sites will probably be tender for several days after tong application. Mention that he'll also feel some muscle discomfort in the injured area.
- Observe each pin site carefully for signs of infection before providing care. Note any loose pins, swelling, redness, or purulent drainage. When necessary to ensure proper assessment and care, use hair clippers to trim the patient's hair around the pin site.
- Put on sterile gloves; then gently wipe each pin site with a cotton-tipped applicator dipped in cleaning solution to loosen and remove crusty drainage. Begin at the pin site and work out from the area. Repeat the procedure, using a fresh applicator to ensure thorough cleaning and to avoid cross-contamination.
- Wipe each pin site with an applicator dipped in 0.9% sodium chloride solution to remove excess cleaning solution.
- Next, wipe each pin site with a povidone-iodine applicator to prevent infection.
- Discard all pin-site cleaning materials.

Care of infected pin sites

- Apply a povidone-iodine wrap as ordered, using fine-mesh gauze strips or 4" × 4" gauze pads cut into strips.
- Soak the strips in a sterile basin of povidone-iodine solution or 0.9% sodium chloride solution; then squeeze out the excess solution.
- Wrap one strip securely around each pin site. Leave the strip in place to dry until you provide care again. (Removing the dried strips aids debridement and helps clear the infection.)

Cautions

Before cleaning pin sites, make sure your patient isn't allergic to povidone-iodine solution. Avoid digging into the pin sites with the applicator because this will cause further tissue injury.

If you suspect a pin has loosened or slipped, don't turn the patient until the doctor examines the skull tongs and fixes them as needed. If the pins pull out, immobilize the patient's head and neck with sandbags or apply a hard cervical collar. Then carefully remove the traction weights. Apply manual traction to the patient's head by placing your hands on each side of the mandible and pulling very gently while maintaining proper alignment. After you've stabilized the alignment, have someone send for the doctor immediately. Remain calm and reassure the patient. Once traction is reestablished, take your patient's neurologic vital signs.

Monitoring and aftercare

- Check the traction apparatus at the start of each shift, then as necessary (for example, after the patient changes position). Make sure the rope hangs freely and the weights never rest on the floor or become caught under the bed.
- Monitor your patient for signs and symptoms of a loose pin, such as persistent pain, redness, or drainage at the pin site. Also suspect a loose pin if the patient reports hearing or feeling the pin move.
- Take vital signs at the start of each shift, then as necessary (for example, after turning or transporting the patient).
- Assess cranial nerve function, which may be impaired by pin placement. Note any asymmetry, deviation, or atrophy.
- Monitor the patient's respirations closely. Note any signs of respiratory distress, such as unequal chest expansion and an irregular or altered respiratory rate or pattern. Keep suction equipment handy.
- To promote turning without disrupting vertebral alignment, place the patient on a turning frame. Establish a turning schedule to help prevent complications of immobility.
- Document the date, time, and type of pin-site care and the patient's response to the procedure. Note any signs or symptoms of infection. Record the patient's vital signs and neurologic status.

Mechanical traction

Mechanical traction exerts a pulling force on a part of the body—usually the spine, pelvis, or the long bones of the arms and legs. It may be applied directly to the skin or indirectly to the bones. The doctor orders skin traction if the patient needs light, temporary, or noncontinuous traction. Skeletal traction requires placement of a pin or wire through a bone, which attaches to the traction device for a direct, constant longitudinal pull.

Nursing responsibilities include setting up the basic or Balkan traction frame, maintaining proper traction, preventing complications of immobility, and (with skeletal traction) monitoring pin sites.

Indications

- To reduce fractures
- To treat dislocations
- To correct deformities
- To improve or correct contractures
- To decrease muscle spasms

Contraindications and complications

Skin traction is contraindicated in patients who have severe injuries with open wounds, circulatory disturbances, dermatitis, varicose veins, or an allergy to tape or other skin traction equipment. Skeletal traction is contraindicated in patients with osteomyelitis.

Immobility during traction may result in pressure ulcers, muscle atrophy, weakness, or contractures. It may also cause GI disturbances, urinary problems (such as stasis), respiratory problems (such as hypostatic pneumonia), and circulatory problems (including blood pooling and thrombophlebitis).

Equipment

Selection of equipment varies according to the frame, but you'll always need a trapeze with clamp and a wall bumper or roller.

Claw-type basic frame

102″ (259-cm) horizontal plain bar • two 66″ (168-cm) vertical swivel-clamp bars • two upper-panel clamps • two lower-panel clamps

I.V.-type basic frame

102″ horizontal plain bar • 27″ (69-cm) vertical double-clamp bar • two 36″ (91-cm) horizontal plain bars • 48″ (122-cm) swivel-clamp bar • four 4″ (10-cm) I.V. posts with clamps • cross clamp

I.V.-type Balkan frame

Two 102″ horizontal plain bars • two 27″ vertical double-clamp bars • five 36″ horizontal plain bars • two 48″ vertical swivel-clamp bars • four 4″ I.V. posts with clamps • eight cross clamps

Skeletal traction care

Sterile cotton-tipped applicators • prescribed antiseptic solution • sterile gauze sponges • povidone-iodine solution • antimicrobial ointment

Preparation

- Order materials from the central supply department.
- Explain the procedure to the patient. Emphasize the importance of maintaining proper body alignment after the traction equipment is set up.

Essential steps

The setup procedure varies depending on the type of frame.

Claw-type basic frame

- Attach one lower-panel clamp and one upper-panel clamp to each 66″ swivel clamp bar.
- Fasten one bar to the footboard and one to the headboard by turning the clamp knobs clockwise until they're tight, then pulling back on the upper clamp's rubberized bar until it's tight.
- Secure the 102″ horizontal plain bar atop the two 66″ vertical swivel-clamp bars, making sure the clamp knobs point up.
- Using appropriate clamps, attach the trapeze to the horizontal bar about 2″ (5 cm) from the head of the bed.

I.V.-type basic frame

- Attach one 4″ I.V. post with clamp to each end of both 36″ horizontal plain bars.
- Secure an I.V. post in each I.V. holder at the bed corners. Using a cross clamp, fasten the 48″ vertical swivel-clamp bar to the middle of the horizontal plain bar at the foot of the bed.
- Fasten the 27″ vertical double-clamp bar to the middle of the horizontal plain bar at the head of the bed.
- Attach the 102″ horizontal plain bar to the tops of the two vertical bars, making sure the clamp knobs point up.
- Using the appropriate clamp, attach the trapeze to the horizontal bar about 2″ from the head of the bed.

I.V.-type Balkan frame

- Attach one 4″ I.V. post with clamp to each end of two 36″ horizontal plain bars.
- Secure an I.V. post in each I.V. holder at the bed corners.
- Attach a 48″ vertical swivel-clamp bar, using a cross clamp, to each I.V. post clamp on the horizontal plain bar at the foot of the bed.
- Fasten one 36″ horizontal plain bar across the midpoints of the two 48″ vertical swivel-clamp bars, using two cross clamps.
- Attach a 27″ vertical double-clamp bar to each I.V. post clamp on the horizontal bar at the head of the bed.
- Using two cross clamps, fasten a 36″ horizontal plain bar across the midpoints of two 27″ vertical double-clamp bars.

• Clamp a 102″ horizontal plain bar onto the vertical bars on each side of the bed, making sure the clamp knobs point up.
• Use two cross clamps to attach a 36″ horizontal plain bar across two overhead bars, about 2″ from the head of the bed.
• Attach the trapeze to this 36″ horizontal bar.

All frames
• Attach a wall bumper or roller to the vertical bars at the head of the bed.

Cautions
With skeletal traction, make sure protruding pins or wire ends are covered with cork to prevent them from tearing the bedding or injuring the patient.

When ordered, apply weight slowly and carefully to avoid jerking the affected extremity. To avoid injury in case the ropes break, arrange the weights so they don't hang directly over the patient.

Monitoring and aftercare
• Perform a neurovascular check before and after placement of traction and every 4 hours thereafter.
• Inspect traction equipment to ensure the correct line of pull.
• Inspect the ropes for fraying, which can eventually cause them to break.
• Show the patient how much movement he's allowed and instruct him not to readjust the equipment. Tell him to report any pain or pressure from the traction.
• Make sure the ropes are positioned properly in the pulley tract to maintain the correct angle of traction.
• Tape all rope ends above the knot to prevent tampering and slippage.
• Inspect the equipment regularly to make sure the traction weights hang freely. Weights that touch the bed, floor, or each other reduce the amount of traction.
• Check the patient for proper body alignment every 2 hours.
• Provide skin care, encourage deep-breathing and coughing exercises, and assist with ordered range-of-motion exercises for unaffected extremities.
• Check the pin sites and surrounding skin regularly.
• Clean the pin sites and surrounding skin with a sterile cotton-tipped applicator dipped in the ordered cleaning solution.
• Document the type and amount of traction used daily and the patient's response to the procedure. Record equipment inspections and patient care, including routine neurologic checks, skin condition, and respiratory status. Also document the condition of the pin sites.

Continuous passive motion

Continuous passive motion (CPM) uses an electrically powered or manually operated machine to move a joint automatically through its normal range of motion for an extended period. This ensures that the joint receives the optimal range of motion comfortable for the patient and that the joint capsule, muscles, and ligaments receive continuous stimulation.

Nursing responsibilities include setting up the machine and positioning the patient. You must also monitor the patient's response to therapy and his comfort level during the procedure, which can prove important to his compliance with treatment. (See *Promoting comfort during CPM,* page 132.)

Indications
CPM is used to provide optimal range of motion after total hip or knee replacement, internal fixation, or removal of the synovial membrane in the knee or another major joint (such as the shoulder or elbow).

Contraindications and complications
There are no contraindications. Joint instability, effusion from hyperextension, and even joint dislocation can occur if the device and patient aren't carefully monitored.

Equipment
CPM machine • sheepskin pad • skin powder

ADVANCED EQUIPMENT

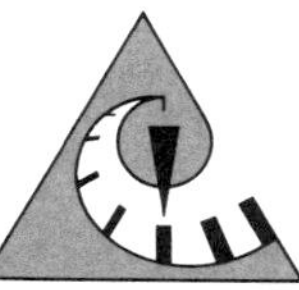

Promoting comfort during CPM

Continuous passive motion (CPM) can seem threatening to a patient who's recently undergone trauma and surgical pain. To help your patient adapt to this device and thus speed his recovery, provide the following comfort measures:
- Medicate the patient before the procedure, if ordered.
- Apply a light layer of powder to the surface of the machine that touches the skin. This will reduce surface friction.
- Cover the affected extremity with a sheet or light blanket to provide privacy and warmth.
- Provide diversionary activities for the patient while he's in the device.

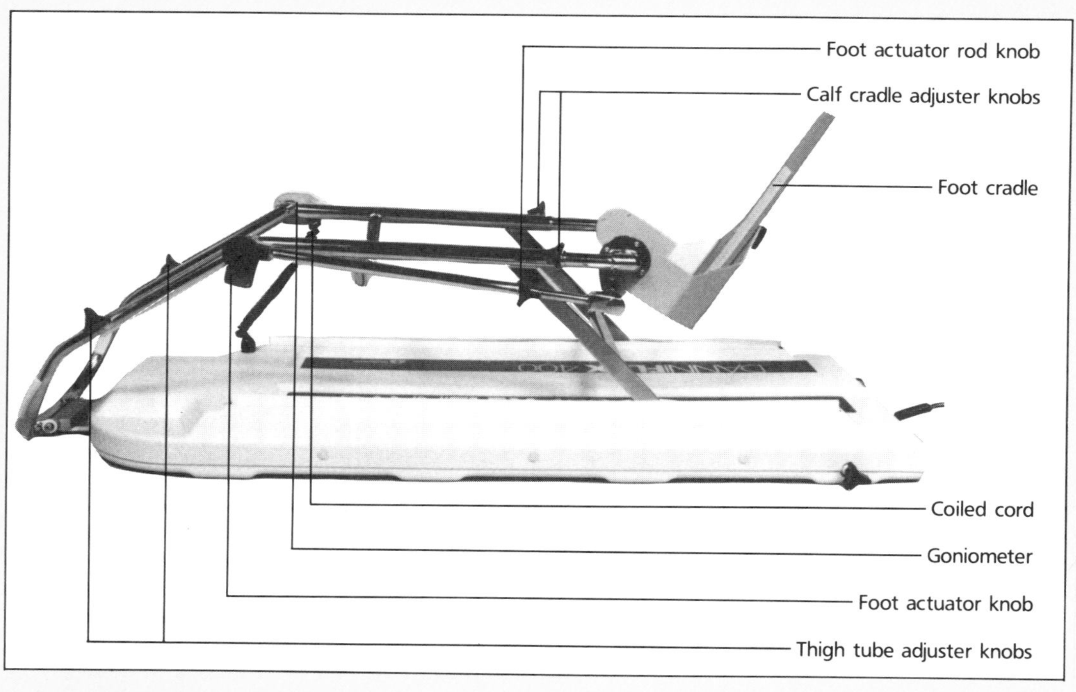

Preparation

- Explain the procedure to the patient. Reassure him that the degree of movement will be tolerable and will be advanced according to his tolerance of the procedure.
- Administer a mild analgesic, if ordered.
- Assemble the equipment, making sure the sheepskin is clean and dry.

Essential steps

- Assess the patient's degree of mobility.
- Attach the machine to the patient's bed and set the degree of flexion and extension, as prescribed.
- Place the affected extremity in the device, making sure it's well supported. Apply skin powder where the extremity and the machine meet.
- Smooth out the sheepskin so that it's wrinkle-free.

- Fasten the safety straps of the device, securing the affected extremity in the frame.
- Run the machine through one cycle and double-check the degree of flexion and extension. Adjust as necessary.
- Restart the machine and continue operation, as ordered.

Cautions

Check the doctor's order before selecting the degree of flexion and extension. Allow time for the patient to ask questions.

Initiate therapy slowly because the mechanical nature of the treatment may intimidate the patient. Stop the device if the patient complains of pain.

Monitoring and aftercare

- Monitor the patient's tolerance of the procedure.
- Note any swelling or change in the appearance of the joint after the procedure.
- Assess the skin for areas of abrasion where movement with the device occurs.
- Document the time, duration, and limits of CPM. Record the patient's tolerance of the procedure.

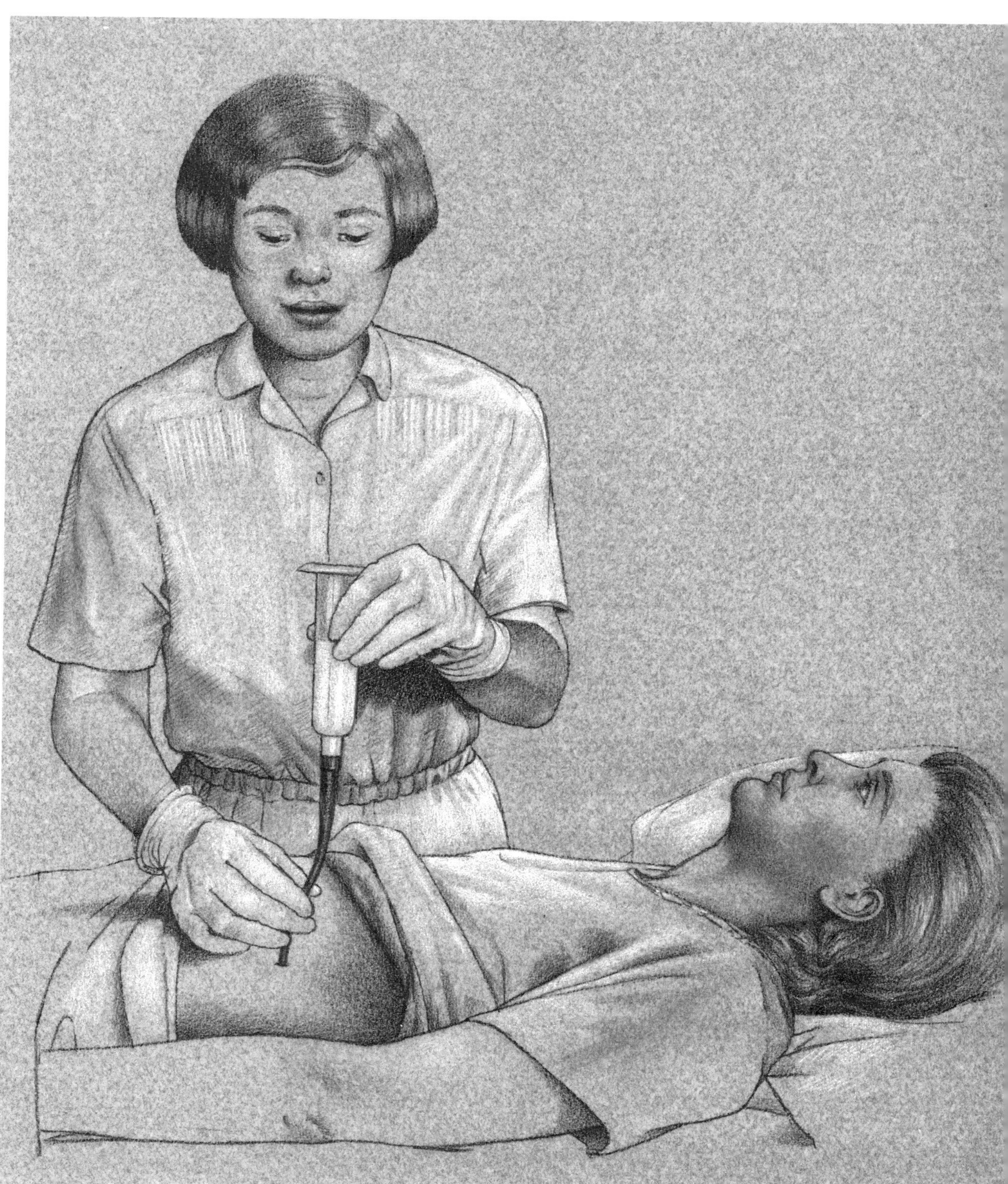

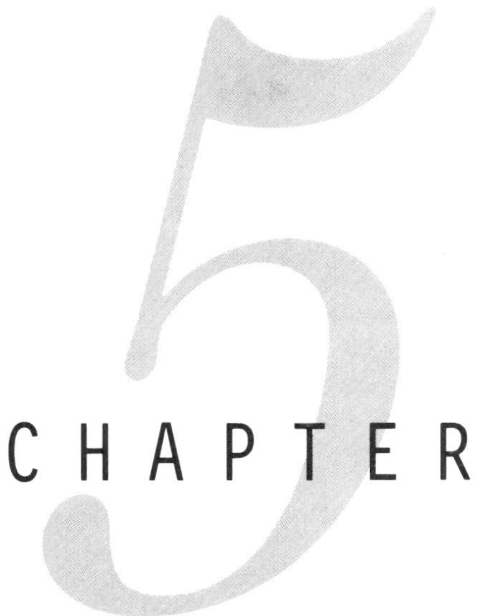

CHAPTER

Gastrointestinal, renal, and urologic procedures

As the site of digestion, the GI system helps fuel the body's major organs by supplying cells with essential nutrients, such as glucose, amino acids, and fatty acids. The renal and urologic systems also directly affect the overall functioning of the body. Because they produce, transport, collect, and excrete urine, any dysfunction of these systems can impair fluid, electrolyte, and acid-base balance and the elimination of waste.

Because GI, renal, and urologic conditions vary widely, so do the procedures that treat them. This chapter focuses first on the placement and maintenance of GI tubes and esophageal tubes. A GI tube may be prescribed for various conditions and for patients in several different settings. For example, patients in acute care facilities as well as those in outpatient, rehabilitation, or extended care settings may receive GI tubes. Esophageal tubes inserted to control hemorrhage from varices are used most commonly for acutely ill patients.

Renal and urologic procedures are discussed next. To restore or improve renal or urologic function, treatment usually involves temporary or permanent insertion of a urinary, peritoneal, or vascular catheter or tube. Catheterization also allows monitoring of the renal and urologic systems and aids in diagnosing dysfunction. Two renal and urologic procedures are presented in this chapter: peritoneal dialysis and continuous arteriovenous hemofiltration.

Whether you're called upon to insert a nasogastric tube, instill nutrients through a gastrostomy button, or perform peritoneal dialysis on a patient with renal failure, you'll need thorough, up-to-date knowledge of how best to perform the procedure. And because some procedures may prove uncomfortable or embarrassing to the patient, you'll also need to remain alert to the patient's emotional needs. Helping the patient undergoing these procedures maintain his sense of dignity, while at the same time eliciting his cooperation, requires a skillful blend of compassion and judgment.

Nasogastric tube insertion and removal

Inserting a nasogastric (NG) tube requires close observation of the patient and verification of proper tube placement. Most NG tubes have a radiopaque marker at the distal end so that the tube's position can be verified by X-ray. Special measures must be taken to make sure that the tube doesn't move. (See *Securing an NG tube*.) Removing the tube requires careful handling to prevent injury or aspiration.

The most common NG tubes are the Levin tube, which has one lumen, and the Salem sump tube, which has two lumens, one for suction and drainage and a smaller one for ventilation. Air flows through the vent lumen of the Salem sump tube continuously. This protects the delicate gastric mucosa by preventing a vacuum from forming should the tube adhere to the stomach lining. Other types of NG tubes include the Moss tube, which has a triple lumen and is usually inserted during surgery, and wide-bore gastric tubes, such as the Ewald, Levacuator, and Edlich tubes. (See *Types of NG tubes*, page 138.)

Indications

• Uncontrolled vomiting preoperatively or postoperatively
• Drug or poison ingestion
• Upper GI bleeding
• Analysis of gastric contents
• Administration of medications or nutrients

Contraindications and complications

NG tube use is contraindicated in patients with facial fractures or basilar skull fractures. If these fractures are unstable, tube insertion and manipulation can worsen them. Certain fractures may make insertion difficult or block insertion. The doctor decides if the need for a tube outweighs the potential problems.

Potential complications of prolonged intubation with an NG tube include skin erosion at the nostril, sinusitis, esophagitis, esophagotracheal fistula, gastric ulceration, and oral infection. Additional complications that may result from suction include electrolyte imbalances and dehydration. Bradycardia may occur during insertion or removal of an NG tube as a result of vagal stimulation.

Equipment

For inserting an NG tube

Tube (usually #14, #16, or #18 French for an adult) • towel or linen-saver pad • facial tissues • emesis basin • penlight • 1″ or 2″ nonallergenic tape • gloves • water-soluble lubricant • cup or glass of water • straw (if appropriate) • stethoscope • tongue blade • catheter-tip syringe, bulb syringe, or irrigation set • safety pin • rubber band • suction equipment (as ordered) •optional: metal clamp, ice, warm water, large basin or plastic container, waterproof marking pen

SKILL TIP

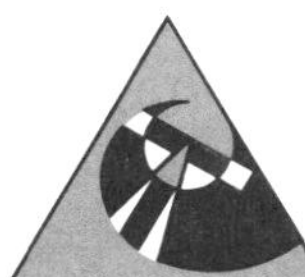

Securing an NG tube

After inserting a nasogastric (NG) tube, you'll need to take steps to make sure that the tube remains properly positioned. If you're not using a prepackaged product that secures and cushions the NG tube at the nose, you have other options.

One option is to secure the NG tube to the patient's nose with nonallergenic tape. You'll need about 4" (10 cm) of 1" tape. Split one end of the tape up the center about 1½" (4 cm). Make tabs on the split ends (by folding sticky sides together). Stick the uncut tape end on the patient's nose so that the split in the tape starts about ½" (1 cm) to 1½" from the tip of her nose, as shown below. Crisscross the tabbed ends around the tube. Then apply another piece of tape over the bridge of the nose to secure the tube.

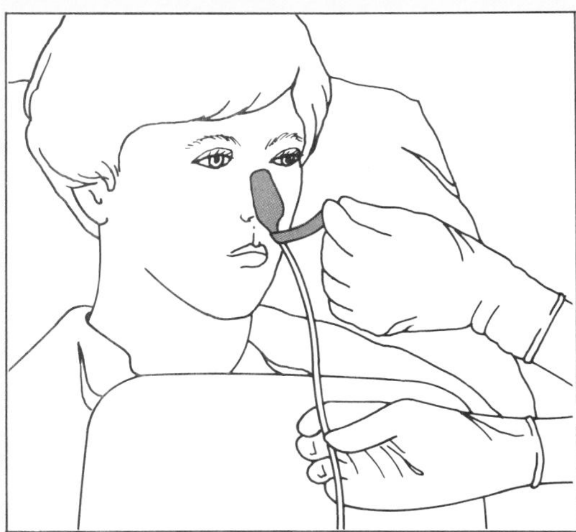

Another option is to use a Coverlet dressing to anchor the tube in place. First, swab the patient's nose with a liquid adhesive to help the dressing adhere. Then place the wide end of the dressing over the bridge of the patient's nose and wrap the smaller end around the tube, as shown below. The dressing won't irritate the patient's nose and is less expensive than a box of regular nasal tube fasteners.

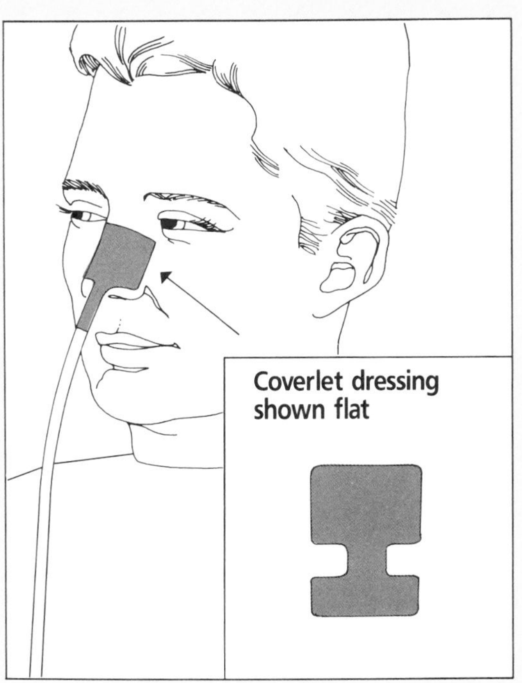

For removing an NG tube
Stethoscope • catheter-tip syringe • 0.9% sodium chloride solution • towel or linen-saver pad • clamp (optional)

Preparation

• Explain the procedure to the patient to ease his anxiety and promote cooperation.
• Before insertion, tell the patient that he may experience nasal discomfort, gagging, and watery eyes. Emphasize that swallowing will ease the tube's advancement. Agree on a signal that the patient can use if he needs you to stop briefly during the procedure.
• Gather all necessary equipment.
• Wash your hands and put on gloves.
• Inspect the tube for defects, such as rough edges or partially closed lumens.
• Check the tube's patency by flushing it with water.
• To ease insertion, increase a stiff tube's flexibility by coiling it around your gloved fingers

Types of NG tubes

The doctor will choose the type and diameter of nasogastric (NG) tube that best suits the patient's needs, which may include lavage, aspiration, enteral therapy, or stomach decompression. Common choices include the Levin, Salem sump, and Moss tubes.

Levin tube

This rubber or plastic tube has a single lumen, a length of 42" to 50" (107 to 127 cm), and holes at the tip and along the side.

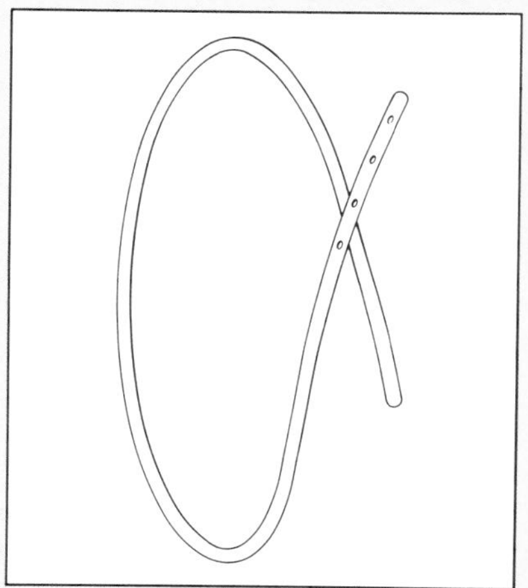

Salem sump tube

This double-lumen tube is made of clear plastic and has a blue sump port (pigtail) that allows atmospheric air to enter the patient's stomach. Thus, the tube floats freely and doesn't adhere to or damage gastric mucosa. The larger port of this 48" (122-cm) tube serves as the main suction conduit. The tube has openings at the sides and the tip; markings at 45, 55, 65, and 75 cm; and a radiopaque line to verify placement.

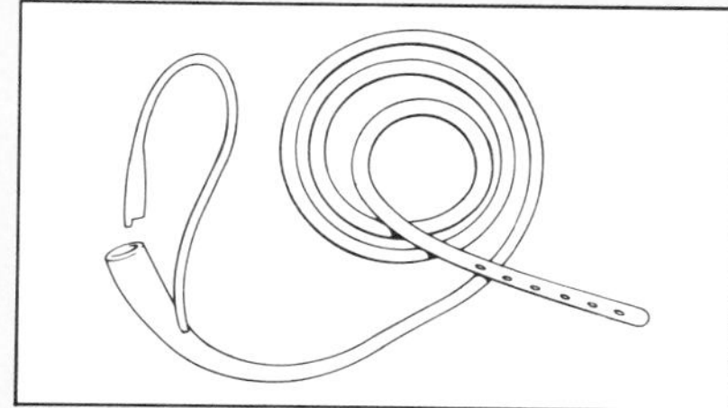

Moss tube

This tube is plastic and has a radiopaque tip and three lumens. The first, positioned and inflated at the cardia, serves as a balloon inflation port. The second is an esophageal aspiration port. The third is a duodenal feeding port.

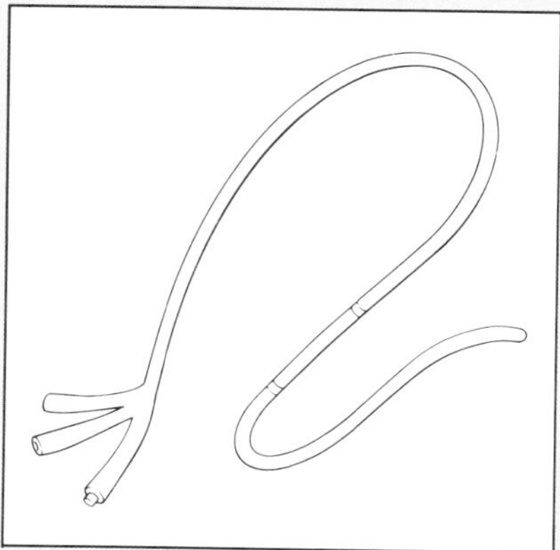

If you need to deliver a large volume of fluid rapidly through a gastric tube (such as when irrigating the stomach of a patient with profuse gastric bleeding or poisoning), a wide-bore tube usually serves best. Typically inserted orally, wide-bore tubes, such as those shown below, stay in place only long enough to complete the lavage and evacuate stomach contents.

Ewald tube

In an emergency, use this single-lumen plastic tube with several openings at the distal end to aspirate large amounts of gastric contents quickly.

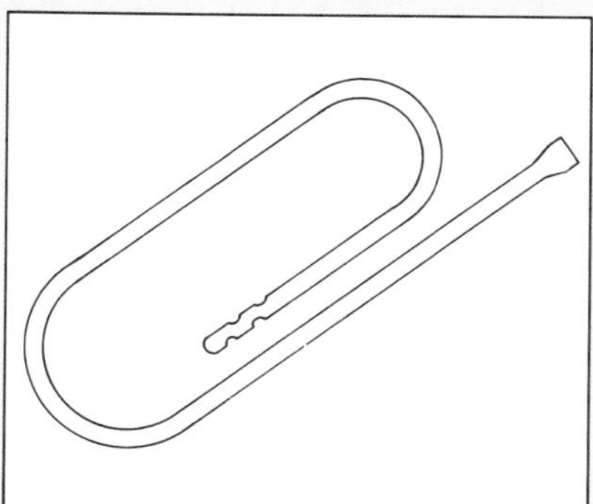

Levacuator tube

The Levacuator tube is plastic and has two lumens. The larger lumen serves to evacuate gastric contents, whereas the smaller lumen allows for the instillation of an irrigant.

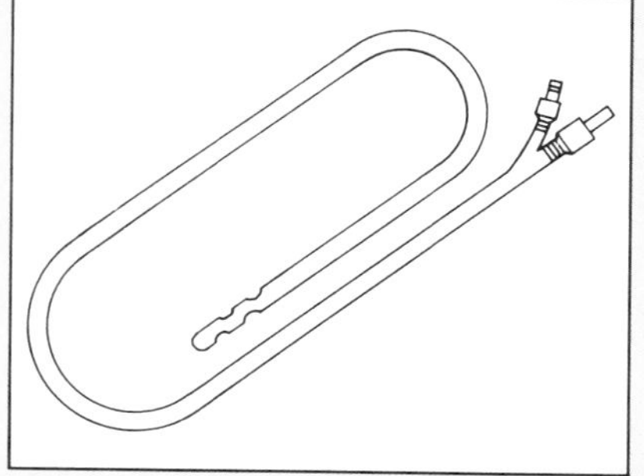

Edlich tube

This single-lumen plastic tube has four openings near the closed distal tip. A funnel or syringe may be connected at the proximal end. Like the Ewald tube, the Edlich tube is used to aspirate large amounts of gastric contents quickly.

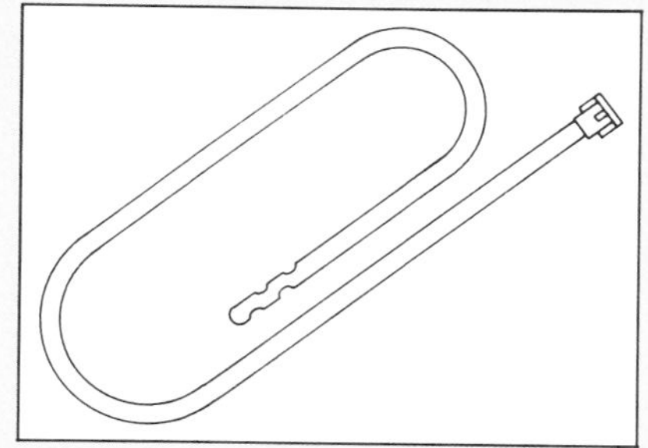

for a few seconds or by dipping it into warm water.

Essential steps

The following measures will facilitate NG tube insertion and removal.

To insert an NG tube

• After providing privacy, help the patient into high Fowler's position unless contraindicated.

• Stand at the patient's right side if you're right-handed or at his left side if you're left-handed to ease insertion.

• Drape a towel or linen-saver pad over the patient's chest to protect his gown and bed linens from spills.

• Have the patient gently blow his nose to clear his nostrils.

• Place the facial tissues and emesis basin within the patient's reach.

• Help the patient face forward with his neck in a neutral position.

• Determine how long the NG tube must be to reach the stomach. (See *Measuring NG tube length.*)

• To determine which nostril will allow easier access, use a penlight and inspect for a deviated septum or other abnormalities. Assess airflow in both nostrils by occluding one nostril at a time while the patient breathes through his nose. Choose the nostril with the better airflow.

• Lubricate the first 3″ (8 cm) of the tube with a water-soluble gel to minimize injury to the nasal passages. Using a water-soluble lubricant prevents lipid pneumonia, which may result from aspiration of an oil-based lubricant or from accidental slippage of the tube into the trachea.

• Instruct the patient to hold his head straight and upright, if appropriate.

• Grasp the tube with the end pointing downward, curve it if necessary, and carefully insert it into the more patent nostril.

• Aim the tube downward and toward the ear closer to the chosen nostril. Advance it slowly to avoid pressure on the turbinates and resultant pain and bleeding.

• When the tube reaches the nasopharynx, you'll feel resistance. Instruct the patient to lower his head slightly to close the trachea and open the esophagus. Then rotate the tube 180 degrees toward the opposite nostril to redirect it so that the tube won't enter the patient's mouth.

• Unless contraindicated, offer the patient a cup or glass of water with a straw. Direct the patient to sip and swallow as you slowly advance the tube. This helps the tube pass into the esophagus. If you aren't using water, ask the patient to swallow.

• To ensure proper tube placement, use a tongue blade and penlight to examine the patient's mouth and throat for signs of a coiled section of tubing (especially in an unconscious patient).

Measuring NG tube length

To determine how much of a nasogastric (NG) tube you need to insert, hold the end of the tube at the tip of the patient's nose. Extend the tube to the patient's earlobe and then down to the xiphoid process, as shown below. Mark this distance on the tubing with tape. The average tube length for an adult ranges from 22″ to 26″ (56 to 66 cm).

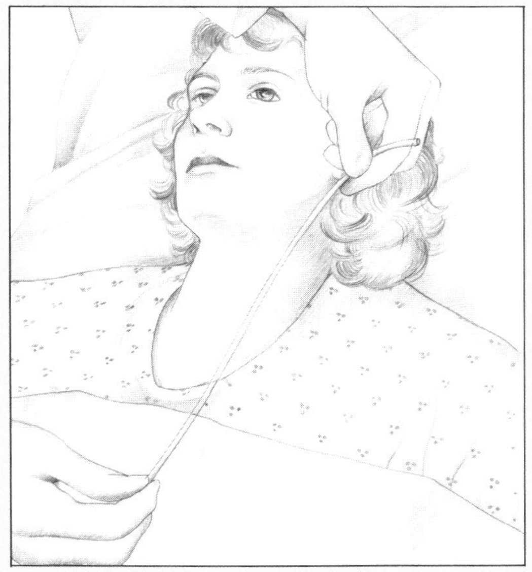

SKILL TIP

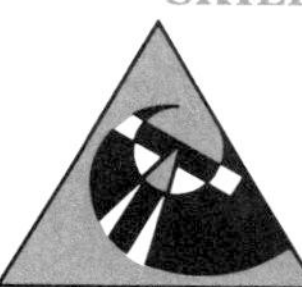

Fitting a face mask with an NG tube

A patient with a nasogastric (NG) tube and an oxygen mask may be uncomfortable if the mask presses on the tube. Some face masks contain holes specially designed for NG tubes. If your patient doesn't have such a mask, solve the problem by cutting a small slit on the top of the face mask after it's positioned on the patient's face. Make sure you still have a good seal on the mask by taping the slit. Then place the mask under the NG tube, as shown here, so that the tube rests on top of it. This will allow the equipment to fit well together and make your patient more comfortable.

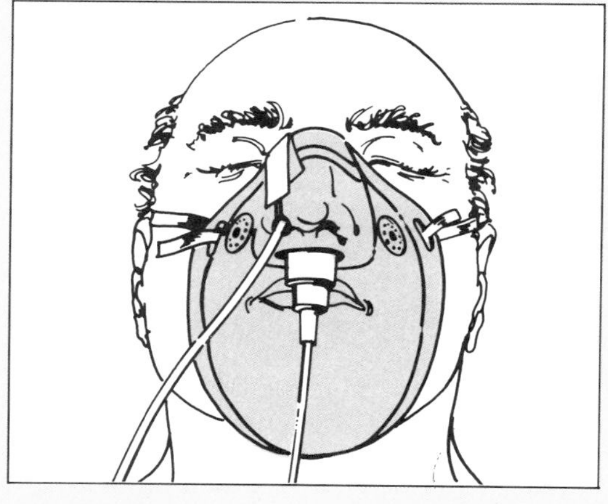

• As you carefully advance the tube and the patient swallows, watch for respiratory distress signs, which may mean that the tube is in the bronchus and must be removed immediately.
• Stop advancing the tube when the tape mark reaches the patient's nostril.
• Attach a catheter-tip or bulb syringe to the tube, and try to aspirate stomach contents. If you do not obtain stomach contents, position the patient on his left side to move the contents into the stomach's greater curvature, and aspirate again.
• If you still can't aspirate stomach contents, advance the tube 1″ to 2″ (2.5 to 5 cm) and try again.
• Next, inject 5 to 10 cc of air into the tube. At the same time, auscultate for air sounds with your stethoscope placed over the epigastric region. You should hear a whooshing sound if the tube is patent and properly positioned in the stomach.
• You'll need X-ray verification of all tube placements.
• Secure the tube as needed to prevent migration and ensure patient comfort.
• To reduce discomfort from the weight of the tube, tie a slip knot around the tube with a rubber band, and secure the rubber band to the patient's gown with a safety pin. Or wrap another piece of tape around the end of the tube and leave a tab. Then fasten the tape tab to the patient's gown with a safety pin.
• You may have to reduce discomfort if the face mask presses on the NG tube. (See *Fitting a face mask with an NG tube.*)
• Attach the tube to suction equipment, if ordered, and set the designated suction pressure.

To remove an NG tube
• Assess bowel function by auscultating for peristalsis or flatus.
• Help the patient into semi-Fowler's position. Then drape a towel or linen-saver pad across the patient's chest to protect his gown and bed linens from spills.
• Using a catheter-tip syringe, flush the tube with 10 ml of 0.9% sodium chloride solution to ensure that the tube doesn't contain stomach contents that could irritate tissues during tube removal.
• Untape the tube from the patient's nose, and unpin it from his gown.
• Clamp the tube by folding it in your hand.
• Ask the patient to hold his breath to close the epiglottis. Then withdraw the tube gently and steadily. When the distal end of the tube reaches the nasopharynx, which is evident when the patient begins to gag, you can pull it quickly.
• If possible, immediately cover and remove the tube because its sight and odor may nauseate the patient.
• Assist the patient with thorough mouth care.

Cautions

While advancing the tube, observe for signs that it has entered the trachea, such as choking or breathing difficulties in a conscious patient and cyanosis in an unconscious patient or a patient without a cough reflex. If these signs occur, remove the tube immediately. Allow the patient to rest; then try to reinsert the tube. When confirming tube placement, never place the tube's end into a container of water; if the tube is incorrectly placed in the trachea, the patient could aspirate water.

Also, don't tape the tube to a patient's forehead. The resulting pressure on the nostril could cause necrosis.

Monitoring and aftercare

After insertion

- Record the type and size of the NG tube and the date, time, and route of insertion. Note the type and amount of suction, if used, and describe the drainage, including the amount, color, character, consistency, and odor. Also document how the patient tolerated the procedure.
- Monitor the patient for nausea, vomiting, and abdominal distention; any of these signs usually indicates an obstructed tube. If the signs continue after vigorous irrigation of the tube, remove the NG tube and insert a new one.

After removal

- Record the date and time of removal and the patient's tolerance of the procedure.
- Monitor the patient for signs and symptoms of GI dysfunction, including nausea, vomiting, abdominal distention, and food intolerance. Such findings may necessitate tube reinsertion.

Nasogastric tube care

Providing effective NG tube care requires consistent monitoring of the patient and the equipment. Monitoring the patient involves checking drainage from the NG tube and assessing GI function. Monitoring the equipment involves verifying correct tube placement and irrigating the tube to prevent mucosal damage and to ensure patency.

Specific care varies only slightly for the most commonly used NG tubes: the single-lumen Levin tube and the double-lumen Salem sump tube.

Indications

- To confirm tube placement
- To instill fluid
- To prevent mucosal damage
- To maintain proper tube function
- To aspirate stomach contents

Contraindications and complications

The only contraindication for NG tube care would be a doctor's order that the tube not be irrigated, aspirated, or repositioned.

Epigastric pain and vomiting may result from a clogged or improperly placed tube. Any NG tube—the Levin tube in particular—may migrate and aggravate ulcers or esophageal varices, causing hemorrhage. Perforation may result from aggressive intubation. Intubation can also cause nasal skin breakdown and discomfort. If suction is applied to the NG tube, the removal of body fluids and electrolytes may result in dehydration and electrolyte imbalances. Vigorous suction may also damage the gastric mucosa and cause significant bleeding. Aspiration pneumonia may result from gastric reflux.

Equipment

Irrigant (0.9% sodium chloride solution or sterile water) • irrigation set with bulb syringe • 60-ml catheter-tip syringe • suction equipment • mouth care swabs or toothbrush and toothpaste • 1" or 1½" nonallergenic tape • water-soluble lubricant • gloves • stethoscope • towel or linen-saver pad • petroleum jelly • emesis basin

Preparation

- Gather all equipment and take it to the patient's bedside.
- Explain the procedure to the patient and provide privacy.
- Check the suction equipment for proper function and correct setting. If the doctor doesn't

Giving drugs through an NG tube

When giving drugs through a nasogastric (NG) tube, follow these simple steps for safe, accurate drug administration:

- Always verify NG tube placement before administering any drug. Do this by aspirating stomach contents and by instilling air through the tube while you listen to the epigastric area with your stethoscope.
- Check the length of tubing from the patient's nose to the distal end. It should match the length of tubing that was documented in the patient's chart after tube placement.
- Examine the oropharynx. If you see coiled tubing, gently remove the tube immediately—it could obstruct the airway.
- When you're sure the tube is placed correctly, flush it with 15 to 30 ml of water (5 to 10 ml for children) before giving drugs.
- Don't crush timed-release, enteric-coated, or slow-release drugs that must be administered by NG tube.
- If you're giving several drugs, administer each one separately and flush the feeding tube with at least 5 ml of water (3 ml for children) between medications. This rule applies even if you're using an NG tube with a Y-port. Although the tube has two external ports, it has only one internal lumen, so fluids given together would mix.
- When you're finished giving the drugs, flush the tube with 15 to 30 ml of water (5 to 10 ml for children). Don't neglect this important final step or the tube may clog.

specify the setting, follow the manufacturer's directions. A Levin tube usually calls for low intermittent suction and a Salem sump tube for low continuous suction.

Essential steps

- Wash your hands and put on gloves.

To check NG tube placement

- Use the catheter-tip or bulb syringe to inject 5 to 10 cc of air into the suction lumen of the tube. At the same time, auscultate for air sounds with your stethoscope placed over the epigastric region.
- If you are working with tubes other than Levin tubes, move the syringe to the suction lumen of the tube and aspirate. Stomach contents should flow up the tube and into the syringe.

To irrigate the NG tube

- Review the ordered irrigation schedule (usually every 4 hours).
- Check NG tube placement, using the method described above.
- Place a towel or linen-saver pad under the NG tube.
- Measure the ordered amount of irrigant (usually 30 ml) in the bulb syringe or the 60-ml catheter-tip syringe to maintain accurate intake and output.
- Disconnect the tube from the suction equipment.
- Slowly instill the irrigant into the suction lumen of the NG tube.
- Gently aspirate the solution with the bulb syringe or the catheter-tip syringe. Gentle aspiration prevents excessive pressure on the delicate gastric mucosa or on a suture line.
- Reconnect the NG tube to the suction equipment after you complete the irrigation.
- Record any difference between the amount of solution injected and the amount aspirated as intake on the intake and output record.

To instill a solution through the NG tube

- Place a towel or linen-saver pad on the patient's chest; then check NG tube placement.
- Measure the ordered amount of solution (usually 30 ml) in the bulb syringe or the 60-ml catheter-tip syringe.
- Disconnect the tube from the suction equipment.
- Inject the solution into the tube but don't aspirate it.
- Note the amount of instilled solution as intake on the intake and output record.
- Reattach the tube to suction as ordered.

To administer medications through the NG tube

- Place a towel or linen-saver pad on the patient's chest and then check NG tube placement. (See *Giving drugs through an NG tube.*)
- Next, irrigate the NG tube with 30 ml of irrigant.
- Draw up the prepared medication into the bulb syringe or catheter-tip syringe, and inject it into the suction lumen of the NG tube.
- Instill 30 ml of irrigant into the tube to ensure that all medication has cleared the tube and entered the stomach.
- Wait 30 minutes, or as ordered, before reconnecting the suction equipment. This allows sufficient time for the medication to be absorbed.

Cautions

Don't clamp the vent lumen on a Salem sump tube at any time while suction equipment is in use. Doing so will create a vacuum and pull the gastric mucosa against the end of the NG tube, causing mucosal trauma. Also, don't reposition any tube that was inserted during surgery, to avoid tearing gastric or esophageal sutures.

Monitoring and aftercare

- Assess the patient's bowel sounds regularly (every 4 to 8 hours) to monitor GI function.
- Provide mouth care once per shift or as needed, using mouth care swabs or a toothbrush and toothpaste. Coat the patient's lips with petroleum jelly to prevent dryness.
- Check the tape that secures the tube every 2 to 4 hours because perspiration or nasal secretions may loosen the tape.
- Clean and inspect the skin at the nostrils, and apply fresh tape daily and as needed.
- If no drainage appears, check the suction equipment for proper function and settings. Separate the tube from the suction source.
- Check the suction equipment by placing the suction tubing in a container of solution. If the suction source drains the solution, check the NG tube for patency. (Include the amount of solution drawn from the container as intake on the intake and output record.)
- A malfunctioning NG tube may be clogged or incorrectly positioned. Attempt to irrigate the tube, reposition the patient, or rotate and reposition the tube unless it was inserted during surgery or is ordered not to be repositioned.
- If the patient has a Salem sump tube, watch for gastric reflux in the vent lumen when pressure in the stomach exceeds atmospheric pressure. If this occurs, assess the suction equipment for proper functioning. Then, irrigate the NG tube and instill 30 cc of air into the vent lumen. Don't attempt to stop reflux by clamping the vent lumen.
- Unless contraindicated, elevate the patient's torso more than 30 degrees to keep the vent lumen above his midline and to prevent a siphoning effect that may cause reflux of gastric contents into the vent lumen.
- Document tube placement confirmation (usually every 4 to 8 hours). Note times of tape changes and the condition of the nostrils. Record the time of each irrigation or instillation. Keep a precise record of fluid intake and output, including instilled solutions and medications as intake and all drainage as output. Inspect and document the color, consistency, odor, and amount of gastric drainage at least every 8 hours. (Normal gastric secretions have a mucoid consistency and are colorless or appear yellowish green from bile.)
- Test gastric drainage for occult blood according to the protocol at your hospital, and report any positive results. Also report any drainage with a coffee-bean color because this may also indicate bleeding.

Esophageal tube insertion and removal

Used to control hemorrhage from esophageal or gastric varices, an esophageal tube is inserted nasally or orally and advanced into the esophagus or stomach. Although a doctor usually inserts and removes the tube, you may be asked to remove it in an emergency.

All esophageal tubes have a gastric balloon. Once the tube is in place, the gastric balloon is inflated and drawn tightly against the cardia of the stomach. Most tubes also have an esophageal balloon that can be inflated to control esophageal bleeding. (See *Types of esophageal tubes.*)

Indications

An esophageal tube controls hemorrhage from gastric or esophageal varices.

Contraindications and complications

Use of an esophageal tube is contraindicated in patients who have peptic ulcer disease, gastric or esophageal tumors, or gastric or esophageal perforation.

Acute airway obstruction may develop during tube placement if the tube enters the trachea instead of the esophagus. Esophageal rupture may occur during intubation or esophageal balloon inflation. Esophageal rupture may also result if the gastric balloon accidentally inflates in the esophagus. Nasal tissue necrosis and aspiration of oral secretions may also complicate the patient's condition.

Equipment

Esophageal tube • NG tube (if using a Sengstaken-Blakemore tube) • two suction sources • basin of ice • irrigation set • 2 liters of 0.9% sodium chloride solution • two 60-ml catheter-tip syringes • water-soluble lubricant • ½″ or 1″ adhesive tape • stethoscope • foam nose guard • Yankauer tonsil-tip catheter • four rubber-shod clamps (two clamps and two plastic plugs for a Minnesota tube) • anesthetic spray (as ordered) • traction equipment (football helmet or a basic frame with traction rope, pulleys, and a 1-lb [0.45-kg] weight) • 60-ml luer-tip syringe • stopcocks • mercury aneroid manometer • Y-connector (for Sengstaken-Blakemore tube) • basin of water • cup of water with straw • scissors • gloves • gown • goggles • waterproof marking pen • penlight • sphygmomanometer • labels

Preparation

- Keep the football helmet at the patient's bedside or attach traction equipment to the bed so that either is readily available after tube insertion.
- Prepare the suction sources. Turn one source to full suction, and attach a Yankauer tonsil-tip catheter. Open the irrigation set and fill the container with 0.9% sodium chloride solution. Place all equipment within reach.
- Test the balloon for air leaks. Using the 60-ml syringe, inflate the gastric balloon with 300 cc of air and the esophageal balloon with 50 to 100 cc of air. Submerge the balloons in a basin of water. If no bubbles appear in the water, the balloons are intact. Remove them from the water and deflate them. Clamp the tube lumens or insert plastic plugs (included in the kit) so that the balloons stay deflated during insertion.
- To prepare the Minnesota tube, connect the mercury aneroid manometer to the gastric pressure monitoring port. Note the pressure when the balloon fills with 100, 200, 300, 400, and 500 cc of air.
- Check the aspiration lumens for patency, and make sure that they're labeled according to their purpose. If they aren't identified, label them carefully with the waterproof marking pen.
- Chill the tube in a basin of ice to stiffen it and facilitate insertion, as ordered.

Essential steps

To insert an esophageal tube

- Wash your hands and put on gloves, a gown, and goggles for protection from splashing blood. The doctor does the same.
- Assist the patient into semi-Fowler's position, and turn him slightly toward his left side. This position promotes stomach emptying and helps prevent aspiration.
- Explain that the doctor will inspect the patient's nostrils for patency.
- Measure the length of tubing to be inserted by holding the balloon tip at the patient's ear and bringing the tube forward to his nose. Mark this point on the tube (usually the 50-cm mark) with a waterproof pen.
- Tell the patient that the doctor will spray his posterior pharynx (throat) and nostril with an anesthetic to minimize discomfort and gagging during intubation.
- Have the Yankauer suction equipment ready if the patient begins to vomit.
- Apply water-soluble lubricant to the tip of the tube to facilitate insertion.

Types of esophageal tubes

When working with patients who have esophageal tubes, keep in mind the features of the most common types.

Sengstaken-Blakemore tube

This triple-lumen, double-balloon tube has a gastric aspiration lumen, which allows you to obtain drainage from below the gastric balloon and to instill medication.

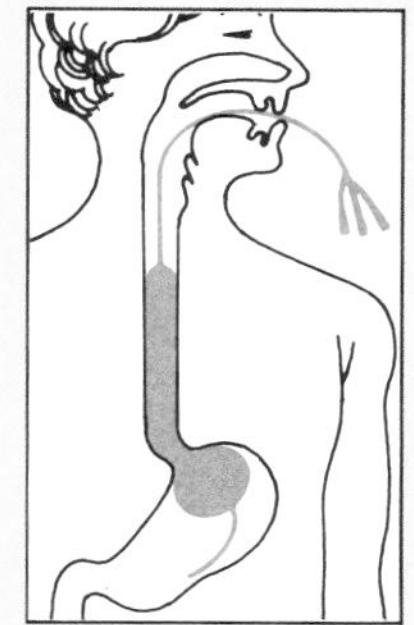

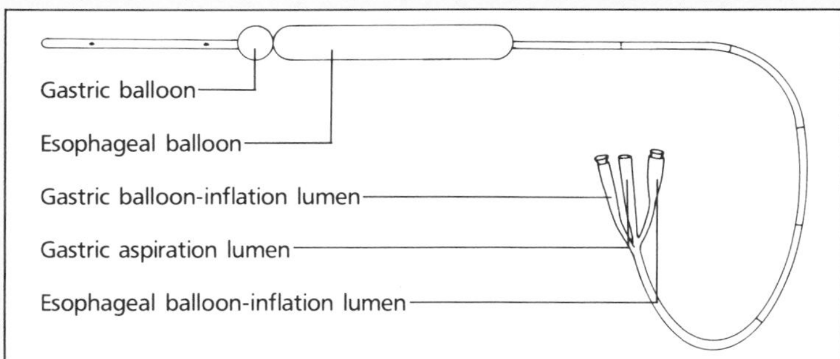

Linton tube

This triple-lumen, single-balloon tube has a lumen for gastric aspiration and one for esophageal aspiration. Additionally, the Linton tube reduces the risk of esophageal necrosis because it doesn't have an esophageal balloon.

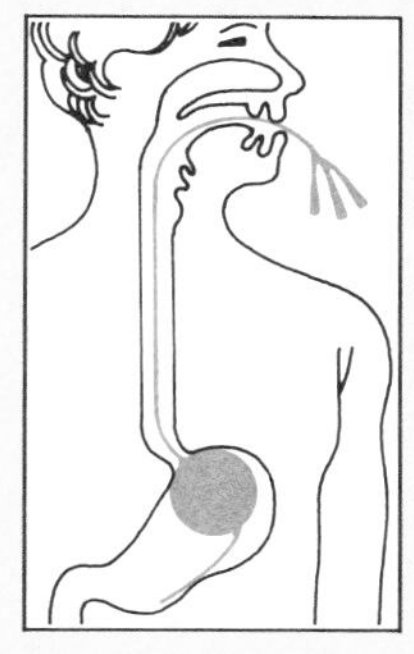

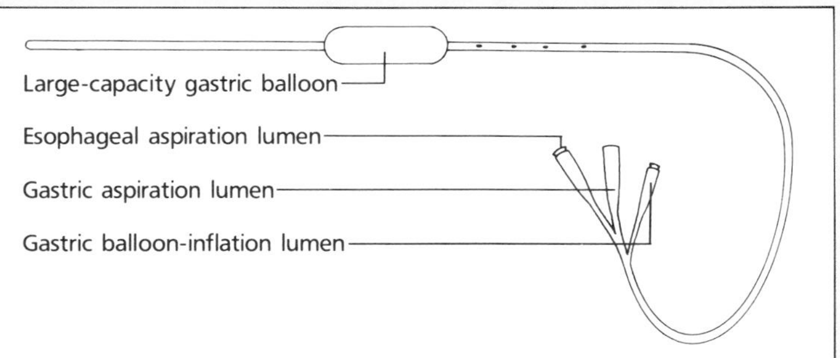

Minnesota esophagogastric tamponade tube

This esophageal tube has four lumens and two balloons. The device provides pressure-monitoring ports for both balloons without the need for Y-connectors. One lumen is used for gastric aspiration, the other for esophageal aspiration.

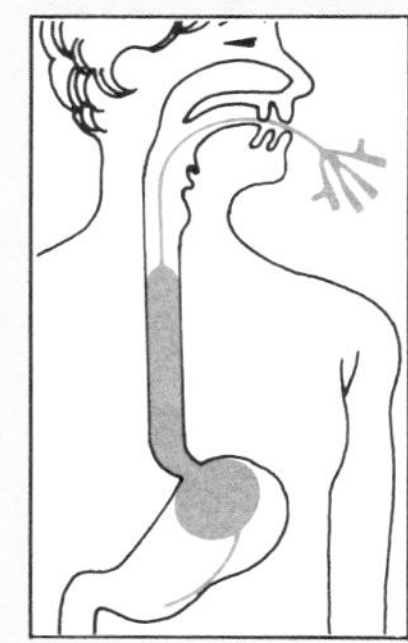

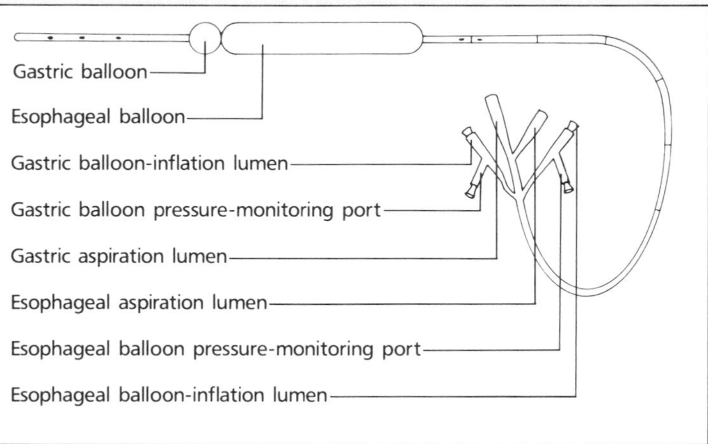

• Monitor the patient's blood pressure, heart rate, and respirations every 5 minutes during insertion.
• The doctor passes the tube through the more patent nostril. Direct the patient to swallow when he senses the tip of the tube in the back of his throat. If he needs water to help him swallow, give him the cup of water with a straw. Swallowing helps to advance the tube into the esophagus. (If the tube is inserted orally, the doctor will direct the patient to swallow immediately.)
• As the patient swallows, the doctor quickly advances the tube to the previously marked point on the tube.
• To confirm tube placement, the doctor aspirates stomach contents through the gastric aspiration lumen. He also injects air with a 60-ml catheter-tip syringe into the gastric aspiration lumen while auscultating the stomach for the whooshing or gurgling sound of the injected air.
• Next, attach a 60-ml luer-tip syringe and a stopcock to the gastric balloon. The doctor then partially inflates the gastric balloon with 50 cc of air, clamps it with a rubber clamp, and orders an abdominal X-ray to confirm correct tube placement.
• After X-ray verification of correct tube placement, the doctor irrigates the stomach with 30 ml of 0.9% sodium chloride solution injected into the gastric aspiration lumen. He then empties the stomach as completely as possible to prevent regurgitation of gastric contents when the balloon inflates further.
• The doctor fully inflates the gastric balloon, using 250 to 500 cc of air for the Sengstaken-Blakemore tube and 700 to 800 cc of air for the Linton tube. He then clamps the gastric balloon port with a rubber-shod clamp. If he's using a Minnesota tube, he connects the pressure-monitoring port for the gastric balloon lumen to the mercury aneroid manometer and inflates the balloon in 100-cc increments until he fills it with up to 500 cc of air. As he introduces the air, he monitors the intragastric balloon pressure to make sure the balloon stays inflated. Then he clamps the ports.
• The doctor gently pulls the tube upward until he feels resistance, indicating that the inflated balloon is firmly at the gastroesophageal junction and exerting pressure on the cardia of the stomach.
• At this point, place the foam nose guard around the area where the tube emerges from the nostril and tape the nose guard in place around the tube.
• With the nose guard secured, traction can be applied to the tube with a traction rope and a 1-lb (0.45-kg) weight, or the tube can be pulled gently and taped securely to the face guard of a football helmet. (See *Securing an esophageal tube.*)
• With pulley-and-weight traction, lower the head of the bed to 25 degrees to produce countertraction.
• Perform gastric lavage through the gastric aspiration lumen with 0.9% sodium chloride solution (iced or tepid) until the return fluid is clear. This will provide a baseline to determine the effectiveness of tamponade therapy.
• Attach one of the suction sources to the gastric aspiration lumen to empty stomach contents, prevent vomiting, and allow observation of the gastric contents for blood.
• If the doctor inserted a Sengstaken-Blakemore or Minnesota tube, he will inflate the esophageal balloon to compress esophageal varices and control bleeding.

One way to do this with a Sengstaken-Blakemore tube involves attaching a Y-connector to the esophageal lumen. Then the doctor attaches a sphygmomanometer inflation bulb to one end of the Y-connector and the mercury aneroid manometer to the other end. Next, he inflates the esophageal balloon until the pressure gauge ranges between 30 and 40 mm Hg. Then he clamps the tube with a rubber-shod clamp.

Another way of inflating the esophageal balloon is to insert a four-way stopcock into the esophageal balloon port. Then the doctor attaches the sphygmomanometer to the opposite end of the stopcock and a 60-ml luer-tip syringe (with the barrel withdrawn to the 50-ml mark) to the remaining stopcock port. The stopcock is opened between the esophageal balloon port, the sphygmomanometer, and the syringe. The doctor inflates the balloon to 30 or 40 mm Hg. The balloon will accommodate up to 100 cc of air. When the balloon is inflated to the appropriate pressure, the doctor clamps the esophageal balloon port with a rubber-shod clamp.

To inflate the esophageal balloon on a Minnesota tube, the doctor attaches the mercury aneroid manometer directly to the esophageal pressure-monitoring outlet. Then, using the 60-ml syringe and pushing the air slowly into the esophageal balloon port, he inflates the balloon until the pressure gauge ranges between 35 and 45 mm Hg.

• Set up esophageal suction to prevent accumulation of secretions that may cause vomiting and pulmonary aspiration since swallowed secretions can't pass into the stomach if the patient has an inflated esophageal balloon in place. For a Linton or Minnesota tube, attach a suction source to the esophageal aspiration port. For a Sengstaken-Blakemore tube, advance an NG tube through the other nostril into the esophagus to the point where the esophageal balloon begins and attach the suction source.

To remove the esophageal tube

• The doctor deflates the esophageal balloon (preferably after 12 to 24 hours) by aspirating all the air from the esophageal balloon port with a syringe. If bleeding does not recur within 6 to 24 hours, as ordered, he'll remove the traction from the gastric tube.

• The doctor may order an additional observation period of 12 to 24 hours, keeping the gastric balloon inflated but without traction. If bleeding does not recur, the doctor will aspirate all of the air from the gastric balloon port with a syringe and remove the tube. The gastric balloon is always deflated just before removing the tube because the balloon may migrate up into the pharynx and obstruct the airway, causing asphyxiation.

Cautions

After intubation, tape scissors to the head of the bed. If the patient develops cyanosis or other signs of airway obstruction, cut across all lumens (ports) while holding the tube at the nose and then quickly remove the tube.

Securing an esophageal tube

To help prevent the gastric balloon from slipping down or away from the cardia of the stomach, secure an esophageal tube to a football helmet. Tape the tube, as shown, to the face guard.

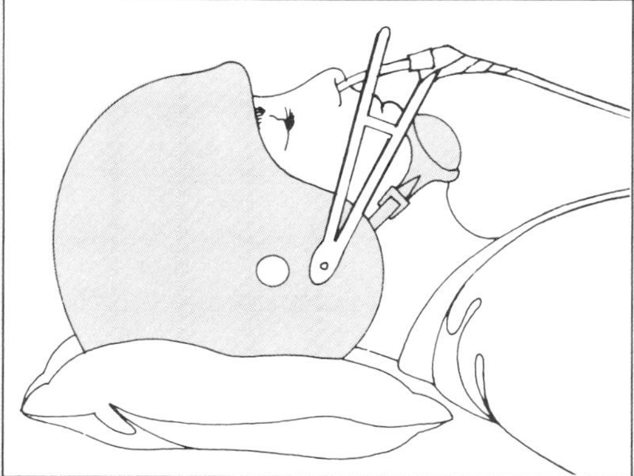

To remove the tube quickly, unfasten the chin strap and pull the helmet slightly forward. Cut the tape and the gastric balloon and esophageal balloon lumens. Be sure to hold onto the tube near the patient's nostril.

Monitoring and aftercare

• Keep in mind that the intraesophageal balloon pressure varies with respirations and esophageal contractions. Baseline pressure is the important pressure.

• Record the date and time of tube insertion and removal as well as the name of the doctor who performed the procedures. Document the intragastric balloon pressure for the Minnesota tube and the amount of air injected into the gastric balloon port for the Sengstaken-Blakemore, Linton, and Minnesota tubes. Note the amount of fluid used for gastric irrigation and the color, consistency, and amount of gastric return both before and after lavage.

Esophageal tube care

Although a doctor inserts an esophageal tube, the nurse cares for the patient during and after intubation. Typically, the patient is in the intensive care unit for close observation and constant care.

The patient who has an esophageal tube in place must be observed closely for possible esophageal rupture because varices weaken the esophagus. Additionally, possible traumatic injury from intubation or esophageal balloon inflation increases the chance of rupture.

Indications

- To observe for esophageal rupture
- To monitor balloon pressure
- To maintain suction
- To measure gastric drainage

Contraindications and complications

If the gastric balloon deflates, the gastric or esophageal balloon may move upward into the trachea, causing an acute airway obstruction. Pressure from prolonged balloon inflation can cause esophageal or gastric mucosal ulceration. Esophageal rupture (indicated by sudden back pain, upper abdominal pain, unstable vital signs, and fluid in the mediastinum) may also occur while an esophageal tube is in place. Nasal irritation, erosion and necrosis can result from tube pressure on the nose.

Equipment

Mercury aneroid manometer • two 2-liter bottles of 0.9% sodium chloride solution • irrigation set • cotton-tipped applicators • water-soluble lubricant • mouth care swabs and mouthwash • oropharyngeal suction apparatus • several #12 French suction catheters or a Yankauer tonsil-tip catheter • gloves • foam nose guard • traction weights or football helmet • scissors • labels

Preparation

- Bring all necessary equipment to the patient's bedside, and explain to him the purpose of the procedure.
- Open the irrigation set and the bottles of 0.9% sodium chloride solution. Prepare the mouth care supplies, and check to make sure that the suction sources are adjusted to the proper setting.

Essential steps

- Provide privacy. Wash your hands and put on gloves.
- Monitor the patient's vital signs every 15 minutes to 1 hour, as ordered. A sudden decrease in blood pressure and increase in heart rate may indicate GI hemorrhage or esophageal rupture.
- If the patient has a Sengstaken-Blakemore or Minnesota tube, check the pressure of the esophageal balloon every 1 to 2 hours to detect any leaks in it and to verify the set pressure.
- Label all lumens for easy identification.
- Maintain drainage from gastric and esophageal aspiration lumens, and keep suction at low settings or as ordered. This is important because fluid accumulating in the stomach may cause the patient to regurgitate the tube, and fluid accumulating in the esophagus may lead to vomiting and aspiration.
- Irrigate the gastric aspiration lumen every 2 to 4 hours, as ordered, using the irrigation set and 0.9% sodium chloride solution. Frequent irrigation keeps the tube from clogging.
- Inject air into the esophageal aspiration lumen or the Salem sump tube as needed to maintain patency.
- To prevent pressure ulcers, clean the patient's nostrils and apply a water-soluble lubricant with cotton-tipped applicators. Put the nose guard on the patient.
- Provide frequent mouth care to relieve dryness from mouth breathing.
- Use #12 French catheters or a Yankauer tonsil-tip catheter to provide gentle oral suctioning as needed to help remove secretions.
- Offer emotional support. Keep the patient as quiet as possible and administer a sedative if ordered.
- Elevate the head of the bed to 25 degrees to provide countertraction for the weights. Ensure that the traction weights hang freely from the foot of the bed at all times. If traction is being provided by a football helmet, elevate the head of the bed 30 to 45 degrees.

Cautions

If using traction, be sure to release the tension before deflating any balloons. If weights and pulleys supply traction, remove the weights. If a football helmet supplies traction, untape the esophageal tube from the face guard before deflating the balloons.

Monitoring and aftercare

• Tape scissors to the head of the bed so you can cut the tube quickly to deflate the balloons if asphyxiation occurs. When performing this emergency intervention, hold the tube firmly and close to the nostril before cutting.
• Make sure that the patient stays in bed while the tube is in place. Never roll the patient from side to side when pulleys and weights are being used for traction. Instead, lift him in the direction of the pulley for such procedures as bed making, using the bedpan, or positioning for X-ray studies.
• Keep the gastric balloon port clamped at all times when using esophageal tubes. Unclamp the esophageal balloon port on a Sengstaken-Blakemore or Minnesota tube only to check esophageal balloon pressures or to periodically relieve pressure from the mucosa, as ordered.
• Record the esophageal pressures, and note when the balloons are deflated and by whom. Document vital signs, the condition of the patient's nostrils, routine care, and any drugs administered.
• Record the color, consistency, and amount of gastric returns. Document gastric port irrigations, and maintain accurate intake and output records. Document any complications and your subsequent interventions.

Gastric lavage

After poisoning or a drug overdose, especially in patients who have central nervous system depression or an inadequate gag reflex, gastric lavage flushes the stomach and removes ingested substances through an NG tube.

For patients with gastric or esophageal bleeding, lavage with tepid or iced water or 0.9% sodium chloride solution may be used to stop bleeding. However, some controversy exists over the effectiveness of iced lavage for this purpose. (See *Is iced lavage effective?*)

Gastric lavage is usually performed in the emergency department or intensive care unit by a doctor, a gastroenterologist, or a nurse; however, the wide-bore lavage tube is almost always inserted by a gastroenterologist. Correct NG tube placement is essential, because instilling fluid into a tube that has been misplaced in the patient's trachea can be fatal.

Is iced lavage effective?

Although an iced irrigant is widely used for gastric lavage when treating acute GI bleeding, some experts question the effectiveness of the practice. Here's why.

To begin with, iced irrigating solutions stimulate the vagus nerve, which triggers increased hydrochloric acid secretion. This, in turn, stimulates gastric motility, which can irritate the bleeding site.

Some doctors prefer using unchilled 0.9% sodium chloride solution (which may prevent rapid electrolyte loss) or even water if the patient must avoid sodium.

Indications

• Poisoning
• Drug overdose
• Gastric or esophageal bleeding

Contraindications and complications

Gastric lavage is contraindicated in patients who have ingested a corrosive substance (such as lye, ammonia, or mineral acids) because the NG tube may perforate the already compromised esophagus.

Vomiting and subsequent aspiration, the most common complication of gastric lavage, occurs more often in groggy patients than alert ones. Bradyarrhythmias also may occur. After iced lavage especially, the patient's body temperature may drop, thereby triggering cardiac arrest.

Equipment

Lavage setup (two graduated containers for drainage, three pieces of large-lumen rubber tubing and a Y-connector or a piece of Y-type tubing, and a clamp) • 2 to 3 liters of irrigant (either 0.9% sodium chloride solution or tap water, as ordered) • I.V. pole • basin of ice (if ordered) • Ewald tube or any large-lumen NG tube (typically #36 to #40 French) • water-soluble lubricant • stethoscope • ½″ nonallergenic tape • 60-ml bulb syringe or catheter-tip syringe • gloves • towel or linen-saver pad • Yankauer tonsil-tip catheter • suction apparatus • labeled specimen container • laboratory request form for specimen • norepinephrine • charcoal tablets (optional)

Preparation

- Explain the procedure to the patient.
- Set up the lavage equipment. First connect one of the three ends of the large-lumen Y-type tubing to the irrigant container.
- Attach a second end of the Y-type tubing to one of the drainage containers. (Later, you'll connect the third end of the tubing to the patient's NG tube.)
- Clamp the tube leading to the irrigant.
- Chill the irrigant in the basin of ice.
- Suspend the entire setup from the I.V. pole, hanging the irrigant container at the highest level. (See *Gastric lavage setup.*)
- Lubricate the end of the NG tube with the water-soluble lubricant. Prepare the suction apparatus.

Essential steps

- Provide privacy and wash your hands. Put on gloves.
- Drape the towel or linen-saver pad over the patient's chest to protect his gown and bed linens from spills.
- After insertion of the NG tube (usually performed by the doctor), check the tube's placement by injecting 5 to 10 cc of air into the tube with the bulb syringe and then auscultating the patient's abdomen with a stethoscope. If the tube is in place, you'll hear the sound of air entering the stomach.
- Secure the NG tube nasally or orally, and make sure the irrigant inflow tube on the lavage setup is clamped. Connect the unattached end of this tube to the NG tube.
- Allow the stomach contents to empty into the drainage container before instilling any irrigant.
- If you're using a syringe irrigation set, aspirate stomach contents with a 60-ml bulb or catheter-tip syringe before instilling the irrigant.
- Begin lavage by instilling about 250 ml of irrigant, 60 ml at a time.
- Clamp the inflow tube and unclamp the outflow tube to allow the irrigant to flow out.
- Measure the outflow amount.
- Repeat the inflow-outflow cycle until returned fluids appear clear. This signals that the stomach no longer holds harmful substances or that the bleeding has stopped.
- To control GI bleeding, the doctor may order continuous irrigation of the stomach with an irrigant and administration of a vasoconstrictor such as norepinephrine. After the stomach absorbs the norepinephrine, the portal system delivers the drug directly to the liver, where it's metabolized. This prevents the drug from circulating systemically and initiating a hypertensive response.

  The doctor may use an alternate drug delivery method, directing you to clamp the outflow tube for a prescribed period after instilling the irrigant and the vasoconstrictor and before withdrawing it. This allows the gastric mucosa time to absorb the drug.
- Assess the patient's vital signs, urine output, and level of consciousness (LOC) every 15 minutes.

Cautions

If the amount of drainage falls significantly short of the amount of irrigant instilled, reposition the tube until sufficient solution flows out.

Never leave a patient alone during gastric lavage. Observe him continuously for any changes in LOC, and monitor his vital signs frequently because the natural vagal response to intubation can depress the patient's heart rate.

When aspirating the stomach for ingested poisons or drugs, be sure to save the contents in a labeled container to send to the laboratory for analysis. If ordered, after lavage to remove poisons or drugs, mix charcoal tablets

Gastric lavage setup

When using a Y-type lavage setup, attach the irrigant to one end of the Y-connector and the drainage bag to the other end. Then attach the Y-connector tube to the patient's nasogastric tube. Hang the equipment from the I.V. pole with the irrigant container at the highest level, as shown below.

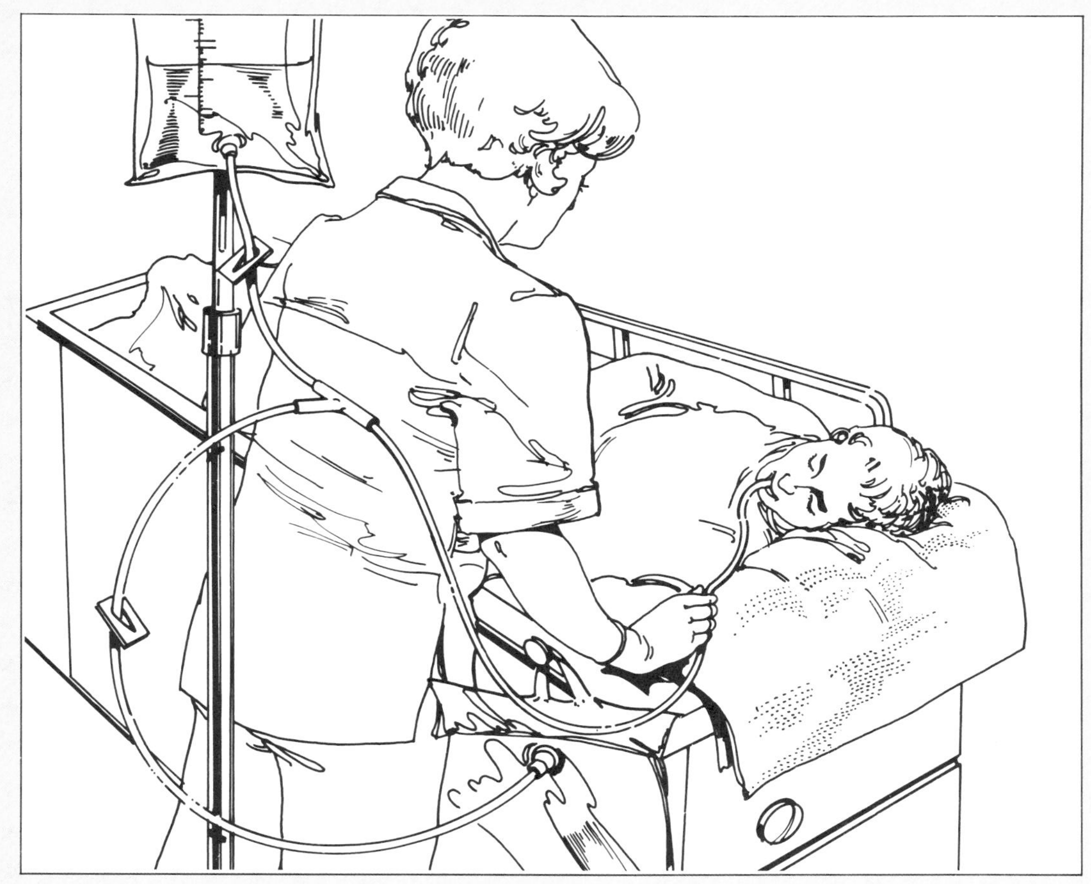

with the irrigant (whether it's 0.9% sodium chloride solution or tap water) and administer the mixture through the NG tube. The charcoal will absorb any remaining toxic substances. The tube may be clamped temporarily, allowed to drain via gravity, attached to intermittent suction, or removed.

Monitoring and aftercare

• Keep tracheal suctioning equipment nearby, and watch closely for airway obstruction caused by vomiting or excess oral secretions. You may need to suction the oral cavity frequently during gastric lavage to ensure a patent airway and prevent aspiration. For the same reasons, and if he doesn't exhibit an adequate gag reflex, the patient may require an endotracheal tube before the procedure.

• When performing gastric lavage to stop bleeding, keep precise intake and output records to determine the amount of bleeding. If the patient is having large volumes of fluid instilled and withdrawn, you may need to measure his serum electrolyte and arterial blood gas levels during or after lavage.
• Record the date and time of lavage, the size and type of NG tube used, the volume and type of irrigant, and the amount of drained gastric contents. Record this information on the intake and output record sheet, and include your observations, such as the color and consistency of drainage.
• Keep precise records of the patient's vital signs and LOC, any drugs instilled through the NG tube, the time the tube was removed, and how well the patient tolerated the procedure.

Feeding tube insertion and removal

Inserting a feeding tube nasally or (sometimes) orally into the stomach or duodenum allows a patient who can't or won't eat to receive nourishment. The feeding tube also permits supplemental feedings in a patient who has an exceptionally high nutritional requirement or decreased oral intake. Typically, the procedure is performed by a nurse. The preferred feeding route is nasal, but the oral route may be used for patients with such conditions as a deviated septum or a head or nose injury. The doctor may order duodenal feeding when the patient can't tolerate gastric feeding or when gastric feeding is likely to produce aspiration.

Feeding tubes differ somewhat from standard NG tubes. Made of silicone, rubber, or polyurethane, feeding tubes have smaller diameters and greater flexibility than NG tubes. This reduces oropharyngeal irritation, necrosis from pressure on the tracheoesophageal wall, distal esophageal irritation, and discomfort from swallowing. To facilitate passage, some feeding tubes are weighted with tungsten; others need a guide wire to keep them from curling in the back of the throat. Small-bore tubes usually have radiopaque markings and a water-activated coating that provides a lubricated surface.

Indications

Insert a feeding tube for long-term (more than 7 days) tube feeding or medication administration.

Contraindications and complications

Obstruction of or trauma to the oropharyngeal or esophageal anatomy contraindicates the use of a small-bore feeding tube. The absence of bowel sounds or a possible intestinal obstruction contraindicates administering enteral feedings.

Prolonged intubation may lead to skin erosion at the nostril, sinusitis, esophagitis, esophagotracheal fistula, gastric ulceration, and oral and pulmonary infections.

Equipment

For insertion

Feeding tube (#6 to #18 French, with or without guide wire) • linen-saver pad • gloves • nonallergenic tape • water-soluble lubricant • cotton-tipped applicators • skin protectant • penlight • small cup of water with straw • emesis basin • 10-ml syringe • stethoscope

During use

Mouthwash, toothpaste, or mild salt solution • nonallergenic tape • water-soluble lubricant • cotton-tipped applicators

For removal

Linen-saver pad • bulb syringe

Preparation

Gather all necessary equipment, including the proper size feeding tube. Explain the procedure to the patient, and provide privacy.

Essential steps

• Wash your hands and put on gloves.
• Assist the patient into semi-Fowler's or high Fowler's position.
• Place a linen-saver pad across the patient's chest to protect his gown and bed linens from spills.

• To determine the length of the tube necessary to reach the stomach, extend the distal end of the tube from the tip of the patient's nose to his earlobe. Then measure from the earlobe to the xiphoid process, and mark the tube with a pen.
• Using a 10-ml luer-tip syringe, flush the feeding tube with water to activate the water-solvent coating and determine the tube's patency.
• Ask the patient to hold the emesis basin if possible.

To insert the tube nasally
• Using the penlight, assess nasal patency.
• Lubricate the tip of the tube with a small amount of water-soluble lubricant. Then insert the lubricated tip of the tube into the nostril, and direct it along the nasal passage toward the ear on the same side.
• As the tube reaches the nasopharyngeal junction, turn the tube 180 degrees and aim down the esophagus as you advance it.
• Direct the patient to sip water through a straw, if possible, to facilitate the tube's passage.
• Advance the tube to the marking you previously measured.

To insert the tube orally
• Have the patient lower his chin to his chest to close his trachea, and ask him to open his mouth.
• Place the tip of the tube at the back of the patient's tongue. Give the patient some water, and instruct him to sip through the straw and swallow.
• Advance the tube as described above while the patient is swallowing.

To position the tube
• To check tube placement, attach the syringe filled with 10 cc of air to the end of the tube. Gently inject the air into the tube as you auscultate the patient's abdomen with the stethoscope. Listen for a whooshing sound, which signals that the tube is in the stomach. If the tube remains coiled in the esophagus, you'll feel resistance when you inject the air, or the patient may belch. In some cases, X-ray confirmation of placement may be necessary.
• Gently aspirate gastric secretions. Successful aspiration of gastric contents confirms correct tube placement. Measure the gastric secretions and then reinstill them through the tube.
• Tape the tube to the patient's nose, being careful not to distort the nostril, and remove the guide wire.

To advance the tube into the duodenum
• After inserting the tube, position the patient on his right side. This allows gravity to help move the tube through the pylorus.
• Remove the tape marking the tube's length. Then advance the tube 2" to 3" (5 to 8 cm) every hour until an X-ray confirms correct placement in the duodenum. (Keep in mind that an X-ray must confirm correct placement before feeding begins because duodenal feedings can cause nausea and vomiting if accidentally delivered to the stomach.)
• Secure the tube with tape, using skin protectant to prevent irritation and ensure adhesion.

To remove the tube
• Place a linen-saver pad on the patient's chest to protect his gown and linens from spills.
• Flush the tube with air; then clamp or pinch it to prevent fluid aspiration during withdrawal.
• Withdraw the tube quickly but gently. Then promptly cover and discard it.

Cautions
Precise feeding tube placement is especially important because small-bore feeding tubes may slide into the trachea without causing immediate signs or symptoms of respiratory distress. However, the patient will usually cough if the tube enters the larynx. To ensure that the tube clears the larynx, ask the patient to speak. If he can't, the tube is in the larynx. Withdraw the tube immediately and reinsert it.

When aspirating gastric contents, pull gently on the syringe plunger or use a bulb syringe to avoid traumatizing the stomach lining or bowel. If you meet resistance during aspiration, stop the procedure. If the tube coils above the stomach, you'll be unable to aspirate stomach contents. To rectify this, change the patient's position or withdraw the tube a few inches, readvance it, and try to aspirate again.

Never use the guide wire to advance or reposition a tube that is out of place.

Monitoring and aftercare

- Flush the feeding tube every 4 hours with up to 60 ml of 0.9% sodium chloride solution or water to maintain patency.
- Retape the tube at least daily and as needed. Alternate taping the tube toward the inner and outer side of the nose to avoid constant pressure on the same nasal area. Inspect the skin for redness and breakdown.
- Verify tube placement before each feeding. Also, aspirate gastric contents before each feeding and document this in your notes.
- Provide nasal hygiene daily using the cotton-tipped applicators and water-soluble lubricant to remove crusted secretions. Assist the patient with oral hygiene at least twice daily.
- Teach the patient how to administer tube feedings at home, if appropriate. Show the patient or family member how to insert the tube and how to verify tube placement. Help the patient obtain home tube-feeding supplies.
- After tube insertion, document the date, time, tube type and size, site of insertion, verification of placement, and the patient's tolerance of the procedure. Also record the name of the person who inserted the tube. After tube removal, record the date and time and the patient's tolerance of the procedure.

Tube feedings

Because of improvement in methods of delivery as well as formula composition, more and more patients are receiving enteral nutrition. Enteral, or tube, feedings are safe, convenient, and cost effective, and they preserve the physiologic integrity of the bowel.

Tube feeding involves delivery of a liquid feeding formula directly into the stomach (known as gastric gavage), duodenum, or jejunum. Duodenal or jejunal feedings decrease the risk of aspiration because the formula bypasses the pylorus. Because jejunal feedings result in reduced pancreatic stimulation, the patient may require an elemental diet.

Usually, patients receive tube feedings as a continuous infusion. As the patient's tolerance improves, or if the patient requires long-term feeding, a schedule for intermittent gravity-drip feedings or syringe feedings may be established.

Liquid nutrient solutions come in various formulas for administration through an NG tube, a small-bore feeding tube, a percutaneous endoscopic gastrostomy or jejunostomy tube, or a gastrostomy feeding button.

Indications

- Dysphagia
- Esophageal obstruction or injury
- Chronic disease (such as cancer or immunosuppressive disorders) requiring supplemental nutrition
- Conditions prohibiting adequate oral intake (such as unconsciousness or intubation)
- After GI surgery

Contraindications and complications

Tube feedings are contraindicated in patients with complete or suspected gastric or intestinal obstruction or questionable enteral access.

Mechanical, metabolic, or GI complications may result from tube feedings. Mechanical complications include tube malposition or rupture, local trauma from tube insertion, and tube occlusion. Metabolic complications, such as electrolyte imbalances, prerenal azotemia, dehydration, hypoglycemia, and hyperglycemia, may result from improper formula selection. GI complications include nausea, vomiting, abdominal bloating, cramps, diarrhea, and constipation. These symptoms may also result if the formula or administration equipment becomes contaminated with bacteria because of poor hygiene or handling.

The patient also may experience dumping syndrome, in which a large amount of hyperosmotic solution in the duodenum causes excessive diffusion of fluid through the semipermeable membrane and results in diarrhea. In a patient with low serum albumin levels, these symptoms may result from low oncotic pressure in the duodenal mucosa. (See *Managing tube feeding problems.*)

Equipment

For gastric feedings

Feeding formula • graduated container • I.V. pole • 120 ml of water • administration set (gavage bag with tubing and flow regulator clamp, for continuous or gravity-drip feeding) • towel or linen-saver pad • 60-ml bulb syringe or catheter-tip syringe • stethoscope • optional: enteral pump, adapter to connect gavage tubing to feeding bag

For nasal and oral care

Cotton-tipped applicators • lemon-glycerin swabs • petroleum jelly

Preparation

• Tell the patient that he will receive nourishment through the tube, and explain the procedure to him.
• Obtain the correct formula. If the formula was prepared in the dietary department, make sure it has been refrigerated. If you'll be administering a commercial formula that was previously opened, make sure the formula has been refrigerated since opening. Check the date on the formula container, and discard any formula prepared or opened for 24 hours or longer.
• Allow the formula to warm to room temperature before administration. However, never warm it over direct heat or in a microwave oven. Heat may curdle the formula or change its chemical composition; also, hot formula could injure the patient.
• Shake the formula container to mix the solution thoroughly. If you'll be administering a gravity-drip or continuous feeding, pour 60 ml of water into the graduated container. Then, after closing the flow clamp on the administration set, pour the appropriate amount of formula into the gavage bag. Hang no more than a 4- to 6-hour supply at one time to prevent bacterial growth.
• Open the flow clamp on the administration set to remove air from the tubing. This keeps air from entering the patient's stomach and causing distention and discomfort.

COMPLICATIONS

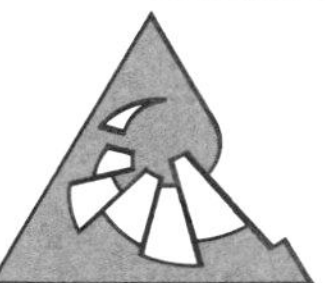

Managing tube feeding problems

Complication	Interventions
Aspiration of gastric secretions	• Discontinue feeding immediately. • Perform tracheal suction of aspirated contents if possible. • Notify the doctor. Prophylactic antibiotics and chest physiotherapy may be ordered. • Check tube placement before feeding to prevent this complication.
Constipation	• Provide additional fluids if the patient can tolerate them. • Administer a bulk-forming laxative. • Increase fruit, vegetable, or sugar content of the feeding.
Electrolyte imbalance	• Monitor serum electrolyte levels. • Notify the doctor. He may want to adjust the formula content to correct the imbalance.
Hyperglycemia	• Monitor blood glucose levels. • Notify the doctor of elevated levels. He may adjust the sugar content of the formula. • Administer insulin if ordered.
Nasal or pharyngeal irritation or necrosis	• Provide frequent oral hygiene, using mouthwash or lemon-glycerin swabs. Apply petroleum jelly to cracked lips. • Change the tube's position, for example, by placing the tube in another nostril. Replace the tube if it is encrusted or obstructed.
Vomiting, bloating, diarrhea, or cramps	• Reduce the flow rate of the formula. • Administer metoclopramide to increase GI motility. • Warm the formula. • For 30 minutes after the feeding, position the patient on his right side with his head elevated to facilitate gastric emptying. • Notify the doctor. He may want to reduce the amount of formula being given during each feeding.

HOME CARE

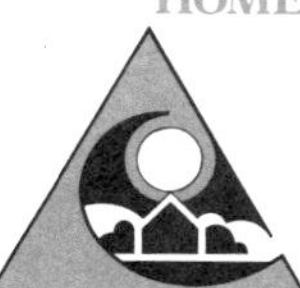

Teaching the patient about tube feedings

If the patient will be receiving tube feedings at home, you'll need to teach the patient and a family member how to administer the feedings before he's discharged. Be sure to cover these issues:
- use of the syringe or bag and tubing
- use of an infusion control device to maintain accuracy
- care of the tube and insertion site
- signs and symptoms to report to the doctor or home care nurse
- measures to take in an emergency.

Tell the patient that he may use an electric blender to mix the formula according to package directions. Caution him to discard any formula not used within 24 hours.

If the formula must remain in the tube for more than 8 hours, tell the patient to use a gavage or pump administration set with an ice pouch to decrease the incidence of bacterial growth.

Tell the patient to use a new bag daily.

Essential steps

- Provide privacy and wash your hands.
- If the patient has a nasal or oral tube, cover his chest with a towel or linen-saver pad to protect his gown and bed linens from spills.
- Assess the patient's abdomen for bowel sounds and distention. Then place the patient in semi-Fowler's or high Fowler's position to prevent aspiration by gastroesophageal reflux and to promote digestion.
- Always make sure that the feeding tube is correctly positioned in the patient's stomach before you give a tube feeding.

To deliver an intermittent gravity-drip feeding

- Remove the cap or plug from the feeding tube. Using the syringe, aspirate and measure residual gastric contents. Reinstill any aspirate obtained.
- Fill the gravity container with the prescribed amount of formula.
- Open the clamp and purge the system of air.
- Connect the gavage bag tubing to the feeding tube, using an adapter if necessary.
- Regulate the drip rate so that the formula will take at least 30 minutes to infuse.
- After all of the formula has infused, flush the tube with 30 to 60 ml of water.
- Wash and thoroughly rinse the feeding container and allow it to dry.
- Leave the patient in semi-Fowler's or high Fowler's position for at least 30 minutes after the feeding.

To deliver a continuous gastric feeding

- Remove the cap or plug from the feeding tube. Using the syringe, aspirate and measure residual gastric contents. Reinstill any aspirate obtained.
- Connect the primed administration set to the feeding tube, using an adapter if necessary.
- Regulate the drip rate according to the package directions, or use an enteral pump if available.
- Flush the feeding tube with 30 to 60 ml of water every 4 hours to maintain tube patency.
- Replace the feeding administration set and irrigation set daily or according to the policy at your hospital.
- Leave the patient in semi-Fowler's or high Fowler's position throughout the feeding.

To deliver a syringe gastric feeding

- Clamp the feeding tube. Remove the plunger or bulb from the syringe, and attach the syringe to the feeding tube.
- Pour the prescribed amount of formula into a graduated container; then pour the formula into the syringe.
- Open the clamp on the feeding tube, and allow the formula to infuse. Regulate the flow by raising or lowering the syringe.
- To prevent air from entering the tube and the patient's stomach, add more formula before the syringe empties.
- Administer the feeding over 30 minutes to prevent stomach distention.
- After administering the appropriate amount of formula, flush the tubing by adding 30 to 60 ml of water to the syringe.
- Next, clamp the feeding tube and remove the

syringe. Cover the end of the feeding tube with a cap or plug to prevent leaking.
• To prevent GI reflux, leave the patient in semi-Fowler's or high Fowler's position for at least 30 minutes after the feeding.
• Rinse all reusable equipment with warm water and dry. Store until the next feeding. Change equipment every 24 hours or according to your hospital's policy.

Cautions

If the patient becomes nauseated or vomits, stop the feeding immediately. The patient may vomit if his stomach becomes distended from overfeeding or delayed gastric emptying.

If the feeding solution won't flow through a bulb syringe, attach the bulb and gently squeeze it to start the flow. Never use the bulb to force formula through the tube.

Monitoring and aftercare

• Allow the patient to brush his teeth or care for his dentures regularly. Also, perform oral hygiene using lemon-glycerin swabs every 4 hours. Use petroleum jelly on dry or cracked lips.
• Clean the patient's nostrils with cotton-tipped applicators, and assess his skin for signs of breakdown.
• Frequently assess the patient's tolerance of the procedure and the formula.
• To maintain patency, flush the feeding tube regularly with water. If the tube becomes obstructed, flush it with warm water or cranberry juice. If necessary, replace the tube.
• Assess the patient's bowel sounds and bowel habits; administer prescribed medications or treatments to relieve constipation or diarrhea. When administering feedings continuously, check the infusion rate every hour.
• Monitor the patient's urine and blood glucose levels to assess glucose tolerance. (A patient with a serum glucose level below 200 mg/dl and without glycosuria is considered stable.) Also monitor serum electrolyte, blood urea nitrogen, and serum glucose levels; serum osmolality; and other pertinent findings to determine the patient's response to therapy and assess his hydration status.
• With duodenal or jejunal feedings, most patients tolerate a continuous drip better than bolus feedings. Bolus feedings can cause hyperglycemia, glycosuria, and diarrhea.
• Until the patient can tolerate the formula, you may need to dilute it to half- or three-quarters strength at first and then increase its potency gradually.
• Teach the patient and a family member how to administer tube feedings at home, if appropriate. Tell them where to obtain the supplies they'll need. (See *Teaching the patient about tube feedings.*)
• Document the amount, rate, route, and method of feeding in the patient's medical record, and note the patient's tolerance of the feeding.

Transabdominal tube care

To access the stomach, duodenum, or jejunum, the doctor may insert a tube through the patient's abdominal wall. The tube can then be used to decompress or drain the stomach or to deliver nutrients or medications. Of course, the patient must have an adequately functioning GI tract for the treatment to be successful.

The tube may be inserted surgically or percutaneously. A gastrostomy or jejunostomy tube may be inserted during intra-abdominal surgery or when percutaneous placement is not possible. The tube may be used for feeding during the immediate postoperative period, or it may provide long-term enteral access. Typically, the doctor will suture the tube in place to prevent gastric contents from leaking onto surrounding skin and to keep the tube from migrating.

In contrast, a percutaneous endoscopic gastrostomy (PEG) tube or a percutaneous endoscopic jejunostomy (PEJ) tube can be inserted endoscopically without the need for a laparotomy or general anesthesia. Safe, simple, and cost effective, PEG is often the procedure of choice. It can be inserted in an endoscopy suite or at the patient's bedside.

After insertion of an abdominal tube for nutrient delivery, the tube is usually attached to gravity drainage overnight. Administration of enteral nutrition can be started 24 hours after tube insertion (or when peristalsis resumes) if no complications occur. Combination PEG-PEJ tubes can decompress or drain the stomach while simultaneously supplying nutrients through the jejunostomy port of the dual tube. After a time, the tube may need replacement, and the doctor may recommend a similar tube, such as a Foley or mushroom catheter, or a gastrostomy button—a skin-level feeding tube.

Your responsibilities in caring for a patient with a transabdominal tube include providing skin care at the tube site, maintaining the feeding tube, and administering feedings. You'll also monitor the patient's response to feedings, adjust the feeding schedule as necessary, and prepare the patient for self-care after discharge.

Indications

For all transabdominal tubes

- Conditions prohibiting adequate oral intake
- Esophageal obstruction or injury
- Gastric distention

For jejunostomy feeding tubes

- Significant gastroesophageal reflux
- Aspiration pneumonia
- Poor gastric emptying
- Gastric outlet obstruction

Contraindications and complications

Contraindications for gastrostomy feeding tubes include gastroesophageal reflux, proven aspiration of gastric contents, high GI fistula, gastric outlet obstruction, and small-bowel obstruction. Mechanical bowel obstruction or a small-bowel fistula contraindicates jejunostomy feeding tube placement. Contraindications for endoscopic placement include obstruction (such as esophageal stricture or duodenal blockage), previous gastric surgery, morbid obesity, and ascites. These conditions would necessitate surgical placement.

Common complications related to transabdominal tubes include GI or other systemic problems, mechanical malfunction, and metabolic disturbances.

Cramping, nausea, vomiting, bloating, and diarrhea may result from a reaction to the medication itself. They may also be caused by a rapid infusion rate; formula contamination, osmolarity, or temperature (too cold or too warm); fat malabsorption; or intestinal atrophy from malnutrition. Constipation may result from inadequate hydration or insufficient exercise.

Systemic problems may be caused by pulmonary aspiration, infection at the tube exit site, or contaminated formula. Perforation and hemorrhage may result from improper tube insertion.

Typical mechanical problems include tube dislodgment, obstruction, or malfunction. For example, a PEG or PEJ tube may migrate if the external bumper loosens. Occlusion may result from incompletely crushed and liquefied medication particles or inadequate tube flushing. Further, the tube may rupture or crack from age, drying, or frequent manipulation.

Equipment

For feeding

Feeding formula • large bulb syringe or catheter-tip syringe • 120 ml of water • 4″ × 4″ gauze pads • prescribed cleaning solution • soap • skin protectant • antibacterial ointment • nonallergenic tape • gravity-drip administration bags • mouthwash, toothpaste, or mild salt solution • sterile gloves • enteral infusion pump (optional)

For decompression

Suction apparatus with tubing or straight drainage collection set

Preparation

- Explain the procedure to the patient, preparing him for surgery or the percutaneous procedure, as indicated.
- Provide privacy.

Essential steps

To perform tube exit site care

- Wash your hands and put on gloves.
- Gently remove the dressing by hand. Never

How to care for a PEG or PEJ site

The exit site of a percutaneous endoscopic gastrostomy (PEG) or percutaneous endoscopic jejunostomy (PEJ) tube requires routine observation and care. Follow these care guidelines:

- Change the dressing daily while the tube is in place.
- After removing the dressing, carefully slide the tube's outer bumper away from the skin about ½" (1 cm).

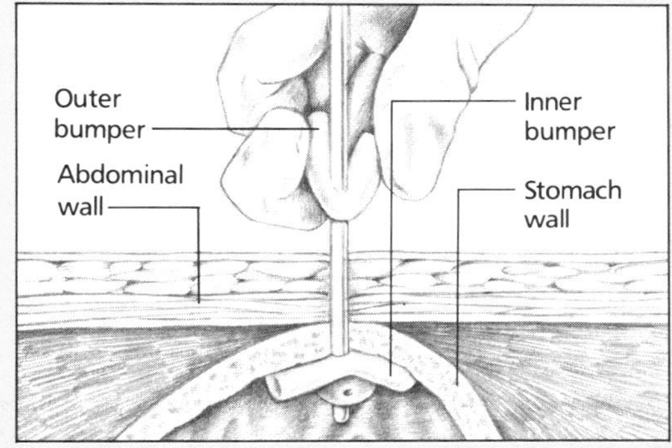

- Examine the skin around the tube. Look for redness and other signs of infection or erosion.
- Gently press the skin surrounding the tube and inspect for drainage, as in the illustration above right. Expect minimal wound drainage right after implantation; however, the drainage should subside in about 1 week.

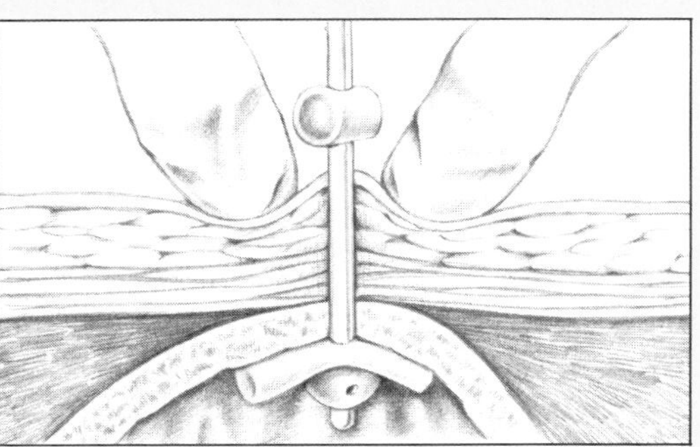

- Inspect the tube for wear and tear. (A tube that wears out will need replacement.)
- Clean the site with the prescribed cleaning solution. Then apply povidone-iodine ointment over the exit site, according to your hospital's guidelines.
- Rotate the outer bumper 90 degrees (to prevent repeating the same tension on the same skin area), and slide the outer bumper back over the exit site.
- If leakage appears at the PEG or PEJ site, or if the patient risks dislodging the tube, apply a sterile gauze dressing over the site. Do not put sterile gauze underneath the outer bumper. Loosening the anchor in this way allows the feeding tube to move about, which could lead to wound abscess.
- Write the date and time of the dressing change on the tape.
- Document care.

cut away the dressing over the catheter because you may inadvertently cut the tube or the sutures holding the tube in place.

- At least daily and as needed, clean the skin around the tube's exit site with a 4" × 4" gauze pad soaked in the prescribed cleaning solution. When the exit site has healed, wash the skin around the site daily with mild soap. Rinse the area with water and pat dry.
- Apply skin protectant, if necessary, and antibacterial ointment to the catheter at the exit site to prevent or treat skin maceration.
- Anchor a gastrostomy or jejunostomy tube to the skin with nonallergenic tape to prevent peristaltic migration of the tube. This also prevents tension on the sutures anchoring the tube in place.
- Coil the tube, if necessary, and tape it to the abdomen to prevent pulling and contamination of the tube. PEG and PEJ tubes have toggle-bolt–like internal and external bumpers that make tape anchors unnecessary. (See *How to care for a PEG or PEJ site.*)

To decompress the stomach

- Connect the PEG port to the suction device with suction tubing or straight gravity drainage tubing. Jejunostomy feedings may be given simultaneously via the PEJ port of the double-lumen tube.

Cautions

If the patient vomits, stop the feeding immediately and assess his condition. Also stop the feeding if he complains of nausea, a feeling of fullness, or regurgitation. Flush the feeding tube and attempt to restart the feeding in 1 hour (measure gastric residual contents first). If the patient develops dumping syndrome (nausea, vomiting, cramps, pallor, and diarrhea), the feedings may have been given too quickly. You may have to decrease the volume or rate of feedings. Control diarrhea resulting from dumping syndrome by using continuous pump or gravity-drip infusions, diluting the feeding formula, or adding antidiarrheal medication.

You can administer most tablets and pills through the tube by crushing them and diluting as necessary. The exceptions are enteric-coated or sustained-released drugs, which lose their effectiveness when crushed. Medications should be in liquid form for administration.

Monitoring and aftercare

- Provide oral hygiene frequently. Clean all surfaces of the teeth, gums, and tongue at least twice daily, using mouthwash, toothpaste, or a mild salt solution.
- To prevent complications, ensure aseptic formula preparation, verification of tube placement, proper tube positioning during feeding, and meticulous skin care. Also, monitor the patient for vitamin and mineral deficiencies, glucose intolerance, and fluid and electrolyte imbalances, which may follow bouts of diarrhea or constipation.
- Document the results of your abdominal assessment, the patient's tolerance for feedings, medication administration, and any complications.
- Instruct the patient and family members or other caregivers in all aspects of enteral feedings, including administering formula, maintaining the feeding tube, and caring for the skin site. Specify signs and symptoms to report to the doctor, such as redness, swelling, tenderness, or purulent discharge at the tube insertion site. Define emergency situations and review actions to take if they occur.
- Tell the patient that when the tube needs replacement, the doctor may insert a gastrostomy feeding button or a latex, indwelling, or mushroom catheter after removing the initial feeding tube. Advise him that, depending on the type of tube inserted, removal of a PEG or PEJ tube may be performed at the bedside or may require an endoscopic procedure. However, once a tract has been established, a nurse may replace a surgically inserted gastrostomy or jejunostomy tube.
- As the patient's tolerance of tube feedings improves, he may wish to try syringe feedings rather than intermittent feedings. If appropriate, teach him how to feed himself by this method.

Gastrostomy feeding button care

The gastrostomy feeding button serves as an alternative feeding device for an ambulatory patient receiving long-term enteral feedings. It may be used to replace the gastrostomy tube, if necessary, and is cosmetically appealing to the patient.

The button has a mushroom dome at one end and two wing tabs and a flexible safety plug at the other end. When inserted into an established stoma, the button lies almost level with the skin, with only the top of the safety plug visible.

The button usually can be inserted into a stoma in less than 15 minutes. The device is easily maintained, reduces skin irritation and breakdown, and poses a smaller risk of dislodgment and migration than an ordinary feeding tube. A one-way, antireflux valve mounted just inside the mushroom dome prevents accidental leakage of gastric contents. The device usually requires replacement after 3 to 4 months, usually because the antireflux valve wears out.

Indications
- Replacement of surgically inserted or percutaneous gastrostomy tubes
- Long-term enteral access in pediatric patients

Contraindications and complications
Contraindications for the feeding button are the same as those for gastrostomy feeding tubes and include gastroesophageal reflux, proven aspiration of gastric contents, high GI fistula, gastric outlet obstruction, and small-bowel obstruction.

Complications include those common to any transabdominal tube, such as GI or other systemic problems, mechanical malfunction, and metabolic disturbances. Cramping, nausea, vomiting, bloating, and diarrhea may result from a reaction to the medication itself. They may also be caused by a rapid infusion rate; formula contamination, osmolarity, or temperature (too cold or too warm); fat malabsorption; or intestinal atrophy from malnutrition. Constipation may result from inadequate hydration or insufficient exercise.

Systemic problems may be caused by pulmonary aspiration, infection at the feeding button site, or a contaminated formula. Mechanical problems include dislodgment, obstruction, or malfunction. Occlusion may result from incompletely crushed and liquefied medication particles or inadequate flushing of the feeding button. Also, the antireflux valve of the feeding button may become lodged in the open position, allowing reflux.

Equipment
Gastrostomy feeding button of the correct size • obturator • water-soluble lubricant • gloves • feeding accessories, including adapter, feeding catheter, feeding syringe or bag, and formula • catheter clamp • cleaning equipment, including water, a syringe, cotton-tipped applicator, and mild soap or povidone-iodine solution • enteral feeding pump (optional)

Preparation
Explain the insertion, reinsertion, and feeding procedure to the patient. Tell him the doctor will perform the initial insertion.

Essential steps
- Wash your hands and put on gloves.
- Attach the appropriate adapter (intermittent or continuous) and feeding catheter to the feeding syringe or bag.
- If you're administering a syringe feeding, clamp the feeding tubing and fill the syringe with 5 to 10 ml of water. (If you're administering a continuous feeding, follow the instructions in "Tube feedings," page 156.)
- Open the safety plug of the feeding button, and attach the adapter and feeding catheter. Elevate the syringe above stomach level, and allow the water to flow in to establish patency.
- Fill the syringe with formula. Adjust the height of the syringe to regulate formula flow. Refill the syringe before it empties to avoid instilling air into the stomach.
- After feeding, flush the device with 10 ml of water and clean the inside of the feeding catheter with a cotton-tipped applicator and water to preserve patency and to dislodge formula or food particles.
- Lower the syringe or bag below the stomach level to allow burping.
- Remove the adapter and feeding catheter. The antireflux valve should prevent gastric reflux.
- Snap the safety plug in place to keep the lumen clean and prevent leakage if the antireflux valve fails.
- Wash the feeding adapter and container in warm, soapy water and rinse them thoroughly.
- Soak the equipment once a week according to the manufacturer's recommendations.

Cautions
If the button pops out during feeding, reinsert it, if possible, and continue feeding. If the patient feels nauseated or vomits after a feeding, use the adapter and feeding catheter to vent the button.

Monitoring and aftercare
- Once daily, clean the peristomal skin with mild soap and water or povidone-iodine solution, and let the skin air-dry for 20 minutes. Also clean the site whenever the formula spills from the feeding bag.

• Rotate the device daily.
• When performing stoma care, note the appearance of the stoma and surrounding skin. Report any signs or symptoms of infection, such as redness, tenderness, swelling, pain, or drainage.
• Document feeding time and duration, the amount and type of feeding formula used, and the patient's tolerance of the procedure. Maintain intake and output records as necessary.
• Before discharge, be sure the patient can insert and care for the gastrostomy feeding button. Teach him or a family member how to reinsert the device by first practicing on a model. Offer written instructions and answer questions on obtaining replacement supplies. Instruct the patient and his family to monitor the insertion site for signs and symptoms of infection.

Peritoneal dialysis

In patients with acute or chronic renal failure, peritoneal dialysis (sometimes called intermittent peritoneal dialysis, or IPD) performs the kidneys' function of removing impurities from the blood. Dialysate—the solution instilled into the peritoneal cavity by a catheter (inflow or infusion)—draws waste products, excess fluid, and electrolytes from the blood across a semipermeable membrane. (See *Setup for peritoneal dialysis.*)

After a prescribed period (called *dwell time* or *equilibration*), the dialysate is drained from the peritoneal cavity, removing impurities with it (drain phase). The dialysis procedure (cycle or exchange) is then repeated, using a new dialysate each time, until waste removal is complete and fluid, electrolyte, and acid-base balance have been restored.

A surgeon inserts the peritoneal catheter in the operating room or at the patient's bedside with a nurse assisting. A specially trained nurse may perform peritoneal dialysis, either manually or using an automatic or semiautomatic cycle machine. (See *Comparing peritoneal dialysis catheters,* page 164.)

Indications

Peritoneal dialysis is performed in patients with acute or chronic renal failure, when combined with severe cardiovascular disease, difficult vascular access, very young age, or diabetes.

Contraindications and complications

Peritoneal dialysis is usually contraindicated in patients who have had extensive abdominal or bowel surgery or extensive abdominal trauma.

The most common complication of peritoneal dialysis is peritonitis. Usually resulting from a break in the integrity of the closed system or from contamination during an exchange or a tubing change, peritonitis also may develop if dialysate leaks from the catheter exit site and flows back into the catheter tract.

Protein depletion may result from the diffusion of blood protein into the dialysate through the peritoneal membrane. As much as ½ oz (15 g) of protein may be lost daily—even more in patients with peritonitis.

Respiratory distress may result when dialysate in the peritoneal cavity increases pressure on the diaphragm, thus decreasing lung expansion.

Constipation is a major cause of inflow-outflow problems; therefore, to ensure regular bowel movements, give a laxative or stool softener as needed.

Excessive fluid loss from the use of 4.25% solution may cause hypovolemia, hypotension, and shock. Excessive fluid retention may lead to blood volume expansion, hypertension, peripheral edema, and even pulmonary edema and congestive heart failure.

Other possible complications include electrolyte imbalance and hyperglycemia (which can be identified by frequent blood tests), exit site or subcutaneous tunnel infections, catheter malfunction, and increased intra-abdominal pressure.

Equipment

All equipment must be sterile. Commercially packaged dialysis kits or trays, which contain all the equipment needed for catheter placement and dressing changes, are available.

For catheter placement and dialysis
Prescribed dialysate (usually in 1- or 2-liter bottles or bags, as ordered) • warmer or heating pad • at least four sterile face masks • medication (such as heparin, potassium chloride, antibiotics, or insulin), if ordered • dialysis administration set with drainage bag • two pairs of sterile gloves • I.V. pole • fenestrated sterile drape • vial of 1% or 2% lidocaine • povidone-iodine sponges • 3-ml syringe with 25G 1″ needle • scalpel (with #11 blade) • peritoneal catheter, as determined by doctor • peritoneal stylet • sutures • nonallergenic tape • povidone-iodine solution (for doctor to prepare abdomen) • precut drain dressings • protective cap for catheter • small, sterile plastic clamp • sterile 4″ × 4″ gauze pads • optional: 10-ml syringe with 22G 1″ needle, protein or potassium supplement, specimen container, label, and laboratory request form

For dressing changes
One pair of sterile gloves • 10 sterile cotton-tipped applicators or sterile 2″ × 2″ gauze pads • povidone-iodine ointment • two precut drain dressings • adhesive tape • povidone-iodine solution • two sterile 4″ × 4″ gauze pads

Preparation

• Bring all equipment to the patient's bedside and explain the procedure.
• Weigh the patient and record his vital signs to establish baseline levels.
• Administer a broad-spectrum antibiotic, as ordered. Commonly ordered antibiotics include ceftriaxone and vancomycin.
• Have the patient try to void. An empty bladder reduces the risk of bladder perforation during insertion of the peritoneal catheter and reduces patient discomfort. If the patient can't void, and if you suspect that his bladder isn't empty, obtain an order for straight catheterization. Also, make sure that the patient isn't constipated. A full bowel increases the risk of bowel perforation during catheter insertion and makes draining dialysate difficult. If the patient is constipated, obtain an order for a laxative or an enema the night before catheter insertion.

Setup for peritoneal dialysis

This illustration shows the correct setup for peritoneal dialysis.

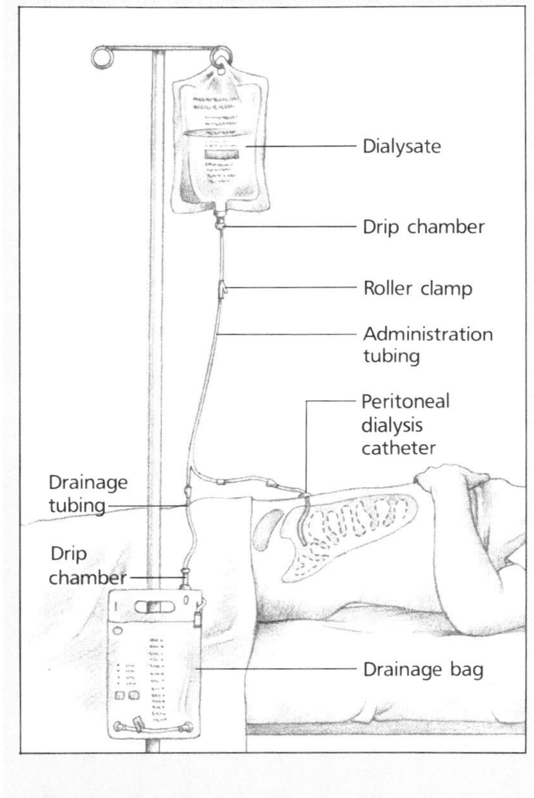

• Make sure that the dialysate is at body temperature. This decreases patient discomfort during the procedure and reduces vasoconstriction of the peritoneal capillaries. Dilated capillaries enhance blood flow to the peritoneal membrane surface, increasing waste clearance into the peritoneal cavity. To warm the solution, place the container in a warmer or wrap it in a heating pad set at 98.6° F (37° C). It should feel tepid. Avoid warming the solution in a water bath, which increases the risk for contamination, or in a microwave oven.
• Add medications, as ordered, to the dialysate just before using the solution. Doctors com-

Comparing peritoneal dialysis catheters

The first step in peritoneal dialysis is the insertion of a catheter to allow instillation of dialysate. The surgeon may insert one of the three different catheters illustrated below.

Tenckhoff catheter

To implant a Tenckhoff catheter, the surgeon inserts the first 6¾" (17 cm) of the catheter into the patient's abdomen. The next 2¾" (7-cm) segment, which may have a Dacron cuff at one or both ends, is embedded subcutaneously. Within a few days after insertion, the patient's tissues grow around the cuffs, forming a tight barrier against bacterial infiltration. The remaining 3⅞" (10 cm) of the catheter extends outside of the abdomen and is equipped with a metal adapter at the tip that connects to dialyzer tubing.

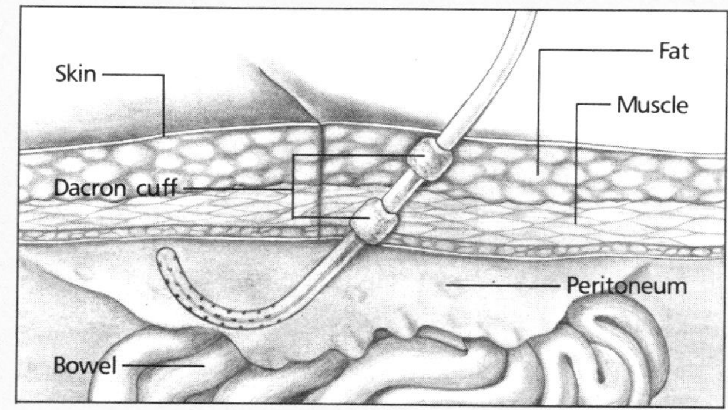

Flanged-collar catheter

To insert this kind of catheter, the surgeon positions its flanged collar just below the dermis so that the device extends through the abdominal wall. He keeps the distal end of the cuff from extending into the peritoneum, where it could cause adhesions.

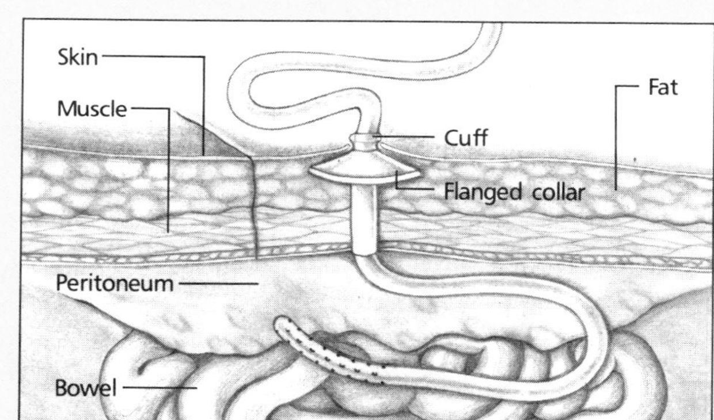

Column-disk peritoneal catheter

To insert a column-disk peritoneal catheter, the surgeon rolls up the flexible disk section of the implant, inserts it into the peritoneal cavity, and retracts it against the abdominal wall. The implant's first cuff rests just outside the peritoneal membrane, and its second cuff rests just beneath the skin. Because this catheter doesn't float freely in the peritoneal cavity, it keeps in-flowing dialysate from being directed at the sensitive organs—which increases patient comfort during dialysis.

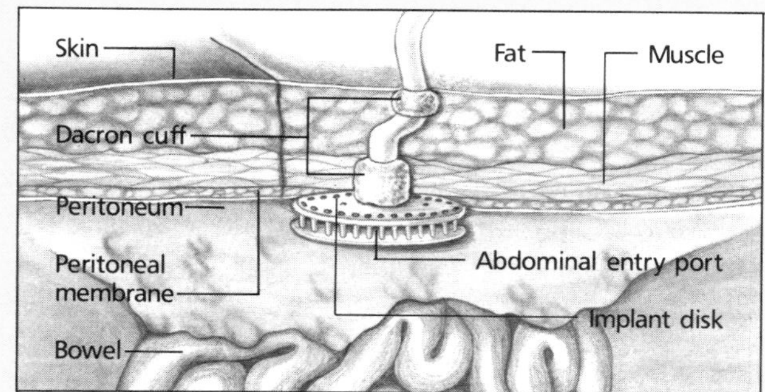

monly order heparin (to decrease fibrin formation), potassium chloride, antibiotics, or insulin. After adding medications, mix the solution well and label the container with the drug, dose, time added, and your initials.

Essential steps

- Place the patient in the supine position, and have him put on a sterile face mask.
- Wash your hands.
- Inspect the warmed dialysate, which should appear clear and colorless.
- Put on a sterile mask.
- Prepare the dialysis administration set.
- Close the clamps on all lines. Place the drainage bag below the patient to facilitate gravity drainage, and connect the drainage line to it. Connect the dialysate infusion lines to the bottles or bags of dialysate.
- Place a povidone-iodine sponge on the dialysate container's port. Cover the port with a dry gauze pad and secure the pad with tape. This must be done with each exchange to help to prevent microorganisms from entering.
- Hang the bottles or bags on the I.V. pole at the patient's bedside. To prime the tubing, open the infusion lines and allow the solution to flow until all lines are primed. Then close all clamps.
- At this point, the doctor puts on a mask and a pair of sterile gloves. He cleans the patient's abdomen with povidone-iodine solution and drapes it with a fenestrated sterile drape.
- Wipe the stopper of the lidocaine vial with a povidone-iodine sponge and allow it to dry. Invert the vial and hand it to the doctor so he can withdraw the lidocaine, using the 3-ml syringe with the 25G 1″ needle.
- The doctor anesthetizes a small area of the patient's abdomen below the umbilicus. He then makes a small incision with the scalpel, inserts the catheter into the peritoneal cavity, using the stylet to guide it, and sutures or tapes the catheter in place.
- Connect the catheter to the administration set, using strict aseptic technique to prevent contamination of the catheter and the solution, which could cause peritonitis.
- Open the drain dressing and the 4″ × 4″ gauze pad packages. Put on sterile gloves. Apply the precut drain dressings around the catheter. Cover them with the gauze pads and tape them securely.
- Unclamp the lines to the patient. Rapidly instill 500 ml of dialysate into the peritoneal cavity to test the catheter's patency.
- Clamp the lines to the patient. Immediately unclamp the lines to the drainage bag to allow fluid to drain into the bag. Outflow should be brisk.
- Having established the catheter's patency, clamp the lines to the drainage bag and unclamp the lines to the patient to infuse the prescribed volume of solution over a period of 5 to 10 minutes. As soon as the dialysate container empties, clamp the lines to the patient to prevent air from entering the tubing.
- Allow the solution to dwell in the peritoneal cavity for the prescribed time (10 minutes to 4 hours). This lets excess fluid, electrolytes, and accumulated wastes move from the blood through the peritoneal membrane and into the dialysate.
- Warm the solution for the next infusion.
- At the end of the prescribed dwell time, unclamp the line to the drainage bag and allow the solution to drain from the peritoneal cavity into the drainage bag.
- Repeat the infusion-dwell-drain cycle immediately after outflow until the prescribed number of fluid exchanges has been completed.
- If a dialysate specimen is ordered, always obtain it during the drain phase of the infusion-dwell-drain cycle. To do this, attach the 10-ml syringe to the 22G 1″ needle and insert it into the injection port of the drainage line, using strict aseptic technique; then aspirate the drainage specimen. Transfer the specimen to its collection container, label it appropriately, and send it to the laboratory with a laboratory request form.
- After completing the prescribed number of exchanges, clamp the catheter, and put on a new pair of sterile gloves and a new sterile mask. Disconnect the administration set from the peritoneal catheter. Place the sterile protective cap over the catheter's distal end. If ordered, instill the prescribed dose of heparin into the peritoneal catheter before applying the cap.

To change dressings

- Explain the procedure to the patient and wash your hands.
- If necessary, carefully remove the old dressings to avoid putting tension on the catheter and accidentally dislodging it and to avoid introducing bacteria into the tract through catheter movement.
- Put on the sterile gloves.
- Saturate the sterile cotton-tipped applicators or the sterile 2″ × 2″ gauze pads with povidone-iodine solution, and clean the skin around the catheter, moving in concentric circles from the catheter site outward. Use a new applicator or pad after each wipe. Remove any crusted material carefully.
- Inspect the catheter site for drainage and the tissue around the site for redness and swelling.
- Apply povidone-iodine ointment to the catheter site with a sterile gauze pad.
- Place two precut drain dressings around the catheter site. Tape the sterile 4″ × 4″ gauze pads over them to secure the dressing. Or apply a large adhesive bandage instead of a gauze dressing.

Cautions

To reduce the risk of peritonitis, use strict aseptic technique during catheter insertion, dialysis, and dressing changes. Masks should be worn by everyone in the room whenever the dialysis system is opened or entered. Change the dressing at least every 24 hours or whenever it becomes wet or soiled. Frequent dressing changes will also help prevent skin excoriation from any leakage.

To prevent respiratory distress, position the patient for maximal lung expansion. Promote lung expansion through turning and deep-breathing exercises. If the patient suffers severe respiratory distress during the dwell phase of dialysis, drain the peritoneal cavity and notify the doctor. Monitor any patient on peritoneal dialysis who's being weaned from a ventilator.

To prevent protein depletion, the doctor may order a high-protein diet or a protein supplement. He will also monitor serum albumin levels.

Dialysate is available in three concentrations: 4.25% dextrose, 2.5% dextrose, and 1.5% dextrose. The 4.25% solution usually removes the largest amount of fluid from the blood because its glucose concentration is highest. If your patient receives this concentration of solution, monitor him carefully to prevent excess fluid loss. Also, some of the glucose in the 4.25% solution may enter the patient's bloodstream, causing hyperglycemia severe enough to require an insulin injection or an insulin addition to the dialysate.

Patients with low serum potassium levels (especially those on hourly exchanges) may require the addition of potassium to the dialysate solution to prevent further losses.

Monitoring and aftercare

- During and after dialysis, monitor the patient and his response to treatment. Monitor his vital signs every 10 to 15 minutes for the first 1 to 2 hours of exchanges, then every 2 to 4 hours or more frequently if necessary. Notify the doctor of any abrupt changes in the patient's condition. Also, examine the outflow fluid (effluent) for color and clarity. (See *Myths and facts about peritoneal dialysis.*)
- Assess fluid balance at the end of each infusion-dwell-drain cycle. Fluid balance is positive if less than the amount infused was recovered; it's negative if more than the amount infused was recovered. Notify the doctor if the patient retains 500 ml or more of fluid for three consecutive cycles or if he loses at least 1 liter of fluid for three consecutive cycles. You can also weigh the dialysate. A 2-liter bag of dialysate weighs approximately 4¾ lb (2.15 kg).
- To further assess fluid balance, weigh the patient daily immediately after the drain phase. Note the time and any variations in the weighing technique next to his weight on the chart. Also measure the patient's abdominal girth daily. Use a permanent marker to identify the measurement area on the patient's skin. Check the patient's skin texture and turgor, the moistness of his mucous membranes, and his extremities or dependent areas for edema every 8 hours.
- If inflow and outflow are slow or absent, check the tubing for kinks. You can also try

Myths and facts about peritoneal dialysis

Myth	Fact
The only reason to warm dialysate before administration is for patient comfort.	Although warmed dialysate helps prevent pain and cramping, warming the fluid to body temperature (not just room temperature) also helps increase urea clearance. To warm dialysate, apply dry heat, such as a heat lamp or heating pad, to the fluid for 2 hours before administration. Avoid using moist heat, which increases the risk of contamination, or placing the dialysate in a microwave oven, which causes uneven warming.
Because patients receiving peritoneal dialysis on a long-term basis have higher-than-normal hematocrit levels, they don't need iron sulfate supplements.	Patients receiving peritoneal dialysis have slightly elevated hematocrit levels because they have less extracellular fluid. However, dialysis does remove iron. Therefore, these patients need iron sulfate supplements.
The color of outflow fluid (effluent) from peritoneal dialysis normally ranges from clear to pale yellow to light amber.	Only clear or pale yellow effluent is normal. Amber fluid suggests occult blood or even a bladder perforation; brown fluid indicates a perforated bowel; milky or opaque fluid suggests peritonitis; and bloody fluid signals abdominal bleeding. Notify the doctor of any of these abnormal findings.
After a peritoneal catheter is inserted, the effluent will be blood-tinged for the first 24 hours.	Although you can expect to see blood-tinged effluent for the first three or four exchanges after catheter insertion, the persistence of blood after that suggests perforation. If the effluent remains blood-tinged, or if it's grossly bloody, suspect bleeding into the peritoneal cavity and notify the doctor.
You needn't be concerned about infection unless the effluent is cloudy.	Although cloudy effluent does indicate infection, it's typically a late sign. Earlier signs and symptoms include abdominal pain, fever, fibrin in the dialysate, and a white blood cell (WBC) count above 10,000/mm^3. If you note these findings, notify the doctor. In turn, the doctor may ask you to obtain a specimen of the effluent for a culture and WBC count. If the WBC count exceeds 100/mm^3, with more than 50% of the cells being neutrophils, suspect infection.

raising the I.V. pole or repositioning the patient to increase the inflow rate. Repositioning the patient, applying manual pressure to the lateral aspects of the patient's abdomen, or administering an enema may also help increase drainage. If these maneuvers fail, notify the doctor. Improper positioning of the catheter or an accumulation of fibrin may obstruct the catheter.

• Patient discomfort at the start of the procedure is normal. If the patient experiences pain during the procedure, determine when it occurs, its quality and duration, and whether it radiates to other body parts. Then notify the doctor. Pain during infusion usually results from a dialysate that's too cool or acidic. Pain may also result from rapid inflow; if that's the case, slowing the inflow rate may reduce the pain. Severe, diffuse pain with rebound tenderness and cloudy effluent may indicate peritoneal infection. Pain that radiates to the shoulder commonly results from air accumulation under the diaphragm. Severe, persistent perineal or rectal pain can result from improper catheter placement.

• The patient undergoing peritoneal dialysis requires a great deal of assistance in his daily care. To minimize his discomfort, perform daily care during the drain phase of the cycle, when the patient's abdomen is less distended. Catheters inserted at the bedside are temporary, so patient activity is limited.

• Record the amount of dialysate infused and drained, any medications added, and the color and character of effluent. Also record the patient's daily weight and fluid balance.

• Avoid using a microwave oven to warm dialysate. But if you must use one, be sure to mix the solution after heating and then manually measure the temperature. Microwave ovens distribute heat unevenly. This means that a bag of dialysate warmed in a microwave oven may feel tepid in one spot but be overheated in another. This overheated solution may injure the patient.

• Use a peritoneal dialysis flowchart to compute total fluid balance after each exchange. Note the patient's vital signs and tolerance of the treatment as well as other pertinent observations. Use a new flowchart every 24 hours.

Continuous arteriovenous hemofiltration

This procedure filters fluid, solutes, and electrolytes from the patient's blood and infuses a replacement solution. Continuous arteriovenous hemofiltration (CAVH) is used to treat patients who have fluid overload but who don't require dialysis. (A similar procedure, continuous arteriovenous filtration and hemodialysis, combines hemodialysis with hemofiltration. Like CAVH, it can also be performed in patients with hypotension and fluid overload.)

The hemofilter used in CAVH, composed of about 5,000 hollow fiber capillaries, filters blood at a rate of about 250 ml/minute and is driven by the patient's arterial blood pressure (a systolic blood pressure of 60 mm Hg is adequate for the procedure). Some of the ultrafiltrate collected during CAVH is replaced with a filter replacement fluid (FRF). This fluid can be lactated Ringer's solution or any solution that resembles plasma. Because the amount of fluid removed is greater than the amount replaced, the patient gradually loses fluid (12 to 15 liters daily).

CAVH carries a much lower risk of hypotension from fluid withdrawal than conventional hemodialysis because it withdraws fluid more slowly—at only 5 to 10 ml/minute (compared with 200 ml/minute or more for hemodialysis). CAVH can be performed in hypotensive patients who require fluid removal, who cannot have peritoneal dialysis, or whose requirements for parenteral nutrition would make fluid volume control problematic. Additionally, CAVH reduces the risk of other complications, including cramps, nausea, vomiting, and headache. And because it withdraws fluid slowly, CAVH makes maintaining a stable fluid volume and regulating fluid and electrolyte balance easier. The procedure costs less than hemodialysis, and the equipment is easier to operate. As a result, CAVH may be performed in a critical care setting and doesn't require the technical expertise of a dialysis nurse.

Indications

• Fluid overload that doesn't respond to diuretics
• Electrolyte and acid-base imbalances
• Acute renal failure, when hemodialysis and peritoneal dialysis are contraindicated

Contraindications and complications

CAVH is contraindicated in patients who have a mean arterial pressure less than 60 mm Hg. Complications include bleeding, hemorrhage, infection, hemofilter occlusion, and thrombosis.

Equipment

CAVH tray • heparin flush solution • occlusive dressings for catheter insertion sites • sterile gloves • sterile mask • povidone-iodine solution • sterile 4" × 4" gauze pads • tape • FRF (as ordered) • infusion pump

Preparation

• Explain the procedure to the patient; then wash your hands. Prime the hemofilter and tubing according to the manufacturer's instructions. Because the filter contains preservatives used in packaging, pay strict attention to the amount of I.V. fluid needed to prime the filter. (See *CAVH setup.*)

• If necessary, help the doctor insert the catheters into the femoral artery and vein, using strict aseptic technique. In some cases, an internal AV fistula or graft or an external AV access may be used instead of the femoral route.)

• If ordered, flush both catheters with heparin flush solution to prevent clotting. Apply occlusive dressings to the insertion sites, and mark the dressings with the date and time. Secure the tubing and connections with tape.

ADVANCED EQUIPMENT

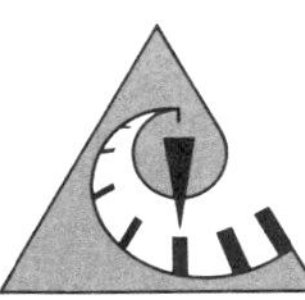

CAVH setup

This illustration shows the correct setup for continuous arteriovenous hemofiltration (CAVH) equipment.

During CAVH, the patient's arterial blood pressure serves as a natural pump, driving blood through the arterial line. A hemofilter removes water and toxic solutes (ultrafiltrate) from the blood. Filter replacement fluid (FRF) is infused into a port on the arterial side; this same port can be used to infuse heparin. The venous line carries the replacement fluid, along with purified blood, to the patient.

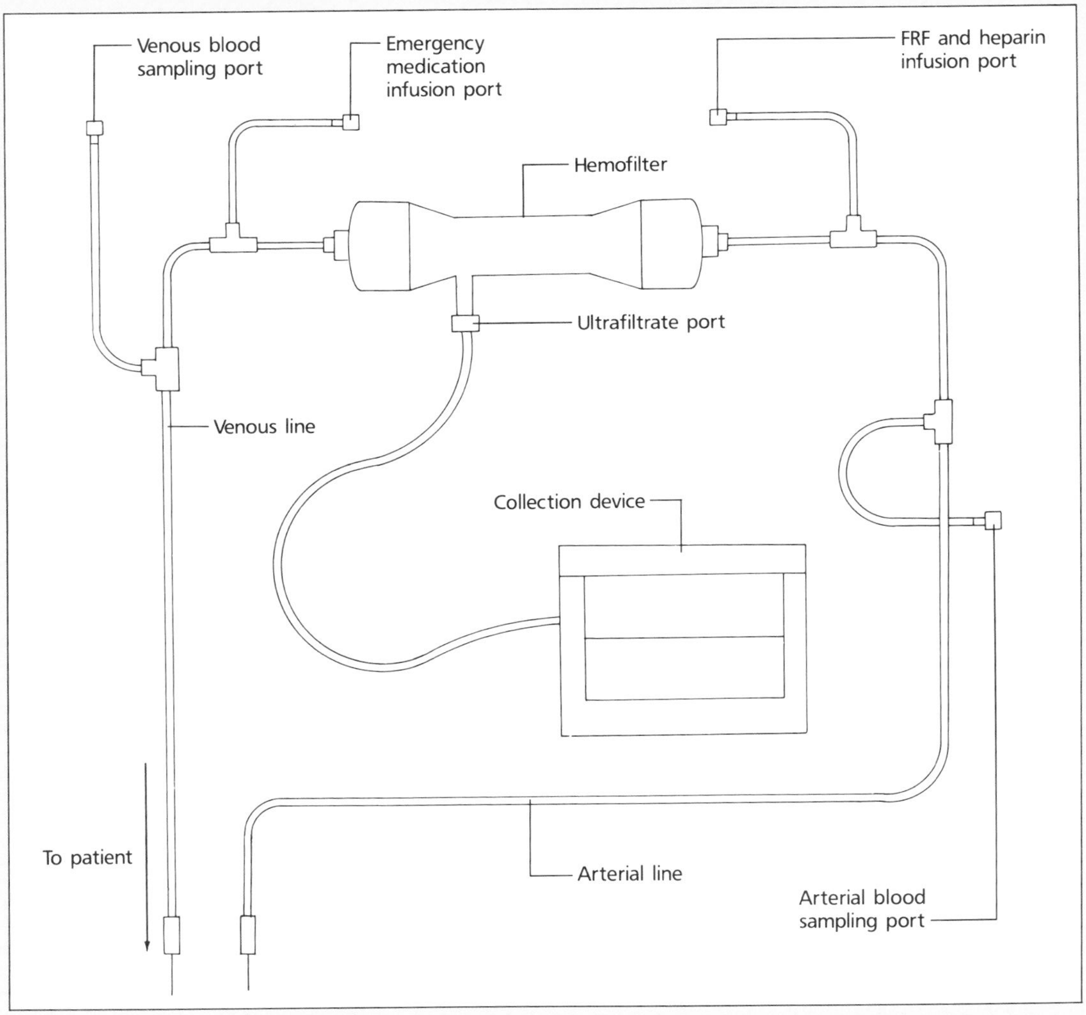

Venous blood sampling port
Emergency medication infusion port
FRF and heparin infusion port
Hemofilter
Ultrafiltrate port
Venous line
Collection device
To patient
Arterial line
Arterial blood sampling port

SKILL TIP

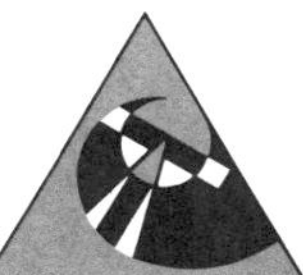

Calculating the right amount of FRF

To calculate the amount of filter replacement fluid (FRF) to infuse into a patient undergoing continuous arteriovenous hemofiltration, you need to know:

- the amount of ultrafiltrate produced during the previous hour
- the patient's other outputs during the previous hour, such as urine, feces, and nasogastric or chest drainage
- the patient's I.V. intake during the previous hour, including total parenteral nutrition, lipids, I.V. drips, medication boluses, heparin infusion (if applicable), and tube feedings
- the net desired hourly fluid loss, as determined by the doctor.

Calculations

Once you've obtained these figures, all you have to do to calculate the amount of FRF is subtract the patient's I.V. intake and desired fluid loss from the total of his ultrafiltrate production and other outputs. The equation would read:

(ultrafiltrate + other outputs)
− (I.V. intake + fluid loss)
= FRF

Let's say, for example, that your patient's ultrafiltrate production during the previous hour was 750 ml, and his other outputs amounted to 60 ml, for a total of 810 ml of output. And let's say that his I.V. intake for the previous hour was 130 ml and his doctor wanted him to lose 100 ml of fluid every hour. Plugging these numbers into the equation would give you:

(750 + 60)
− (130 + 100)
= 580

So, over the next hour, you'd want to infuse a total of 580 ml of FRF. If the patient had received an unusually large amount of I.V. fluids or medications during the previous hour, or if his ultrafiltrate production were very low because of clotting in the hemofilter, the above equation might yield a minimal or negative FRF. In these cases, you can skip the FRF infusion for the next hour or simply continue it at a keep-vein-open rate of 10 ml/hour.

- Assess all pulses in the affected leg before and immediately after catheter insertion. Weigh the patient, take baseline vital signs, and make sure that all necessary laboratory studies have been done (usually electrolyte levels, coagulation factors, complete blood count, and blood urea nitrogen and creatinine levels).

Essential steps

- Put on the sterile gloves and mask. Prepare the connection sites by cleaning them with gauze pads soaked in povidone-iodine solution; then connect them to the exit port of each catheter.
- Connect the arterial and venous lines to the hemofilter, using aseptic technique.
- Turn on the hemofilter, and monitor the blood flow rate through the circuit. The flow rate usually ranges from 500 to 900 ml/hour. Keep the hemofilter at heart level, taping it to the patient's leg if necessary.
- Calculate the amount of FRF every hour or as dictated by your hospital's policy. Then infuse the prescribed amount and type of FRF through the infusion pump into the arterial side of the circuit. (See *Calculating the right amount of FRF.*)

Cautions

Clamping the ultrafiltrate line is contraindicated with some types of hemofilters because pressure may build up in the filter, clotting it and collapsing the blood compartment.

Because blood flows through an extracorporeal circuit during CAVH, the blood in the hemofilter may need to be anticoagulated. To do this, infuse heparin in low doses (usually starting at 500 units/hour) into an infusion port on the arterial side of the setup. Then measure thrombin clotting time or activated clotting time (ACT). This ensures that the circuit, not the patient, is anticoagulated. ACT is normally 100 seconds; during CAVH, keep it between 100 and 300 seconds, depending on the patient's clotting times. If ACT is too high or too low, the doctor will adjust the heparin dose accordingly or write parameters.

Another way to prevent clotting in the hemofilter is not to infuse medications or blood through the venous line. This line may be used in emergencies to infuse I.V. fluids but will slow the return of dialyzed blood to the patient, increasing the risk of clotting. Run infusions through another line if possible.

A third way to help prevent clots in the hemofilter and to prevent kinks in the catheter is to make sure the patient doesn't bend the affected leg more than 30 degrees at the hip. The patient may logroll from side to side with assistance. When helping the patient turn, be sure to move the patient and the hemofilter as a single unit.

Monitoring and aftercare

- Monitor the patient's weight daily and vital signs and hemodynamics at least hourly. If needed, draw specimens for laboratory tests from the ultrafiltrate. To accurately monitor the amount of ultrafiltrate, consider using an infusion pump.
- Inspect the ultrafiltrate during the procedure. It should remain clear yellow, with no gross blood. Pink-tinged or bloody ultrafiltrate may signal a membrane leak in the hemofilter, which would leave the blood compartment open to contamination from bacteria. If a leak is suspected or occurs, notify the doctor so that he can have the hemofilter replaced.
- Assess all pulses in the affected leg at least every hour for the first 4 hours, then every 2 hours thereafter. Also check for signs of obstructed blood flow, such as coolness, pallor, and a weak pulse. Check the groin area on the affected side for signs of hematoma. Also, ask the patient if he has pain at the insertion sites.
- To prevent infection, perform skin care at the catheter insertion sites every 48 hours, using aseptic technique. Cover the sites with an occlusive dressing. Also change the hemofilter and tubing at least every 72 hours.
- Check the connection sites to be sure they're taped securely. Blood loss from a sudden disconnection in the circuit could cause serious complications. Keep four clamps at the bedside at all times to use in an emergency.
- If the ultrafiltrate flow rate decreases, raise the bed to increase the distance between the collection device and the hemofilter. Lower the bed to decrease the flow rate.
- Record the time the treatment began and ended. Also record fluid balance information, times of dressing changes, any complications and subsequent interventions, and the patient's tolerance of the procedure and any medications given. Use a 24-hour flowchart to record fluid balance.

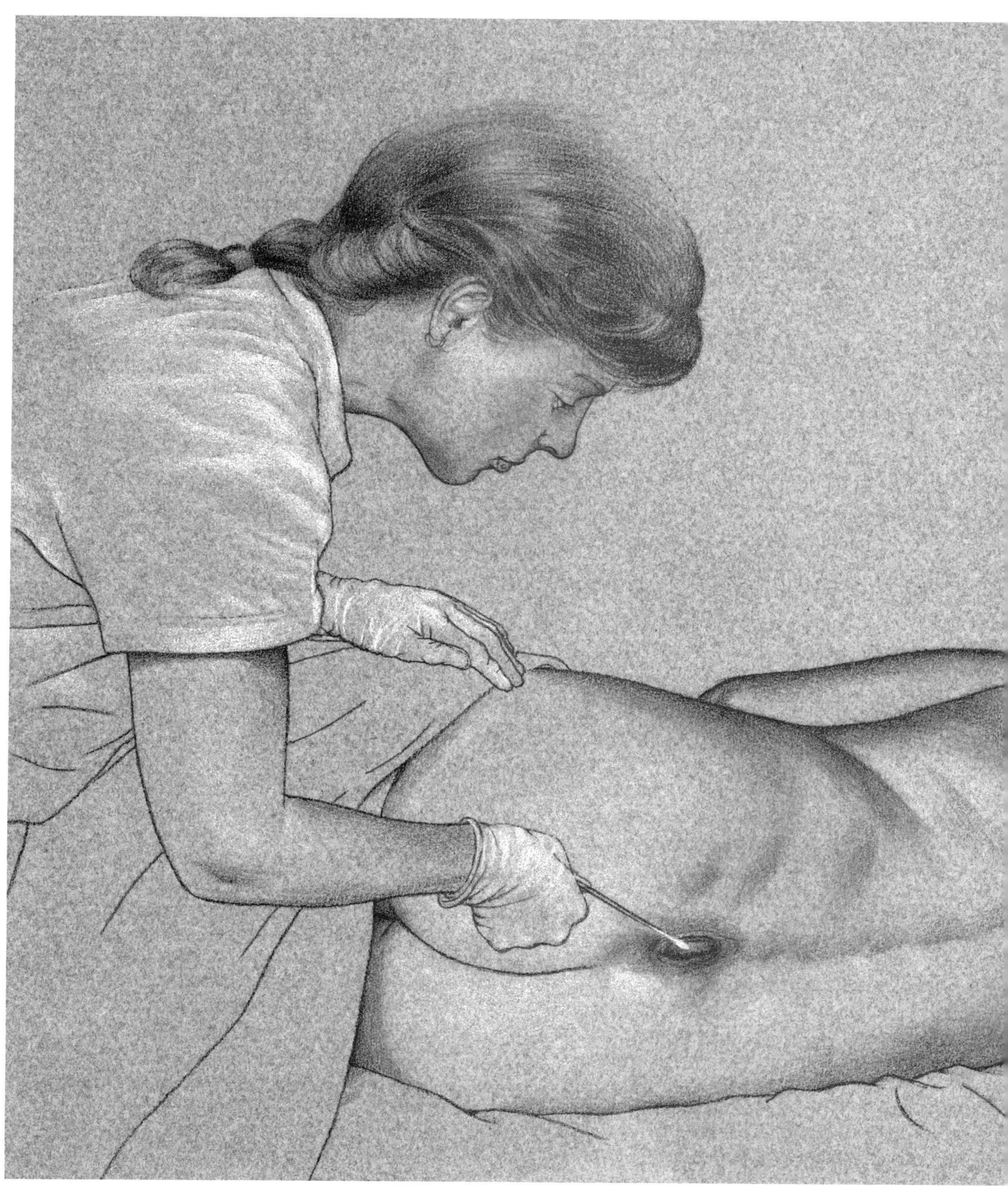

CHAPTER 6

Skin and wound care

The skin has many functions. It protects internal body structures from the environment and potential pathogens. It regulates body temperature and homeostasis and acts as an organ of sensation and excretion. It also helps shape a person's self-image.

That's why meticulous skin care is essential to your patient's overall health. If pressure ulcers, burns, or other lesions compromise his skin integrity, you must take steps to prevent or control infection, promote new skin growth, control pain, and provide emotional support.

The skin serves as the first line of defense against infection. So any threat to its integrity increases the risk of infection. Besides delaying healing, infection can worsen pain and even jeopardize the patient's life. Most burn deaths, for instance, result from complications of infection, not from the burns themselves.

To control infection and avoid introducing new pathogens into an already contaminated wound, you must use sterile technique. You can control infection by washing your hands thoroughly with an antiseptic agent and by using sterile equipment during wound care.

To enhance natural healing, skin wounds need regular dressing changes, thorough cleaning and, if necessary, debridement to remove debris, reduce bacterial growth, and encourage tissue repair. To control pain effectively, you must evaluate your patient's response to pain and adapt your techniques accordingly.

A patient with a disfiguring and painful skin disorder may have to deal with depression, frustration, and anger. Along with physical support, you must provide continuing emotional support as he develops coping mechanisms to adjust to his altered self-image.

This chapter discusses important procedures for skin and wound care. For each procedure, you'll find key information on the indications, contraindications, complications, and necessary equipment. You'll also find out about patient preparation, step-by-step directions for carrying out the procedure, cautions, and patient monitoring and aftercare.

Surgical wound management

When caring for a surgical wound, you carry out procedures that help prevent infection by stopping pathogens from entering the wound. Besides promoting patient comfort, such procedures also protect the skin surface from maceration and excoriation caused by contact with irritating drainage. They also allow you to measure wound drainage to monitor fluid and electrolyte balance.

The two primary methods used to manage a draining surgical wound are dressing and pouching. Dressing is preferred unless caustic or excessive drainage is compromising your patient's skin integrity. Usually, lightly seeping wounds with drains and wounds with minimal purulent drainage can be managed with packing and gauze dressings. Some wounds, such as those that become chronic, may require an occlusive dressing.

A wound with copious, excoriating drainage calls for pouching to protect the surrounding skin. If your patient has a surgical wound, you must monitor him and choose the appropriate dressing.

Dressing a wound calls for sterile technique and sterile supplies to prevent contamination. You may use the color of the wound to help determine which type of dressing to apply. (See *Tailoring wound care to wound color.*) Be sure to change the dressing often enough to keep the skin dry.

Indications

- To help prevent infection
- To protect the skin surface from maceration and excoriation
- To allow measurement of wound drainage
- To enhance patient comfort

Contraindications and complications

Surgical wound care has no contraindications, but a major complication of a dressing change is an allergic reaction to an antiseptic cleaning agent, a prescribed topical medication, or adhesive tape. This reaction may lead to skin redness, rash, excoriation, or infection.

Equipment

Waterproof trash bag • clean gloves • sterile gloves • gown, if indicated • sterile 4" × 4" gauze pads • ABD pads, if indicated • sterile cotton-tipped applicators • sterile dressing set • povidone-iodine swabs • topical medication, if ordered • adhesive or other tape • soap and water • optional: skin protectant; nonadherent pads; collodion spray, acetone-free adhesive remover, or baby oil; sterile 0.9% sodium chloride solution; graduated container; and Montgomery straps, a fishnet tube elasticized dressing support, or a T-binder

For a wound with a drain

Sterile scissors • sterile 4" × 4" gauze pads without cotton lining • sump drain • ostomy pouch or other collection bag • precut tracheostomy pads or drain dressings • adhesive tape (paper or silk tape if the patient is hypersensitive) • surgical mask

Tailoring wound care to wound color

With any wound, promote healing by keeping it moist, clean, and free of debris. If your patient has an open wound (one healing by secondary intention), you can assess how well it's healing by inspecting its color, and use wound color to guide the specific management approach.

Red wounds

Red, the color of healthy granulation tissue, indicates normal healing. When a wound begins to heal, a layer of pale pink granulation tissue covers the wound bed. As this layer thickens, it becomes beefy red. Cover a red wound, keep it moist and clean, and protect it from trauma. Use a transparent dressing (such as Tegaderm or Op-Site), a hydrocolloid dressing (such as DuoDerm), or a gauze dressing moistened with sterile 0.9% sodium chloride solution or impregnated with petroleum jelly or an antibiotic.

Yellow wounds

Yellow is the color of exudate produced by microorganisms in an open wound. When a wound heals without complications, the immune system removes microorganisms. But if there are too many microorganisms to remove, exudate accumulates and becomes visible. Exudate usually appears whitish yellow, creamy yellow, yellowish green, or beige. Water content influences the shade, with exudate appearing darker when dry.

If your patient has a yellow wound, clean it, remove exudate using high-pressure irrigation; then cover it with a moist dressing. Use absorptive products (for example, Debrisan beads and paste) or a moist gauze dressing with or without an antibiotic. You may also use hydrotherapy with whirlpool or high-pressure irrigation.

Black wounds

Black, the least healthy color, signals necrosis. Dead, avascular tissue slows healing and provides a site for microorganisms to proliferate.

You should debride a black wound. After removing dead tissue, apply a dressing to keep the wound moist and guard against external contamination. As ordered, use enzyme products (such as Elase or Travase), surgical debridement, hydrotherapy with whirlpool or high-pressure irrigation, or a moist gauze dressing.

Multicolored wounds

You may note two or even all three colors in a wound. In this case, you'd classify the wound according to the least healthy color present. For example, if your patient's wound is both red and yellow, classify it as a yellow wound.

For pouching a wound

Collection pouch with drainage port • sterile gloves • skin protectant • sterile gauze pads

Preparation

- Explain the procedure to the patient to allay his anxiety.
- Ask the patient about allergies to tapes and dressings.
- Assemble all equipment in the patient's room.
- Check the expiration date on each sterile package and inspect for tears.
- Open the waterproof trash bag and place it near the patient's bed.
- Position the bag to avoid reaching across the sterile field or the wound when disposing of soiled articles.
- Form a cuff by turning down the top of the trash bag to provide a wide opening and to prevent contamination of instruments or gloves by touching the bag's edge.

Essential steps

Removing the old dressing

- Check the doctor's order for specific wound care and medication instructions. Be sure to note the location of surgical drains to avoid dislodging them during the procedure.
- Assess the patient's condition.

• Identify the patient's allergies, especially to adhesive tape, povidone-iodine or other topical solutions, or medications.
• Provide the patient with privacy, and position him as necessary. To avoid chilling him, expose only the wound site.
• Wash your hands thoroughly. Put on a gown, if necessary, to shield your clothing from wound drainage. Then put on clean gloves.
• Loosen the soiled dressing by holding the patient's skin and pulling the tape or dressing toward the wound. This protects the newly formed tissue and prevents stress on the incision. Moisten the tape with acetone-free adhesive remover or baby oil, if necessary, to make the tape removal less painful (particularly if the skin is hairy). Don't apply solvents to the incision because these could contaminate the wound.
• Slowly remove the soiled dressing. If the gauze adheres to the wound, loosen the gauze by moistening it with sterile 0.9% sodium chloride solution.
• Observe the dressing for the amount, type, color, and odor of drainage.
• Discard the dressing and gloves in the waterproof trash bag.

Caring for the wound

• Wash your hands. Establish a sterile field with all the equipment and supplies you'll need for suture-line care and the dressing change, including a sterile dressing set and povidone-iodine swabs. If the doctor has ordered ointment, squeeze the needed amount onto the sterile field. If you're using an antiseptic from an unsterile bottle, pour the antiseptic cleaning agent into a sterile container so you won't contaminate your gloves. Then put on sterile gloves.
• Saturate the sterile gauze pads with the prescribed cleaning agent. Avoid using cotton balls because these may shed fibers in the wound, causing irritation, infection, or adhesion.
• If ordered, obtain a wound culture; then proceed to clean the wound. (See *Obtaining an aerobic wound culture specimen.*)
• Pick up the moistened gauze pad or swab, and squeeze out the excess solution.
• Working from the top of the incision, wipe once to the bottom and then discard the gauze pad. With a second moistened pad, wipe from top to bottom in a vertical path next to the incision.
• Continue to work outward from the incision in lines running parallel to it. Always wipe from the clean area toward the less clean area (usually from top to bottom). Use each gauze pad or swab for only one stroke to avoid tracking wound exudate and normal body flora from surrounding skin to the clean areas. Remember that the suture line is cleaner than the adjacent skin and the top of the suture line is usually cleaner than the bottom because more drainage collects at the bottom of the wound.
• Use sterile cotton-tipped applicators for efficient cleaning of tight-fitting wire sutures, deep and narrow wounds, or wounds with pockets. Because the cotton on the swab is tightly wrapped, it's less likely than a cotton ball to leave fibers in the wound. Remember to wipe only once with each applicator.
• If the patient has a surgical drain, clean the drain's surface last. Because moist drainage promotes bacterial growth, the drain is considered the most contaminated area. Clean the skin around the drain by wiping in half or full circles from the drain site outward.
• Clean all areas of the wound to wash away debris, pus, blood, and necrotic material. Try not to disturb sutures or irritate the incision. Clean to at least 1" (2.5 cm) beyond the end of the new dressing. If you aren't applying a new dressing, clean to at least 2" (5 cm) beyond the incision.
• Check to see that the edges of the incision are lined up properly, and check for signs of infection (heat, redness, swelling, and odor), dehiscence, or evisceration. If you observe such signs or if the patient reports pain at the wound site, notify the doctor.
• Irrigate the wound, as ordered.
• Wash skin surrounding the wound with soap and water, and pat dry using a sterile 4" × 4" gauze pad. Avoid oil-based soap because it may interfere with pouch adherence. Apply any prescribed topical medication.

Obtaining an aerobic wound culture specimen

If the doctor orders an aerobic wound culture specimen, you can help ensure accurate results, asepsis, and patient comfort by following these guidelines when collecting drainage from your patient's wound.

Do's

- Wash your hands and put on disposable gloves. Then remove the old dressing. Note the color, odor, and amount of drainage on it. Put the dressing in a moisture-proof bag.
- Clean the area around the wound with an antiseptic swab, sterile water, or 0.9% sodium chloride solution (according to your hospital's policy) to avoid contaminating the specimen with skin flora. Don't let antiseptic enter the wound.
- Discard your gloves; then open a package of sterile swabs or a commercial kit for an aerobic culture. Put on sterile gloves and open the sterile specimen tube.
- Tell the patient he may feel a tickling sensation when you swab the wound. Then insert the tip of the swab into the wound and gently rotate it, as shown below. Absorb as much exudate as possible.

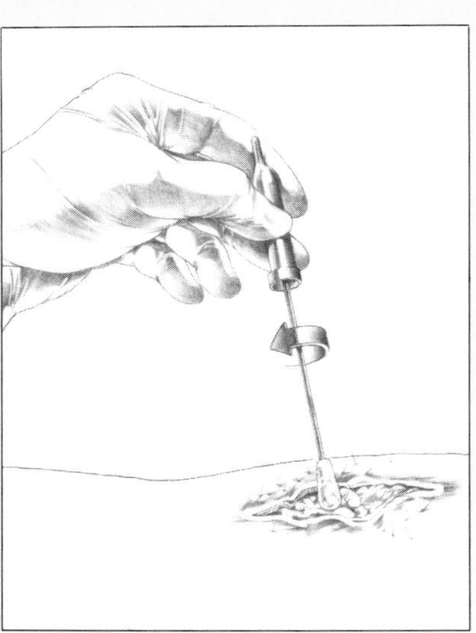

- Insert the swab into the sterile container or culture tube. Cap the container or tube and crush the culture-medium ampule; the culture medium should coat the swab tip. Then close the container or tube securely.

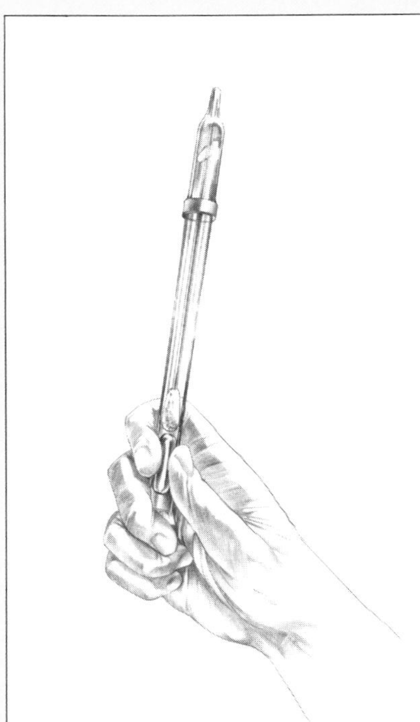

- Label each specimen, noting the exact site it was taken from.
- Clean the wound, as ordered. Then apply a sterile dressing. Send the specimen to the laboratory.

Don'ts

- Be sure not to remove the patient's wound dressing without first assessing whether he needs an analgesic. If he does, give it to him early enough before the dressing change so it will peak at the right time.
- Don't collect the wound culture specimen from old exudate because it may be contaminated with resident bacterial colonies.
- Avoid collecting exudate from the skin, unless it is a separate culture and labeled as such.
- Don't touch the top or outside of the specimen tube with the swab. (The illustration below shows this error in technique.) Those areas should remain free of pathogens that could be spread to others who handle the tube.

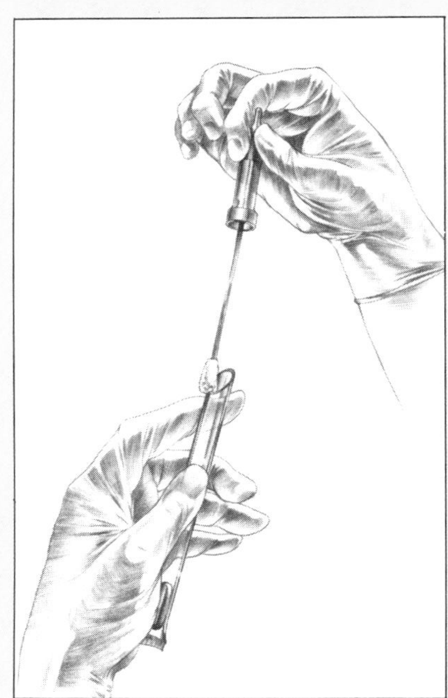

• Apply a skin protectant, if needed.
• If ordered, pack the wound with gauze pads or strips folded to fit. Avoid using cotton-lined gauze pads because cotton fibers can adhere to the wound surface and cause complications. Pack the wound using the wet-to-damp method. Soaking the packing material in solution and wringing it out so it's slightly moist provides a moist wound environment that absorbs debris and drainage. But removing the packing won't disrupt new tissue.

Applying a fresh gauze dressing
• Gently place sterile 4" × 4" gauze pads at the center of the wound, and move progressively outward to the edges of the wound site. Extend the gauze at least 1" (2.5 cm) beyond the incision in each direction, and cover the wound evenly with enough sterile dressings (usually two or three layers) to absorb all drainage until the next dressing change. Use ABD pads to form outer layers, if needed, to provide greater absorbency.
• When the dressing is in place, remove and discard your gloves because the tape may stick to them, making it hard to apply.
• Secure the dressing's edges to the patient's skin with strips of tape to maintain sterility of the wound site. Or secure the dressing with a T-binder or Montgomery straps to prevent skin excoriation that may occur with repeated tape removal necessitated by frequent dressing changes.
• Make sure that the patient is comfortable.
• Properly dispose of the solutions and trash bag, and clean or discard soiled equipment and supplies according to your hospital's policy. If your patient's wound has purulent drainage, don't return unopened sterile supplies to the sterile supply cabinet because this could cause cross-contamination of other equipment.

Dressing a wound with a drain
• Prepare a drain dressing by using sterile scissors to cut a slit in a sterile 4" × 4" gauze pad. Fold the pad in half; then cut inward from the center of the folded edge. Don't use a cotton-lined gauze pad because cutting the gauze opens the lining and releases cotton fibers into the wound. Prepare a second pad the same way.
• Gently press one folded pad close to the skin around the drain so that the tubing fits into the slit. Press the second folded pad around the drain from the opposite direction so that the two pads encircle the tubing.
• Layer as many uncut sterile 4" × 4" gauze pads or ABD pads around the tubing as needed to absorb expected drainage. Tape the dressing in place or use a T-binder or Montgomery straps.

Pouching a wound
• If your patient's wound is draining heavily or if drainage may damage surrounding skin, you'll need to create a pouch.
• Measure the wound. Cut an opening ⅛" (0.3 cm) larger than the wound in the facing of the collection pouch.
• Apply a skin protectant as needed. (Some protectants are incorporated within the collection pouch and also provide adhesion.)
• Make sure that the drainage port at the bottom of the pouch is closed firmly to prevent leaks. Then gently press the contoured pouch opening around the wound, starting at its lower edge, to catch any drainage.
• To empty the pouch, put on gloves, insert the pouch's bottom half into a graduated collection container, and open the drainage port. Note the color, consistency, odor, and amount of fluid. If ordered, obtain a culture specimen and send it to the laboratory immediately. Remember to follow isolation precautions when handling infectious drainage.
• Wipe the bottom of the pouch and the drainage port with a gauze pad to remove any drainage that could irritate the patient's skin or cause an odor. Then reseal the port. Change the pouch only if it leaks or fails to adhere to the skin. More frequent changes are unnecessary and only irritate the patient's skin.

Cautions
If the patient has two wounds in the same area, cover each wound separately with layers of sterile 4" × 4" gauze pads. Then cover both sites with an ABD pad secured to the patient's skin with tape. Don't eliminate the gauze pads

and use only an ABD pad to cover both sites because drainage quickly saturates a single pad, promoting cross-contamination.

When packing a wound, don't pack it too tightly because this compresses adjacent capillaries and may prevent the wound edges from contracting. Avoid using overly damp packing because it slows wound closure from within and increases the risk of infection.

To save time when dressing a wound with a drain, use precut tracheostomy pads or drain dressings instead of custom-cutting gauze pads to fit around the drain. If your patient is sensitive to adhesive tape, use paper or silk tape because these are less likely to cause a skin reaction and will peel off more easily than adhesive tape. Use a surgical mask to cradle a chin or jawline dressing; this provides a secure dressing and avoids the need for shaving the patient's hair.

If ordered, use a collodion spray or similar topical protectant instead of a gauze dressing. Moisture- and contaminant-proof, this covering dries in a clear, impermeable film that leaves the wound visible for observation and avoids the friction caused by a dressing.

If a sump drain isn't adequately collecting wound secretions, reinforce it with an ostomy pouch or other collection bag. Use waterproof tape to strengthen a spot on the front of the pouch near the adhesive opening; then cut a small "X" in the tape. Feed the drain catheter into the pouch through the "X" cut. Seal the cut around the tubing with more waterproof tape; then connect the tubing to the suction pump. This method frees the drainage port at the bottom of the pouch so you don't have to remove the tubing to empty the pouch. If you use more than one collection pouch for a wound or wounds, be sure to record the volume of drainage separately for each pouch. Avoid using waterproof material over the dressing because it reduces air circulation and predisposes the wound to infection from accumulated heat and moisture.

Monitoring and aftercare

- Because many doctors prefer to change the first postoperative dressing themselves to check the incision, don't change the first dressing unless you have specific instructions to do so. If you have no such order and drainage comes through the dressings, reinforce the dressing with fresh sterile gauze. Request an order to change the dressing, or ask the doctor to change it as soon as possible. A reinforced dressing should not remain in place longer than 24 hours because it's an excellent medium for bacterial growth.
- For the recent postoperative patient or a patient with complications, check the dressing every 30 minutes or as ordered. For the patient with a properly healing wound, check the dressing at least once every 8 hours.
- If the dressing becomes wet from the outside (for example, from spilled drinking water, bath water, or urine), replace it as soon as possible to prevent wound contamination.
- Consider all dressings and drains infectious.
- If your patient will need wound care after discharge, provide appropriate teaching. If the patient will be caring for the wound himself, stress the importance of using aseptic technique and teach him how to examine the wound for signs of infection and other wound complications. Also show him how to change dressings, and provide him with written instructions for all procedures to be performed at home.
- Document the date, time, and type of wound management procedure; amount of soiled dressing and packing removed; wound appearance (size, condition of margins, presence of necrotic tissue) and odor (if present); type, color, consistency, and amount of drainage (for each wound); presence and location of drains; any additional procedures, such as irrigation, packing, or application of a topical medication; type and amount of new dressing or pouch applied; and the patient's tolerance for the procedure.
- Document special or detailed wound care instructions and pain management steps on the nursing care plan. Record the color and amount of measurable drainage on the intake and output sheet.

Management of traumatic wounds

Traumatic wounds include abrasions, lacerations, puncture wounds, and amputations. In an abrasion, the skin is scraped, with partial loss of the skin surface. In a laceration, the skin is torn, causing jagged, irregular edges; the severity of a laceration depends on its size, depth, and location. A puncture wound occurs when a pointed object, such as a knife or glass fragment, penetrates the skin. Traumatic amputation refers to removal of a part of the body or a limb or part of a limb.

When caring for a patient with a traumatic wound, first assess his ABCs—airway, breathing, and circulation. It may seem natural to focus on a gruesome injury, but a patent airway and pumping heart take first priority. Once the patient's ABCs are stabilized, you can turn your attention to the traumatic wound. Initial management concentrates on controlling bleeding—usually by applying firm, direct pressure and elevating the extremity. If bleeding continues, you may need to compress a pressure point. (Tourniquets are rarely necessary.) Assess the condition of the wound. Management and cleaning technique usually depend on the specific type of wound and degree of contamination. A large, deep, or obviously dirty wound may require analgesic administration and special procedures, such as debridement and irrigation.

Indications

- To remove bacteria and prevent infection
- To promote healing
- To minimize scarring

Contraindications and complications

Although there are no contraindications, cleaning and care of traumatic wounds may temporarily increase the patient's pain. Excessive, vigorous cleaning may cause further disruption of tissue integrity.

Equipment

Sterile basin • 0.9% sodium chloride solution • sterile 4″ × 4″ gauze pads • sterile gloves • clean gloves • sterile cotton-tipped applicators • dry sterile dressing, nonadherent pad, or petroleum gauze • linen-saver pad • optional: scissors, towel, goggles, mask, gown, 50-ml catheter-tip syringe, surgical scrub brush, antibacterial ointment, porous tape, sterile forceps, sutures and suture set, hydrogen peroxide

Preparation

- Check the patient's medical history for previous tetanus immunization and, if needed and ordered, arrange for current immunization.
- Explain the procedure to the patient and provide privacy.
- Assess the patient's pain. Administer pain medication, if ordered (except intradermally injected local anesthetics, which the doctor administers).
- Place a linen-saver pad under the area to be cleaned.
- Remove any clothing covering the wound. If necessary, cut hair around the wound with scissors to promote cleaning and treatment.
- Assemble needed equipment at the patient's bedside.
- Fill a sterile basin with 0.9% sodium chloride solution.
- Make sure the treatment area has enough light to allow close observation of the wound.
- Depending on the nature and location of the wound, wear sterile or clean gloves to avoid spreading infection.

Essential steps

- Wash your hands.
- Use appropriate protective equipment, such as a gown, mask, and goggles, if spraying or splashing of body fluids is possible.

For an abrasion

- Flush the scraped skin with 0.9% sodium chloride solution.
- Remove dirt or gravel with a sterile 4″ × 4″ gauze pad moistened with 0.9% sodium chloride solution. Rub in the opposite direction from which the dirt or gravel became embedded.
- If the wound is extremely dirty, you may use a surgical brush to scrub it.

• With a small wound, allow it to dry and form a scab. With a larger wound, you may need to cover it with a nonadherent pad or petroleum gauze and a light dressing. Apply antibacterial ointment if ordered.

For a laceration

• Moisten a sterile 4″ × 4″ gauze pad with 0.9% sodium chloride solution. Clean the wound gently, working outward from its center to approximately 2″ (5 cm) beyond its edges. Discard the soiled gauze pad and use a fresh one as necessary.
• Continue until the wound appears clean.
• If the wound is dirty, you may irrigate it with a 50-ml catheter-tip syringe and 0.9% sodium chloride solution. (See "Wound irrigation," page 182.)
• Assist the doctor in suturing the wound edges using the suture kit, or apply sterile strips of porous tape.
• Apply the ordered antibacterial ointment to help prevent infection.
• Apply a dry sterile dressing over the wound to absorb drainage and help prevent bacterial contamination.

For a puncture wound

• If the wound is minor, allow it to bleed for a few minutes before cleaning it.
• For a larger puncture wound, you may need to irrigate it before applying a dry dressing. (See "Wound irrigation," page 182.)
• Stabilize any embedded foreign object until the doctor can remove it. After he removes the object and bleeding is stabilized, clean the wound as you'd clean a laceration or deep puncture wound.

For an amputation

• Apply a gauze pad moistened with 0.9% sodium chloride solution dressing to the amputation site. Elevate the affected part and immobilize it for surgery.
• Recover the amputated part and prepare it for transport to a facility where microvascular surgery is performed. (See *Caring for an amputated part.*)

SKILL TIP

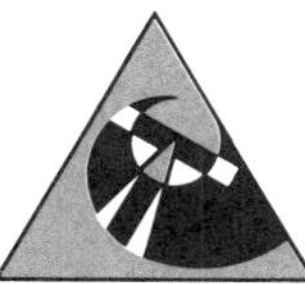

Caring for an amputated part

If your patient has suffered a traumatic amputation, wrap the amputated body part in dry, sterile gauze.

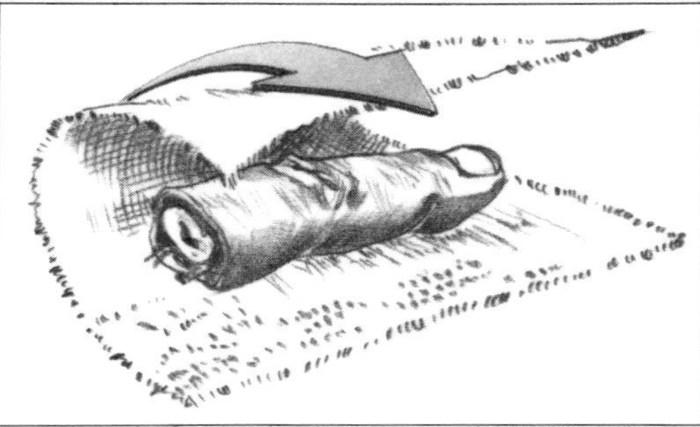

Place the body part in a plastic bag or other waterproof container.

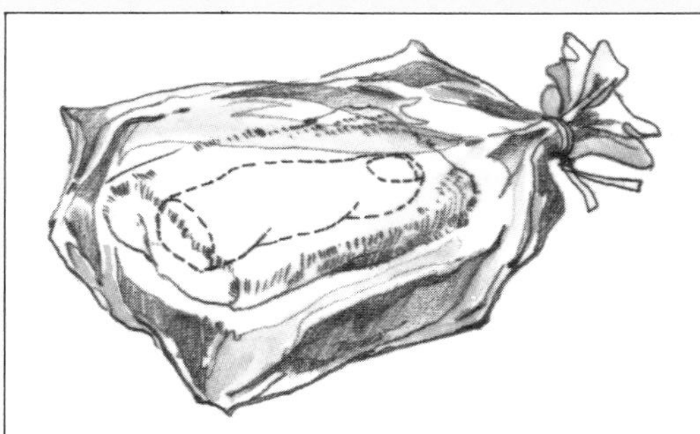

Place this container on a bed of ice—but *don't* bury it in ice.

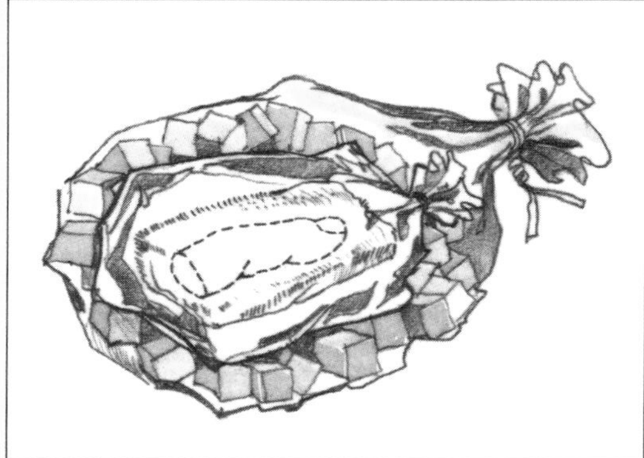

Cautions

Don't use more than 8 pounds per square inch of pressure when irrigating a traumatic wound. High-pressure irrigation can seriously interfere with healing, kill cells, and push bacteria into the tissue.

To clean the wound, you may use hydrogen peroxide, which causes debris to bubble to the surface so that it's easier to clean away. However, *never* instill hydrogen peroxide into a deep wound. Be sure to rinse well after using hydrogen peroxide.

Don't clean a traumatic wound with alcohol because it causes pain and tissue dehydration.

Never use a cotton ball or cotton-filled gauze pad to clean a wound because cotton fibers left in the wound may cause contamination.

Be aware that antiseptics are discouraged for wound cleaning because they can impede healing.

Monitoring and aftercare

• After a wound has been cleaned, the doctor may want to debride it to remove dead tissue and reduce the risk of infection and scarring. If this is necessary, pack the wound with gauze pads soaked in 0.9% sodium chloride solution until debridement.
• Observe for signs and symptoms of infection, such as red warm skin at the site or purulent discharge. Be aware that infection of a traumatic wound can delay healing, increase scar formation, and trigger systemic infection, such as septicemia.
• Observe all dressings. If edema is present, the dressing should not be tight and constrictive. This could impair circulation to the area.
• Recognize that a wound in an area subjected to repeated traumatic injury may require splinting to promote complete healing.
• Teach the patient how to care for his wound. If necessary, inform him when to return to have sutures removed.
• Document the date and time of the procedure, wound size and condition, medication administration, specific wound care measures, and patient teaching.

Wound irrigation

Irrigation cleans tissue and flushes cell debris and drainage from an open wound. Irrigating with an antiseptic or antibiotic solution helps the wound heal properly from the inside tissue layers outward to the skin surface. It also helps prevent premature surface healing over an abscess pocket or infected tract. Using strict sterile technique, you flush the area with the prescribed solution (usually sterile water, 0.9% sodium chloride solution, or an antiseptic solution). After irrigating, you'll usually pack an open wound to absorb additional drainage. (For other techniques you may use to clean a wound, see *Alternative wound cleaning methods.*).

Indications

Wound irrigation is used to clean and flush a deep, open wound.

Contraindications and complications

There are no contraindications, but wound irrigation increases the risk of infection. It may also cause excoriation and increased pain.

Equipment

Sterile irrigation set (basin, container for irrigant, 50- to 60-ml piston syringe) • prescribed irrigating solution • sterile, soft rubber catheter • sterile gloves • gown • goggles, if indicated • mask, if indicated • clean disposable gloves • sterile dressing set or suture set • waterproof pad • emesis basin • sterile gauze and other materials as needed for wound care • waterproof trash bag • sterile petroleum jelly • bath blanket • adhesive tape • Montgomery straps

Preparation

• Explain the procedure to the patient.
• Administer a prescribed analgesic 30 to 45 minutes before starting the procedure.
• Instruct the patient to tell you if any burning or pain occurs during wound irrigation.
• Check the doctor's order for wound irrigation and type of solution.
• Assemble all equipment in the patient's room.
• Check the expiration date on each sterile package and inspect packages for tears.

• Check the sterilization date and the date each bottle of irrigating solution was opened. Don't use any solution that has been open longer than 24 hours.
• Prepare the prescribed irrigating solution using aseptic technique.
• Using a warm-water bath, warm the irrigating solution to 90° to 95° F (32.2° to 35° C).
• Open the waterproof bag and place it near the patient's bed to avoid reaching across the sterile field or the wound when disposing of soiled articles.
• Form a cuff by turning down the top of the trash bag to provide a wide opening and prevent contamination caused by touching the bag's edge.
• Check recent wound assessment findings, including wound size, extent of impaired skin integrity, body temperature elevation, and wound drainage (including amount, color, odor, and consistency). This allows you to assess how the wound has changed since the previous irrigation.
• Assess the patient's comfort level and pain. Discomfort may be related directly to the wound or indirectly to muscle tension or immobility. Medicate the patient for pain according to the doctor's orders.

Essential steps

• Provide privacy.
• Position the patient comfortably to allow irrigating solution to flow by gravity through the wound and into the collection basin. The wound should be vertical to the basin.
• Place a waterproof pad on the bed surface in front of the wound. Place a clean collection basin directly under the wound.
• Wash your hands.
• Prepare a sterile field using the sterile dressing set and supplies.
• Add the sterile basin and pour the estimated volume of warm, sterile irrigating solution. Then set the irrigating syringe in the basin with the solution.
• Place several strips of adhesive tape within reach – but not on the sterile field.
• Put on clean gloves and a gown; then remove the soiled dressing and discard it in a leakproof refuse bag.

Alternative wound cleaning methods

Besides irrigation, you can use a Water Pik or the Dey-Wash device to clean a wound.

Water Pik

The Water Pik's versatility makes it appropriate for cleaning open wounds. You can use it throughout the patient's treatment; the patient can take it home if necessary. A pressure setting allows you to adjust the flow.

The Water Pik has two tips, each with a specific purpose. You use the straight jet tip to deliver a direct stream for loosening and debriding necrotic tissue. For gentle wound cleaning, use the shower-head tip.

Water Pik therapy is contraindicated in patients with wounds of the neck, eyes, or dura and in those with exposed vessels.

Dey-Wash

A new product, Dey-Wash is a sterile saline skin wound cleanser. It saves time and doesn't compromise aseptic technique. Designed for single-patient use, the Dey-Wash canister delivers sterile saline solution in a continuous, 19G-stream at 8 pounds per square inch of pressure. It strikes a balance between stream size and flow rate, cleaning effectively with minimal fluid volume.

Dey-Wash cleans away exudate quickly and effectively, using relatively little fluid and causing little or no fluid pooling. For optimal application, use it at a 45-degree angle, holding the nozzle 6″ (15 cm) from the wound bed.

• Remove and discard the gloves.
• Inspect the wound and make a mental note of the degree of healing, inflammation, and presence of drainage or purulent matter.
• Put on a mask and goggles, if indicated.
• Put on sterile gloves.

To irrigate a wound with a wide opening

• Fill the syringe with irrigating solution.
• Hold the syringe tip 1″ (2.5 cm) above the upper edge of the wound.

SKILL TIP

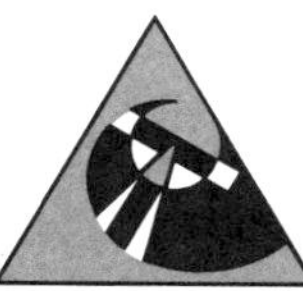

Irrigating hard-to-reach wounds

Limb wounds
You may soak an arm or a leg wound in a large basin of warm irrigating fluid, such as water, 0.9% sodium chloride solution, or an appropriate antiseptic. If necessary, use an agitator to help dislodge bacteria and loosen debris. Rinse the wound several times, if possible, and carefully dispose of the infected liquid. Reserve the equipment you used for that particular patient. After soaking these items in disinfectant, dry and store them.

Trunk or thigh wounds
These wounds can be hard to irrigate. However, a recently developed device can help. It uses Stomahesive and a plastic irrigating chamber applied over the wound. You run warm solution through an infusion set and collect it in a drainage bag. Performing syringe irrigation at the time of dressing is another alternative. Where possible, direct the flow at right angles to the wound and allow the fluid to drain by gravity. You'll need to position the patient carefully, either in bed or on a chair. He may need analgesia during the procedure.

If irrigation isn't possible, you'll have to swab-clean the wound, which is time-consuming. Swab away exudate before using an antiseptic or 0.9% sodium chloride solution to clean the wound, taking care not to push loose debris into the wound. If your hospital's policy permits, use sharp sterile scissors to snip off loose, dead tissue. Never pull it off.

• Flush the wound using slow, continuous pressure. Make sure the solution flows from the clean to the dirty area of the wound so that exudate won't contaminate clean tissue. Collect the dirty exudate in the emesis basin. Continue flushing the wound until the solution draining into the basin is clear.

To irrigate a deep wound with a small opening
• Attach a sterile, soft rubber catheter to a filled irrigating syringe.
• Lubricate the catheter tip with irrigating solution. Gently insert the tip until you feel resistance; then pull out the catheter about ½" (1 cm) to remove the tip from the fragile inner wall of the wound.
• Flush the wound using slow, continuous pressure.
• Pinch off the catheter just below the syringe to prevent aspirating drainage and contaminating the equipment.
• Remove the syringe; then fill and reattach it to the catheter. Repeat the process until the returned fluid is clear. (See *Irrigating hard-to-reach wounds.*)
• Dry the wound edges with sterile gauze.
• Apply packing, if ordered, and a sterile dressing.
• Remove and discard the gloves.
• Secure the dressing with adhesive tape or Montgomery straps.
• Assist the patient to a comfortable position.
• Discard equipment and refuse. Retain the remaining bottle of sterile solution. Mark the date and time of opening on the bottle.
• Wash your hands.

Cautions

Be sure to maintain strict sterile technique, and use only the irrigating solution specified by the doctor because other irrigants may be erosive or otherwise harmful. When using an irritating solution, such as Dakin's solution, apply sterile petroleum jelly around the wound site to protect the skin.

Don't irrigate with a bulb syringe unless a piston syringe isn't available. Using a piston syringe reduces the risk of aspirating drainage.

Follow your hospital's policy regarding wound and skin precautions, as appropriate. Wear a mask and goggles whenever splashing is possible.

Check the patient's history for allergies before administering any new medications with the irrigating solution, to prevent an allergic reaction.

Monitoring and aftercare

• Change the dressing as frequently as ordered.
• Evaluate the patient's skin integrity regularly.
• Inspect the dressing every 4 hours or as or-

dered. Record the amount and type of drainage (if any).

• If your patient will irrigate his wound after discharge, show him or a caregiver how to perform the procedure using strict aseptic technique. Ask for a return demonstration. Also provide written instructions. Instruct the patient or caregiver to wear a mask and goggles if appropriate. Arrange for home health supplies and nursing visits as appropriate. Encourage the patient to eat a well-balanced diet to promote wound healing. Teach him the signs of wound infection, and urge him to contact the doctor if he detects any.

• Document the date and time of irrigation; amount and type of irrigant used; amount and type of wound drainage; appearance of the wound and surrounding skin; any tissue sloughing or exudate; amount, color, consistency, and odor of the returned solution; any skin care performed around the wound; any dressing applied; the patient's tolerance of the procedure; and patient teaching and the patient's level of understanding.

Closed-wound drain management

Typically inserted during surgery when the doctor expects substantial postoperative drainage, a closed-wound drain promotes healing and prevents swelling by suctioning the serosanguineous fluid that accumulates at the wound site. By removing this fluid, the closed-wound drain helps reduce the risk of infection and skin breakdown and decreases the number of dressing changes needed. The most commonly used closed drainage systems are the Hemovac and Jackson-Pratt systems.

A closed-wound drain consists of perforated tubing connected to a portable vacuum unit. The distal end of the tubing lies within the wound and usually leaves the body from a site other than the primary suture line, to preserve the integrity of the surgical wound. The tubing exit site is treated as an additional surgical wound; the drain is usually sutured to the skin.

If the wound produces copious drainage, the closed-wound drain may be left in place longer than 1 week. Drainage must be emptied and measured frequently to maintain maximum suction and prevent strain on the suture line.

Indications

Closed-wound drain management promotes healing and prevents swelling of a wound when significant postoperative drainage is expected.

Contraindications and complications

There are no contraindications, but occlusion of the tubing by fibrin, clots, or other particles can reduce or obstruct drainage. This may cause fluid stasis within the wound, which can lead to infection.

Equipment

Graduated cylinder • sterile laboratory container, if needed • alcohol sponges • sterile gloves • trash bag • sterile gauze pads • antiseptic cleaning agent • prepackaged povidone-iodine swabs

Preparation

• Check the doctor's orders for how often to maintain the closed-wound drain and assess the patient's condition.

• Explain the procedure to the patient, provide privacy, and wash your hands.

• Unclip the vacuum unit from the patient's bed or gown.

Essential steps

• Put on sterile gloves.

• Using aseptic technique, release the vacuum by removing the spout plug in the collection chamber. The container expands completely as it draws in air.

• Empty the unit's contents into a graduated cylinder and note the amount and appearance of the drainage. If diagnostic tests will be performed on the fluid specimen, pour the drainage directly into a sterile laboratory container and send it to the laboratory.

• Using an alcohol sponge and sterile tech-

Using a closed-wound drainage system

The portable closed-wound drainage system draws drainage from a wound site, such as a patient's chest wall after mastectomy, by means of a Y tube.

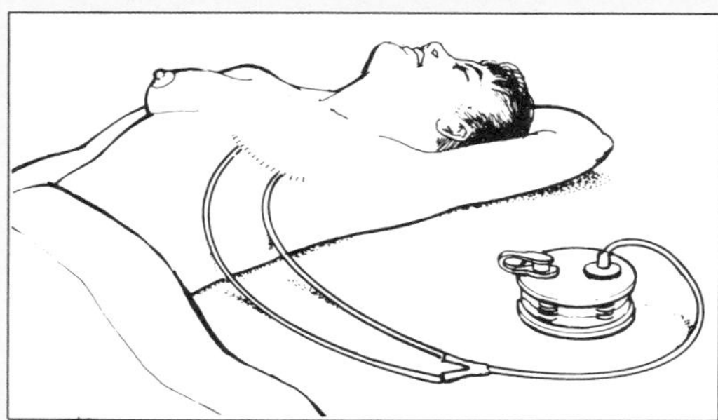

To empty the drainage, remove the plug and empty it into a graduated cylinder. To reestablish suction, compress the drainage unit against a firm surface to expel air and, while holding it down, replace the plug with your other hand.

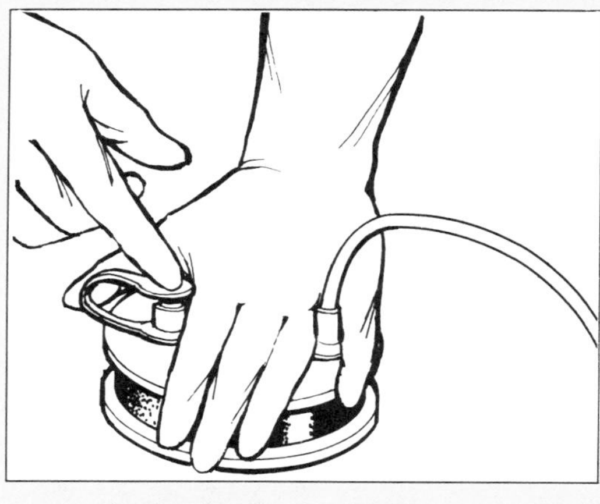

nique, clean the unit's spout and plug.

• To reestablish the vacuum that creates the drain's suction power, fully compress the vacuum unit. With one hand holding the unit compressed to maintain the vacuum, replace the spout plug with your other hand. (See *Using a closed-wound drainage system.*)

• Check the patency of the equipment. Make sure that the tubing is free of twists, kinks, and leaks because the drainage system must be airtight to work properly. The vacuum unit should remain compressed when you release manual pressure. Rapid reinflation signals an air leak; if this occurs, recompress the unit and make sure that the spout plug is secure.

• Secure the vacuum unit to the patient's bedding or, if he is ambulatory, to his gown. Fasten it below wound level to promote drainage. To prevent possible dislodgment, don't apply tension on the drainage tubing when fastening the unit. Remove and discard your gloves and wash your hands thoroughly.

• Observe the sutures securing the drain to the patient's skin, checking for signs of pulling or tearing and for swelling or infection of surrounding skin. Gently clean the sutures with sterile gauze pads soaked in an antiseptic cleaning agent or with a povidone-iodine swab.

• Properly dispose of the drainage, solutions, and trash bag, and clean or discard soiled equipment and supplies according to your hospital's policy.

Cautions

Don't mistake chest tubes for closed-wound drains because the vacuum of a chest tube should never be released.

Monitoring and aftercare

• Empty the system and measure its contents once each shift if drainage has accumulated—more often if drainage is excessive. Removing excess drainage maintains maximum suction and avoids straining the drain's suture line.

• If the patient has more than one closed drain, number the drains so you can record drainage from each site.

• Record the date and time you emptied the system, the appearance of the drain site, and any swelling or signs of infection.

Burn care

A burn injury can result from fire, excessive heat, radiation, electricity, or chemicals. Thermal burns occur from contact with flames, hot liquids, hot metal, and semisolids (such as tar). A direct thermal burn of the respiratory tract, for instance, can follow inhalation of smoke or toxic chemicals. Radiation burns can result from therapeutic radiation sources or industrial accidents involving ionizing radiation. Electrical burns result from electrical current traveling through the body, arcing of electrical current, or the effects of electrical current combined with flames from ignited clothing. Chemical burns typically follow contact with strong acids and alkalies, which destroy tissue by denaturing tissue protein or interfering with cell metabolism.

Burns have multiple effects on the body. Loss of fluid from the wound surface into surrounding tissues causes edema and reduces circulating blood volume. Damage or destruction of red blood cells by heat leads to anemia. Skin destruction allows entry of bacteria and impairs the body's temperature control mechanisms. Loss of water, salts, and proteins from the wound increases the body's metabolic rate.

To help guide treatment, burn injuries are classified by severity. (See *Evaluating burn severity,* page 188.) Estimating the extent of your patient's burns can help determine appropriate treatment and evaluate him for possible transfer to a burn unit. (See *Using the Rule of Nines,* page 189.) Usually, transfer to a burn unit is required for patients with second-degree burns totaling more than 25% of total body surface area (TBSA) in an adult or 20% in a child; third-degree burns involving 10% TBSA or more; burns involving the hands, feet, face, eyes, ears, or perineum; inhalation injury; electrical burn injury; and burns complicated by fracture or other major trauma. Poor-risk patients (such as infants, elderly, and diabetic patients, and those with preexisting heart or renal problems) also require transfer to a burn unit. Victims of major burns can expect to be hospitalized 1 day for each percentage of body surface injured.

Caring for a burn victim may be one of the biggest challenges you'll face as a nurse. Your responsibilities include helping to prevent infection and promote regrowth of burned tissue, maintaining the patient's physiologic stability, providing emotional support to him and his family, and promoting his return to his previous roles and relationships.

Although some burns respond to topical medications and exposure to air (to limit bacterial growth), most need greater protection from the environment. Burn dressings encourage healing by barring bacterial invasion and removing exudate, eschar (hardened, dead tissue), and other debris that host infection. Expect to apply natural or synthetic dressing materials in layers. Typically, the first layer consists of nonadherent, fine-mesh gauze moistened with water, 0.9% sodium chloride solution, or a topical antibacterial agent. Subsequent layers consist of absorptive coarse mesh. You'll usually use an outer, elastic gauze layer to secure the dressings in place. If your patient has a full-thickness, circumferential burn of the chest (which affects respirations by restricting chest movement), expect him to undergo escharotomy.

Indications

Burn care encourages regrowth of burned tissue, prevents infection, and maintains physiologic stability in a patient with a burn injury.

Contraindications and complications

Although burn care has no contraindications, certain complications may occur from the injury. Infection, for instance, is the major complication. Besides increasing wound depth, infection can cause rejection of skin grafts, delay healing, worsen pain, prolong hospitalization, and even lead to death. In fact, over 70% of deaths from burns result from sepsis in the first 5 days—despite such treatment advances as vigorous nutritional support, topical antibacterial therapy, and aggressive wound care.

Signs of infection include a purulent, soupy exudate with a foul odor, which indicates a frank infection; a greenish gray exudate, suggesting *Pseudomonas* infection; blue-black dis-

Evaluating burn severity

To judge the severity of your patient's burn, you'll need to assess its size, depth, and character.

Superficial (first-degree) burn
Does the burned area appear pink or red with minimal edema? Is the area sensitive to touch and temperature changes? If so, your patient most likely has a first-degree, or partial-thickness, burn affecting just one or two skin layers.

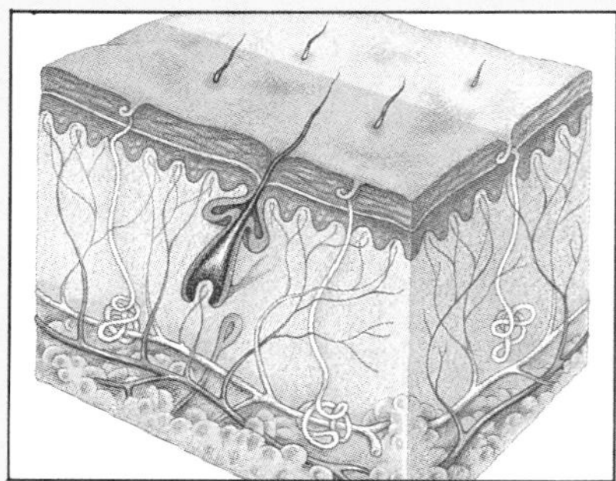

Moderate (second-degree) burn
Does the burned area appear pink or red? Do red areas blanch when you touch them? Does the skin have large, thick-walled blisters with subcutaneous edema? Is the burned area itself firm or leathery? Does touching the burn cause severe pain? If so, your patient has a second-degree, or partial-thickness, burn affecting at least two skin layers.

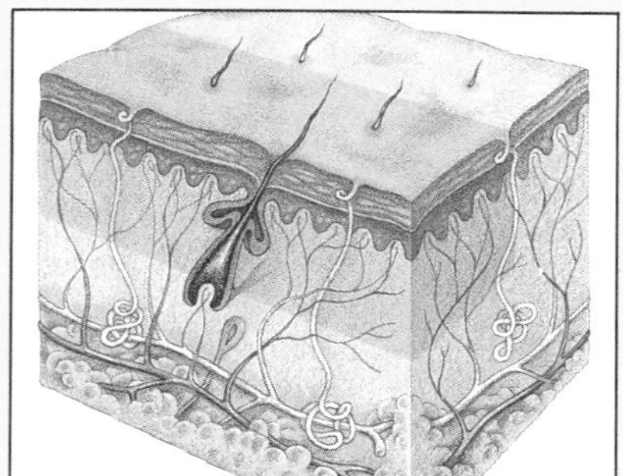

Deep (third-degree) burn
Does the burned area appear waxy white, red, brown, or black? Does red skin remain red with no blanching when you touch it? Is the skin leathery with extensive subcutaneous edema? Is the skin insensitive to touch? If so, your patient has a third-degree, or full-thickness, burn affecting all skin layers.

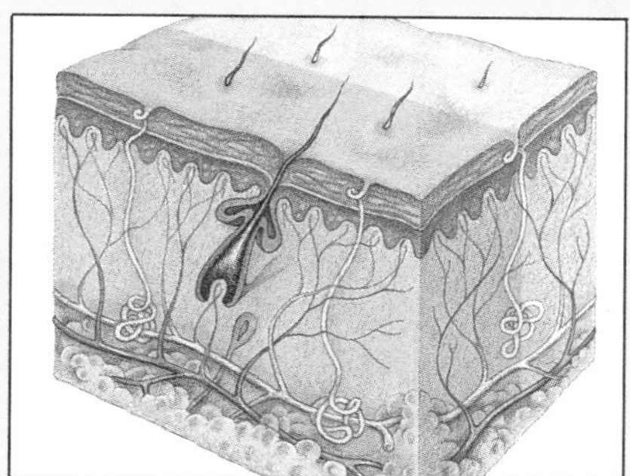

coloration at the wound edges, which may signal septicemia; a white, powdery appearance, which indicates fungal growth; and redness and swelling after the edema stage, which may mean cellulitis. (In contrast, healthy granulation tissue appears clean, pink, and faintly shiny with no exudate.) Typically, body temperature rises 1.8° F (1° C) a few days after a burn; suspect infection if your patient's temperature rises above or falls below this amount.

Hypothermia may occur during dressing changes if the saline solutions for wet-to-dry dressings are not warmed or heat lights aren't used. Pain may occur during dressing changes.

Equipment

Prescribed topical medication • prescribed pain medication • sterile 4″ × 4″ gauze pads • two sterile basins • two pairs of sterile gloves • rolls or sheets of sterile fine-mesh gauze • elastic sterile gauze dressing • dry roller gauze • sterile cotton-tipped applicators • antiseptic cleaning agent • 0.9% sodium chloride solution • sterile towels • sterile blunt scissors • sterile hair clippers • sterile tissue forceps • sterile cotton bath blanket • sterile gowns • masks • surgical cap • heat lamps • tracheostomy ties • impervious trash bags

Preparation

- Administer ordered analgesics about 20 minutes before wound care to promote patient comfort and cooperation.
- Explain the procedure to the patient. Reassure him you'll make every effort to complete the dressing change as painlessly and quickly as possible.
- Turn on overhead lights to help keep the pa-

tient warm, but be careful not to overheat him.
• Assemble equipment on the dressing table.
• Make sure the treatment area has adequate light to allow accurate wound assessment.
• Check equipment packages for tears, which could indicate contamination. Open equipment packages using aseptic technique.
• Arrange supplies on a sterile field in order of use.
• Warm 0.9% sodium chloride solution by immersing unopened bottles in warm water.

Essential steps

To remove a dressing without hydrotherapy

• Put on a gown (a clean one if you're in a burn unit, a sterile one if you're not), mask, and sterile gloves.
• Remove dressing layers down to the innermost fine-mesh layer by cutting the outer dressings with sterile blunt scissors. Lay these dressings open.
• Soak the fine-mesh inner layer with warm 0.9% sodium chloride solution or another ordered solution to ease removal.
• Remove the inner dressing with sterile tissue forceps or your sterile glove.
• Because soiled dressings harbor infectious microorganisms, discard them carefully in an impervious trash bag, according to your facility's policy.
• Gently remove any exudate and old topical medication with a sterile 4″ × 4″ gauze pad moistened with an ordered antiseptic cleaning agent or 0.9% sodium chloride solution.
• Carefully remove all loose eschar with sterile tissue forceps and sterile blunt scissors, if ordered.
• Assess the condition of the wound. The wound should appear clean, with no debris, loose tissue, purulence, inflammation, or darkened edges.
• Before applying a new dressing, remove your gown, gloves, and mask and discard them properly. Then put on a fresh, clean mask, surgical cap, sterile gown, and sterile gloves.

To apply a wet dressing

• Soak the fine-mesh gauze and elastic sterile gauze dressing in a large, sterile basin containing the ordered solution (for example, silver nitrate).
• Wring out the fine-mesh gauze until it's moist (but not dripping) and apply it to the wound. Warn the patient that he may feel

Using the Rule of Nines

You can use the Rule of Nines to estimate how much of your patient's body has been burned. The percentages shown here for the head, arms, and legs represent totals for the anterior and posterior areas.

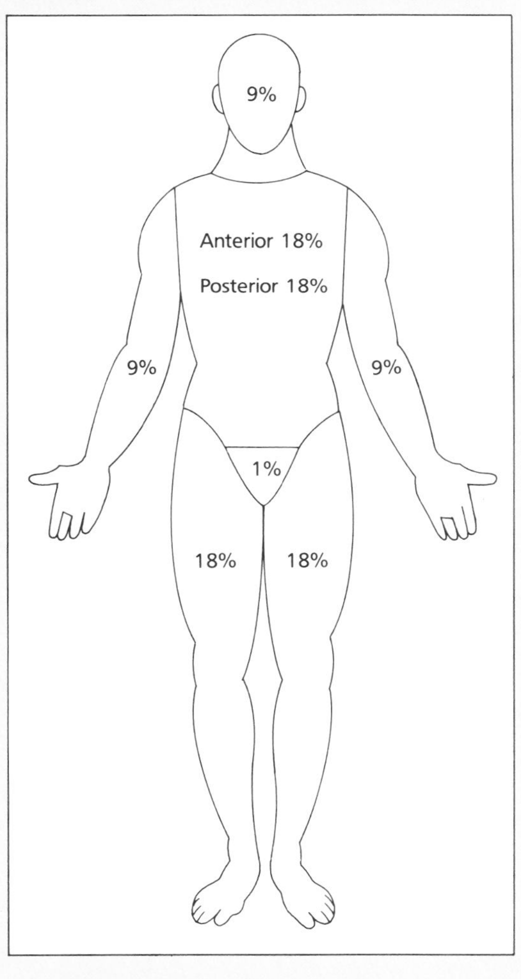

fleeting pain from the solution when you apply the dressing.
• Wring out the elastic sterile gauze dressing, and position it to hold the fine-mesh gauze in place.
• Roll an elastic gauze dressing over the dressing to keep the dressings intact.
• Cover the patient with a sterile cotton bath blanket to prevent chills. Change the blanket if it becomes damp. Use an overhead heat lamp if necessary.
• Change dressings frequently, as ordered, to keep the wound moist—especially if you're using silver nitrate. Silver nitrate becomes ineffective and silver ions may damage tissue if the dressings become dry. (To maintain moisture, some hospital protocols call for irrigating the dressing with 0.9% sodium chloride solution at least every 4 hours through small slits cut into the outer dressing.)

To apply a dry dressing with a topical medication
• Remove old dressings and clean the wound as described above.
• If the fine-mesh gauze doesn't already hold topical medication, apply the ordered medication to the wound in a thin layer (2 to 4 mm thick) with your sterile gloved hand. Then apply fine-mesh gauze over the wound to contain the medication but allow exudate to escape. (If you apply an occlusive dressing, wrap it with an elastic gauze dressing to hold the fine-mesh gauze in place and absorb any drainage.)
• Remember to cut the dressing to fit only the wound area. Don't cover unburned areas.
• Apply several layers of coarse, absorptive gauze. Then cover the entire dressing with an elastic sterile gauze dressing to secure the dressing and prevent evaporation of body fluid.

To provide arm and leg care
• Apply the dressings from the distal to the proximal area to stimulate circulation and prevent constriction. Wind the dressings once around the patient's arm or leg so the edges overlap slightly. Continue wrapping in this way until the dressing covers the wound. Then cut the bandage.
• Apply a dry roller gauze or an elastic gauze bandage to hold the bottom layers in place.

To provide hand and foot care
• Wrap each finger separately with a single layer of fine-mesh gauze to prevent webbing contractures and to allow the patient to use his hand.
• Place the patient's hand in a functional position, and secure this position using a dressing.
• Put gauze between each toe, as appropriate, to help prevent webbing contractures.

To provide chest, abdomen, and back care
• Cover the wound with the fine-mesh gauze and a layer of coarse gauze saturated with the ordered medication.
• Place sterile towels on top of the gauze and pin other sterile towels to the dressing so the bandage wraps around the patient's chest, abdomen, or back. Or wrap the wound area with an elastic sterile gauze dressing to avoid restricting respiratory movements, especially in very young or elderly patients and in those with circumferential injuries.

To provide facial care
• If the patient has scalp burns, use the sterile hair clippers to clip or shave the hair around the burn, as ordered. To prevent contamination of burned scalp areas, clip other hair until it's about 2" (5 cm) long.
• Be sure not to cover the patient's eyes, nostrils, or mouth with the final elastic sterile gauze dressing.

To provide ear care
• Use the sterile hair clippers to clip or shave the hair around the affected ear.
• Remove exudate and crusts with sterile cotton-tipped applicators dipped in 0.9% sodium chloride solution.
• Place a layer of sterile fine-mesh gauze behind the auricle to prevent webbing.

To provide nasal care
- Check the nostrils for inhalation injury, inflamed mucosae, and singed vibrissae.
- Clean the nostrils with sterile cotton-tipped applicators dipped in 0.9% sodium chloride solution.
- Remove crusts.
- Apply the ordered ointments.
- If ordered, place small Plexiglas inserts in the nostrils to prevent contractures.
- If the patient has a nasogastric (NG) tube, use tracheostomy ties to secure it.
- Clean the area around the tube every 4 to 6 hours using the antiseptic cleaning agent.
- Apply sterile fine-mesh gauze and sterile 4" × 4" gauze pads to the burned area. Dampen the pads with the ordered topical medication. (To prevent pooling in the middle ear, don't soak the pads.) Before securing the dressing with a bandage, position the patient's ears normally to avoid damaging auricular cartilage.
- Assess the patient's hearing.

To provide eye care
- Clean the area around the patient's eyes and eyelids with a sterile cotton-tipped applicator and 0.9% sodium chloride solution every 4 to 6 hours, or as needed, to remove crusts and drainage.
- Administer any ordered eye ointments or eyedrops.
- If the patient can't close his eyes, apply lubricating ointments or drops as ordered.
- Be sure to close the patient's eyes before applying eye pads to prevent corneal abrasion. Don't apply topical ointments near the eyes without a doctor's order.

Cautions

If you're administering first aid to a burn victim, be sure to assess for inhalation injury. (See *Assessing for inhalation injury.*)

With all burn patients, take measures to prevent infection, such as using strict aseptic technique, dressing the burn site properly, monitoring and rotating I.V. lines regularly, assessing body system functions, monitoring the patient's emotional status, and avoiding invasive procedures whenever possible. Also ensure appropriate care of indwelling catheters and proper retaping of NG and endotracheal tubes.

To prevent contractures, use careful positioning and regular exercise for burned extremities. This also helps to maintain joint function and minimize deformity. (See *Preventing deformity in the burn patient,* page 192.)

Vascular compromise can occur with circumferential, full-thickness burns of the extremities. To detect this complication, during the first 24 to 36 hours after the injury, assess

Assessing for inhalation injury

When you give first aid to a burn victim, consider the possibility of inhalation injuries. If he has inhaled smoke, hot vapors, or toxic fumes, he may have suffered damage to his tracheobronchial tree and will need prompt medical attention. (The only way to confirm this injury is with fiber-optic bronchoscopy.) So after you've extinguished any flames and checked his ABCs (airway, breathing, and circulation), assess him for an inhalation injury.

If possible, ask the victim (or a bystander) what happened. Was he in an enclosed space during a fire? Maybe he was trapped in a house with little ventilation. Or perhaps the front of his shirt caught fire and he inhaled smoke. In these cases, he may have both upper and lower respiratory tract damage. A victim of a steam explosion who inhales heat and superheated water vapor may suffer upper respiratory tract damage.

Note whether the victim has burns on his face or neck. Look for singed nasal hairs or eyebrows and soot on the face and in the nasopharynx and oropharynx. Does his breath smell of smoke or any of the chemicals involved? Is he wheezing, coughing up carbonaceous sputum, or showing other signs of respiratory distress, such as stridor?

Facial and circumferential neck burns may cause edema within 1 hour. If the victim has such burns, be sure to tell emergency care responders when they arrive. Depending on how long it will take to get him to an emergency department, they may decide to intubate him to prevent airway occlusion from the edema.

COMPLICATIONS

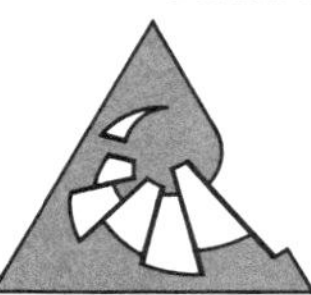

Preventing deformity in the burn patient

When caring for a burn patient, take steps to prevent contractures and preserve joint function so that deformity doesn't develop. Use this chart to choose the right positioning based on the specific area burned.

Burned area	Potential deformity	Preventive positioning	Nursing interventions
Neck	• Flexion contracture of neck • Extensor contracture of neck	• Extension • Prone with head slightly raised	• Remove pillow from bed. • Place pillow or rolled towel under upper chest to flex cervical spine. Or apply cervical collar.
Axilla	• Adduction and internal rotation • Adduction and external rotation	• Shoulder in external rotation and 100- to 130-degree abduction • Shoulder in forward flexion and 100- to 130-degree abduction	• Use an I.V. pole, bedside table, or sling to suspend arm. • Use an I.V. pole, bedside table, or sling to suspend arm.
Pectoral region	• Shoulder protraction	• Shoulders abducted and externally rotated	• Remove pillow from bed.
Chest or abdomen	• Kyphosis	• As for pectoral region, with hips neutral (not flexed)	• Don't use pillow under head or legs.
Lateral trunk	• Scoliosis	• Supine; affected arm abducted	• Put pillows or blanket rolls at sides.
Elbow	• Flexion and pronation	• Arm extended and supinated	• Use an elbow splint, arm board, or bedside table.
Wrist	• Flexion • Extension	• Splint in 15-degree extension • Splint in 15-degree flexion	• Apply a hand splint. • Apply a hand splint.
Fingers	• Adhesions of extensor tendons, loss of palmar grasp	• Metacarpophalangeal joints in maximum flexion; interphalangeal joints in slight flexion; thumb in maximum abduction	• Apply hand splint; wrap fingers separately.
Hip	• Internal rotation, flexion, and adduction; possible joint subluxation if contracture is severe	• Neutral rotation and abduction; maintain extension by prone position	• Put pillow under buttocks (if supine) or use trochanter rolls or knee or long leg splints.
Knee	• Flexion	• Maintain extension	• Use knee splint with no pillow under legs.
Ankle	• Plantar flexion if foot muscles are weak or their tendons are divided	• 90-degree dorsiflexion	• Use footboard or ankle splint.

your patient every hour for the five Ps: pain, paresthesia, pallor, paralysis, and pulselessness. Elevate the affected extremity to the level of the heart to aid venous return and arterial flow.

Don't administer I.M. pain medications to a patient with a burn of more than 30% TBSA. After a burn, fluid moves from the vascular to the interstitial spaces. Regardless of the I.M. injection site, essentially all of the drug remains in the interstitial space, providing no pain relief. Later, when the fluid moves back into the vascular system, respiratory depression may occur.

If your patient has a chemical burn, tailor initial care to the type of chemical involved. (See *Chemical burns: Special considerations.*)

Ileus and stress ulcers may occur in patients with burns of more than 20% TBSA. To help prevent ileus, an NG tube is inserted until bowel sounds are normal and gastric secretions decrease. To help prevent stress ulcers, monitor your patient's gastric acidity at least every 2 hours, and keep the pH above 5.0.

Renal failure results from the presence of myoglobin and hemochromogens in the blood, especially after an electrical burn or a deep burn involving muscle tissue. Myoglobin and hemochromogens result from the breakdown of muscle tissue and red blood cells, respectively. Increased myoglobin, which gives urine a bloody to port-wine color, can cause renal tubular damage.

Be aware that hypothermia may follow a burn because excessive skin loss impairs body temperature regulation. During initial care of a burn of less than 30% TBSA, you may cool the affected area with water at room temperature, as ordered. For a burn of more than 30% TBSA, this measure is contraindicated because it may cause systemic hypothermia (burned tissue can't act as a thermal insulator). To help prevent hypothermia and excessive metabolic stress, keep your patient warm during dressing changes by using heat lamps, warmed solutions, and warmed linens. (See *Myths and facts about burn care,* page 194.)

Because blisters protect underlying tissues, you should leave them intact as long as they

Chemical burns: Special considerations

How you intervene for a patient with a chemical burn depends on the chemical involved. Here are some special precautions you should take for four types of chemical burns you may see.

Dry lime

Don't wash the burn site with water right away because this would create a corrosive liquid. Instead, brush dry lime from your patient's skin, hair, and clothing. Wash the site with water only after brushing lime off the body and removing contaminated clothing and jewelry. Be sure to use a continuous flow of running water for at least 20 minutes.

Hydrofluoric acid

Used in glass etching, this chemical has a fluoride ion that rapidly penetrates soft tissue, causing liquefaction of cellular membranes and decalcification of bone. A hydrofluoric acid burn requires irrigation with water, then local subcutaneous injection of 10% solution of calcium gluconate. Calcium gluconate administration can prevent loss of bone and soft tissue and markedly decrease pain.

Phenol

Used in sanitizers and disinfectants, phenol is an acidic alcohol that is highly corrosive and can damage blood vessels. First, irrigate the affected area with copious amounts of water. Then wash it with alcohol, which increases phenol's solubility and allows you to flush more rapidly.

White phosphorus

For a burn with this chemical, you must irrigate with copious amounts of water and then debride to remove particles. When these particles are exposed to air, they may spontaneously ignite. So after they're removed, they must be kept underwater. This type of injury may require irrigation with 1% copper sulfate solution.

Myths and facts about burn care

Myth: By applying cold 0.9% sodium chloride solution dressings or flushing burns with cool water, you can minimize swelling and reduce pain.
Fact: Cooling may anesthetize a minor burn, but it's contraindicated for large burns. Burned skin loses its ability to act as a thermal insulator, so systemic hypothermia may occur. Keep the patient with a large burn as warm as possible to conserve body heat.

Myth: You may need to withhold oxygen from some patients with chronic obstructive pulmonary disease (COPD) who've suffered carbon monoxide poisoning. Otherwise, they may stop breathing.
Fact: Oxygen is always indicated to reverse the effects of carbon monoxide poisoning. At 100% oxygen, the patient's carbon monoxide level decreases by about one-half in just 40 minutes. You'd have to wait 4 hours for the same effect with room air (20% oxygen). Some COPD patients may stop breathing when given high percentages of oxygen because their respiratory systems are stimulated by low oxygen tension. (Normally, blood carbon dioxide levels control breathing.) But oxygen is nonetheless indicated to reverse carbon monoxide poisoning. If the patient stops breathing, be prepared to assist ventilation. Have a manual resuscitation bag readily available.

Myth: You can estimate the extent of damage from an electrical burn by examining the surface burn on the patient's skin.
Fact: An electrical burn is deceptive. You'll usually see just small burns where the current entered and exited, literally exploding through the skin. But you should assume the patient has suffered deep tissue damage.

don't impede the patient's joint motion, become infected, or cause discomfort.

Early wound closure and elastic pressure garments help minimize scarring. The garments approximate capillary pressure over the healing surface and reduce the bulk of hypertrophic scars by enhancing collagen fiber lysis and slowing its synthesis through decreased tissue circulation and cell hypoxia. An adult may wear the garment for up to 12 months; a child, for 18 months. Silicone sheets, used experimentally as coverings for hypertrophic scars, seem to speed scar resolution, possibly by reducing oxygen content and hastening wound maturation.

Fluid loss, a major concern in burn patients, is caused by destruction of the epidermis and by volume shifts from the intravascular to the extravascular compartments. Normally functioning epidermis prevents the loss of fluid, electrolytes, and proteins from the body. The resulting fluid shifts are directly proportional to burn depth and extent (as reflected by fluid replacement formulas). Fluid replacement should begin at the scene of the injury, usually with lactated Ringer's solution. The optimal fluid contains salt but no glucose because a burn injuries commonly cause glucose intolerance. Fluids can be administered orally to patients with small burns. However, patients with deep burns of more than 20% TBSA usually have intestinal ileus, making the oral route unacceptable.

Make sure your patient receives a tetanus toxoid vaccine.

Monitoring and aftercare

- Monitoring a burn is a complex process that involves assessment of all body systems. You must also monitor your patient's emotional and psychological status.
- During the first 24 to 36 hours, check every hour for the five Ps.
- Initially, use the patient's hematocrit value to evaluate the effectiveness of fluid replacement.
- Monitor urine output every hour for the first 48 to 72 hours. For an adult, consider an output of 0.5 to 1 ml/kg adequate.

HOME CARE

Caring for a burn injury

You can help your burn patient make a successful transition from the hospital to home by teaching him or a caregiver to follow these wound and skin care guidelines after discharge.

Wound care

- Clean the bathtub, shower, or wash basin thoroughly before using these items for wound care to help prevent infection.
- Use mild soap and warm water to wash the wound (unless ordered otherwise). To remove topical creams, scales, or loose skin, apply gentle abrasion with a clean washcloth and pat the skin dry with a clean towel.
- Check the burn for signs of infection and call the doctor if you think infection is present. Apply a new dressing, following the instructions provided before discharge.
- If you're using a splint, wash it with soap and cold water to prevent wound infection.
- To enhance healing, consume adequate carbohydrates and proteins. Eat three well-balanced meals and three between-meal snacks daily. Include one protein source with each meal and snack.

Skin care

- Be aware that regenerated skin tissue is delicate and needs protection. Avoid bumping or scratching it.
- You may wash the new skin with mild soap and water, but apply lotions sparingly and only if they contain no alcohol or perfume.
- Wear clothing that doesn't restrict movement or cause abrasion. Launder clothes in a mild detergent.
- Don't expose new skin to strong sunlight or such irritants as paint, solvent, strong detergent, or antiperspirants.
- Take cool baths or apply ice packs to relieve itching.
- Avoid ingesting substances that cause peripheral vasoconstriction, such as tobacco, alcohol, and caffeine.
- To minimize scar formation, you may need to wear a pressure garment as instructed—usually for 23 hours a day, for 6 months to 1 year. Suspect that the garment is too tight if it causes coldness, numbness, or discoloration (cyanosis) of the fingers or toes or if its seams and zippers leave deep, red impressions in the skin that last more than 10 minutes after removing the garment.

- Use an indwelling urinary catheter only during initial treatment, if ordered.
- Obtain the patient's baseline weight as soon as possible to help calculate his fluid and nutritional needs. Thereafter, weigh the patient daily.
- Measure the patient's serum electrolyte levels every 3 to 4 hours initially.
- Monitor calorie counts and protein intake. Be aware that a burn patient may require up to 5,000 calories/day.
- Begin discharge planning as soon as your patient is admitted to the hospital, to help smooth his transition from the burn unit to the home. To encourage therapeutic compliance, prepare him to expect scarring, teach him about wound management and pain control, and urge him to follow the prescribed exercise regimen. Provide encouragement and emotional support. You should also teach family members or caregivers how to encourage, support, and care for the patient. (See *Caring for a burn injury.*)

Cardiovascular monitoring

- Expect your patient's heart rate to increase during the first few hours after a burn (from hypovolemia), then to remain elevated (from increased metabolic demands).
- Anticipate reduced blood pressure (from hypovolemia). If your patient's blood pressure doesn't increase after fluid administration, the doctor may order invasive monitoring.

• Monitor your patient for arrhythmias, which may stem from hypoxemia, acidosis, hypovolemia, electrolyte imbalance, or cardiac injury (common after an electrical burn). Arrhythmias may resemble those associated with myocardial infarction.
• When placing electrodes to monitor your patient's electrocardiogram, you may use a topical antibacterial agent as a conducting agent if you can't find any unburned areas to place them.

Invasive hemodynamic monitoring
• Expect a central venous pressure (CVP) of 0 to 5 mm Hg in a patient with a severe burn. A CVP that rises rapidly above 12 mm Hg usually indicates heart failure.
• Be aware that a pulmonary artery catheter is used only when absolutely necessary. When caring for the catheter, use strict aseptic technique.
• Anticipate extremely low cardiac output immediately after a severe burn. However, the patient's cardiac output should rise within 12 to 18 hours.
• Right atrial pressure will range from 1 to 10 mm Hg and pulmonary capillary wedge pressure will range from 4 to 5 mm Hg.

Respiratory monitoring
• Monitor the patient's respiratory rate and characteristics every 15 minutes for 2 hours, then every 2 hours.
• Obtain a chest X-ray on admission and daily, as ordered.
• Ensure good pulmonary hygiene. Turn the patient regularly, and encourage coughing and deep-breathing exercises. Suction as needed and as ordered.

Neurologic monitoring
• Conduct a thorough neurologic assessment every hour. A victim of major burns should be awake, alert, and oriented unless heavily medicated. If the patient becomes agitated, restless, or hostile in the first 3 hours after a burn injury, suspect hypovolemia. Its neurologic signs include decreased orientation and increased drowsiness. If the patient becomes uncooperative, always consider pain as the cause.

Bacteriologic monitoring
• With a burn of less than 20% TBSA, obtain cultures if the patient has signs or symptoms of infection. With larger burns, obtain routine cultures two to three times weekly to assess for sepsis.
• Monitor the patient's white blood cell count to detect sepsis.

Biological dressings

Biological dressings provide a temporary covering for burn wounds and clean granulation tissue. In some cases, they're used to temporarily secure fresh skin grafts and protect graft donor sites.

Providing immediate coverage for a clean wound, a biological dressing decreases evaporative fluid and protein loss, protects exposed nerve endings, decreases heat loss, lowers the body's metabolic rate, and provides a bacterial barrier. It also enhances reepithelialization by maintaining a moist environment for healing and is used to debride untidy wounds after eschar formation. It permits better assessment of the patient's readiness for autografting; once the dressing starts to adhere with minimal exudate, the site is considered ready for permanent grafting.

A biological dressing may be made of any material that promotes healing and rapid adherence to the wound bed or that helps prepare the wound for permanent autograft coverage. Common materials include skin obtained from a living or recently deceased (within 4 hours of death) human (homografts or allografts), or from animals of other species (heterografts or xenografts); amnion from the human placenta; and synthetic material. The most common synthetic dressing used today is Biobrane, a knitted elastic flexible nylon fabric bonded to a thin, Silastic, semipermeable membrane coated with dermal collagen. Omniderm, a newer product, is producing good results. (See *Comparing biological dressings.*)

Comparing biological dressings

Type	Description and uses	Nursing considerations
Cadaver (homograft)	• Obtained at autopsy up to 24 hours after death • Available as fresh, cryopreserved homografts in tissue banks nationwide • Applied by the doctor to debride an untidy wound • Provides protection, especially to granulation tissue after escharotomy • May be used in some patients as a test graft for autografting • Covers excised wounds immediately	• Observe for exudate. • Watch for signs of rejection. • As needed, remove the gauze dressing every 8 hours to observe the graft.
Pigskin (heterograft or xenograft)	• Comes fresh or frozen in rolls or sheets • Applied by the nurse • Can cover and protect debrided untidy wounds, mesh autografts, clean (eschar-free) partial-thickness burns, and exposed tendons	• Reconstitute the frozen form with 0.9% sodium chloride solution 30 minutes before use. • Cover with a gauze dressing or leave exposed to air, as ordered. • Watch for signs of rejection. • Note that pigskin dressings are typically changed every 2 to 5 days.
Amniotic membrane (homograft)	• Available from the obstetric department; must be sterile and come from an uncomplicated birth • Is bacteriostatic and thus doesn't require antimicrobials • Applied by the doctor to clean wounds only • May be used to protect partial-thickness burns or (temporarily) granulation tissue before autografting	• The membrane will be changed every 48 hours. • Cover the membrane with a gauze dressing or leave exposed, as ordered. • If you apply a gauze dressing, change it every 48 hours.
Biobrane (biosynthetic membrane)	• Comes in sterile, prepackaged sheets in various sizes and in glove form for hand burns • Applied by the nurse • Used to cover donor graft sites, superficial partial-thickness burns, debrided wounds awaiting autograft, and meshed autografts • Provides significant pain relief	• Leave the membrane in place for 3 to 14 days, possibly longer. • Don't use this dressing to prepare a granulation bed for subsequent autografting.
Omniderm (polyurethane membrane)	• Available in mesh or unmeshed form • Applied by the nurse • Serves as a barrier to the external environment but is permeable to oxygen and molecules (such as those in antibiotics) • Can be used as a postgraft dressing or as a temporary dressing when burns are excised	• Observe for exudate. • You may leave the dressing in place for 7 to 10 days.

Indications

• To promote early closure of partial-thickness and full-thickness burns
• To secure skin grafts and protect graft donor sites

Contraindications and complications

There are no contraindications for a biological dressing. Infection may develop under a biological dressing. Observe the wound for signs of infection during dressing changes. If wound drainage appears purulent, remove the dressing, clean the area with 0.9% sodium chloride solution or another prescribed solution, and apply a fresh biological dressing.

An allergic reaction may occur. Allograft rejection may manifest as an inflammatory reaction and may lead to sloughing of the graft. (However, in most uses, biological dressings are changed frequently enough to prevent rejection.)

Equipment

Ordered analgesic • cap • mask • two pairs of sterile gloves • sterile or clean gown • shoe covers • biological dressing • 0.9% sodium chloride solution • sterile basin • 18″ × 18″ fine-mesh gauze (impregnated with a topical medication, if ordered) • sterile elastic gauze dressing • stockinette or elastic bandage • sterile forceps • sterile scissors • sterile hemostats

Preparation

- Place the biological dressing in the sterile basin (or open the Biobrane package).
- Using aseptic technique, open the sterile dressing packages.
- Arrange the equipment on the dressing cart, and keep the cart within easy access.
- Ensure adequate lighting in the treatment area to allow accurate wound assessment and dressing placement.
- Provide privacy.
- Explain the procedure to the patient to allay his fears and promote cooperation.
- Administer the prescribed analgesic I.M. 20 minutes before the procedure or I.V. immediately before the procedure.

Essential steps

- Wash your hands and put on the cap, mask, gown (clean if in a burn unit, sterile if not), shoe covers, and sterile gloves.
- Clean and debride the wound to reduce bacteria. Then put on a fresh pair of sterile gloves.
- Place the dressing directly on the wound surface. Apply a pigskin dressing dermal (shiny) side down; apply a Biobrane dressing nylon-backed (dull) side down.
- Roll the dressing directly onto the skin, if applicable.
- Place dressing strips so that the edges touch but don't overlap. Use sterile forceps if necessary.
- Smooth out the dressing, eliminating folds and wrinkles by rolling out the dressing with the hemostat handle, forceps handle, or your sterile-gloved hand to cover the wound completely and ensure adherence.
- Use sterile scissors to trim the dressing around the wound so that it fits the wound without overlapping adjacent areas.
- Place 18″ × 18″ fine-mesh gauze (impregnated with a topical medication, if ordered) over the biological dressing to avoid disturbing it during the first dressing change.
- Cover the 18″ × 18″ fine-mesh gauze with an elastic gauze dressing to hold the biological dressing in place.
- Place a stockinette over the entire area or wrap the area with an elastic bandage to protect and secure the dressing layers.
- Position the patient comfortably.
- Remove the dressing cart. Take off your gloves, gown, mask, cap, and shoe covers. Discard disposable items according to hospital policy.

Cautions

Handle the dressing as little as possible to ensure proper placement and decrease the risk of infection. Most biological dressings are opaque, making observation of the wound bed difficult. Early adherence of the dressing typically signals a healthy wound bed. However, if you suspect infection, remove a portion of the dressing to allow inspection. You may cover this area immediately with another biological dressing.

Be aware that the use of biological dressings for donor sites is controversial.

Monitoring and aftercare

- If your patient will be discharged with a biological dressing, instruct him to avoid disturbing it. Inform him that the dressing will slough off in 7 to 10 days or when the wound heals. If the dressing isn't covered, teach him to observe the wound daily for redness, swelling, blisters, drainage, and separation of the dressing from the burn. Instruct him to notify the doctor if signs of infection develop.

• Document the time and date of dressing changes. Note the areas of application, adherence quality, and purulent drainage or other infection signs. Also record the patient's tolerance of the procedure.

Mechanical debridement

Mechanical debridement involves removing necrotic tissue by mechanical, chemical, or surgical means to allow underlying healthy tissue to regenerate. Procedures used for mechanical debridement include irrigation, hydrotherapy, and excising dead tissue with forceps and scissors. If your patient requires immediate debridement, the doctor may use a carbon dioxide laser; this procedure may take place in a specially prepared room.

Burn wound debridement removes eschar. This prevents or controls infection, promotes healing, and prepares the wound surface to receive a graft. Ideally, you should debride the wound daily when changing the dressing. Frequent, regular debridement helps prevent significant blood loss resulting from more extensive and forceful debridement. It also reduces the need for extensive debridement done under anesthesia.

The debridement method you'll use depends on various factors, including the type and extent of your patient's injury and his overall condition. (The following descriptions of equipment, preparation, and essential steps apply to the forceps-and-scissors excision method performed at the patient's bedside. For details on other methods, see *Other wound debridement methods,* page 200.)

Indications

Mechanical debridement promotes regeneration of underlying healthy tissue in patients with complex burn wounds or wounds requiring immediate attention.

Contraindications and complications

Mechanical debridement is contraindicated in patients with closed blisters over partial-thickness burns.

Because burns damage or destroy the protective skin barrier, infection may develop despite aseptic techniques and equipment.

Some blood loss may occur if debridement exposes an eroded blood vessel or if you accidentally cut a vessel. Fluid and electrolyte imbalances may result from loss of exudate during the procedure.

Equipment

Ordered analgesic • two pairs of sterile gloves • two gowns or aprons (clean if you're in a burn unit, sterile if not) • mask • cap • sterile scissors • sterile forceps • sterile 4″ × 4″ gauze pads • sterile solutions and topical medications, as ordered • hemostatic agent (as ordered) • needle holder and gut suture with needle (to control hemorrhage)

Preparation

• Assemble all supplies. Check expiration dates on sterile solutions and medications. Inspect for tears in sterile packages, which may indicate contamination.
• Explain the procedure to the patient to allay his fears and promote cooperation. Teach him distraction and relaxation techniques, as possible, to minimize discomfort.

Essential steps

• Provide privacy.
• Administer an analgesic 20 minutes before debridement, or give an I.V. analgesic immediately before the procedure.
• Keep the patient warm. To prevent chilling and fluid and electrolyte loss, expose only the area to be debrided.
• Wash your hands and put on a cap, mask, gown or apron (clean if in a burn unit, sterile if not), and sterile gloves.
• Remove the burn dressings and clean the wound. Usually, 0.9% sodium chloride solution is used for wound cleaning.
• Remove your gown or apron and dirty gloves, and change into another gown or apron (clean if in a burn unit, sterile if not) and sterile gloves.
• Lift loosened edges of eschar with the sterile forceps. Use the blunt edge of the sterile scissors or forceps to probe the eschar. Cut dead

Other wound debridement methods

Besides the forceps-and-scissors method you perform at the patient's bedside, a wound can be debrided using a wet-to-dry dressing, irrigation (see "Wound irrigation," page 182), hydrotherapy, or chemical or surgical means.

Wet-to-dry dressing

Gather a sterile bowl, sterile gauze, Kling gauze, wetting solution, an outer dressing, two pairs of sterile gloves, and tape. Loosen and lift the outer layer of the old dressing; then discard it. Clean the wound well.

Open the wrapper of the sterile bowl and use it as a sterile field. Open the sterile gauze and put it into the bowl. Pour enough wetting solution into the bowl to dampen the gauze. Then open the outer dressing and drop it onto the sterile field.

Put on sterile gloves and gently remove the dressing that has adhered to the wound. Discard the old dressing and gloves. Then put on fresh sterile gloves.

Remove the gauze from the bowl and wring out excess moisture. Place the moistened gauze over the wound and gently pack it in. Then apply the outer dressing and remove your gloves. Secure the dressing with tape or wrap it with Kling gauze.

Hydrotherapy

Before starting, clean and disinfect the tub, room, and equipment to prevent cross-contamination. Place a liner in the tub, then fill the tub with water warmed to 98° to 104° F (36.7° to 40° C). Add the prescribed chemicals, which may include sodium chloride (to maintain isotonicity and prevent dialysis and irritation), potassium chloride (to prevent potassium loss), calcium hypochlorite detergent (to help prevent infection), and an anti-foaming agent. Make sure the room is warm enough to keep the patient from being chilled.

Gather the same equipment and supplies used for bedside debridement. (See "Mechanical debridement," page 199.) Then measure and record the patient's vital signs. If possible, weigh him to obtain a baseline weight. If the dressing is to be changed, remove and discard the outer dressing. Leave the inner dressing in place.

Help the patient into the tub. (If he isn't ambulatory, use a plinth and hydraulic lift system.) After he soaks for 3 to 5 minutes, remove the rest of the gauze dressings. If ordered, place the agitator in the water and turn it on.

Clean all unburned areas and provide general hygiene. Then gently scrub the burned areas with gauze pads or sponges to remove topical agents, exudates, necrotic tissue, and other debris. Debride the wound as described in "Mechanical debridement."

Limit hydrotherapy to 20 or 30 minutes, to prevent hypothermia and fluid and electrolyte imbalance. When the treatment is completed, spray-rinse the patient's entire body to remove any remaining debris. Pat dry unburned areas of his body, working quickly to prevent chilling. Then transport him to the dressing area to perform further debridement, if necessary. Apply sterile dressings.

Help the patient dress and escort him back to his room. Take his vital signs and weight to detect any fluid loss. Document the condition of the wound.

Chemical debridement

Gather a dextranomer, 4" × 4" gauze sponges, a transparent plastic dressing, a rubber bulb and syringe, 0.9% sodium chloride solution, and a sterile container.

Gently irrigate the wound and surrounding tissues with 0.9% sodium chloride solution to remove any dextranomer remaining from the previous application. Blot the area, leaving it slightly moist.

Pour the dextranomer into the wound, forming a layer at least 3 mm thick. Cover the wound with gauze sponges and apply the transparent plastic dressing.

Between dressing changes, monitor the dextranomer's color through the plastic dressing. When it turns from white to gray or yellow (usually after 6 to 8 hours), it's time for a new application.

Watch for and report viable, nonoozing granulation tissue, which signals the need for less frequent chemical debridement. Expect to see some inflammation from the dextranomer. If it's widespread or if signs of infection appear, notify the doctor immediately.

Surgical wound debridement

This procedure is done in the operating room by a doctor. Your role is to conduct standard preoperative and postoperative monitoring and to stay alert for blood loss, which can quickly progress to hypovolemic shock. Also monitor the patient for signs and symptoms of septicemia.

tissue from the wound with the scissors. Leave a 1/4" (0.5-cm) edge on the remaining eschar to avoid cutting into viable tissue.

- Because debridement removes only dead tissue, bleeding should be minimal. If bleeding occurs, apply gentle pressure on the wound with sterile 4" × 4" gauze pads. Then apply the hemostatic agent, as ordered. If bleeding persists, notify the doctor and maintain pressure on the wound until he arrives. Excessive bleeding or spurting vessels may call for ligation.
- Perform additional procedures, such as applying topical medications and dressing replacements, as ordered.

Cautions

Before debridement, consult your state's nurse practice act and your hospital's policy to make sure you're permitted to perform the procedure.

Debride no more than a 4" (10-cm) square area at one time. Limit the procedure time to 20 minutes or less, if possible.

Be aware that repeated pressure can cause injury to the wound bed. Chemical injury can occur with agents that are cytotoxic to granular tissue.

Work with an assistant, if possible, to complete this painful procedure as quickly as possible. Acknowledge the patient's discomfort and provide emotional support.

Monitoring and aftercare

- Ensure good nutrition, which is essential to wound healing. The patient may need enteral supplements or parenteral nutrition.
- Don't order supplies in large volumes because wound care often requires therapeutic modifications.
- Document the date and time of wound debridement, the area debrided, and the solutions and medications used. Describe the condition of the wound, noting signs of infection or skin breakdown. Also record the patient's tolerance of and reaction to the procedure. Note indications for additional therapy.

Pressure ulcer care

Pressure ulcers are lesions caused by unrelieved pressure applied to the skin. Such pressure impairs circulation, depriving tissues of oxygen and other life-sustaining nutrients and damaging the skin and underlying structures. Untreated, pressure ulcers can lead to serious infection.

Most pressure ulcers develop over bony prominences, where friction and shearing forces combine with pressure to break down skin and underlying tissues. Common ulcer sites include the sacrum, coccyx, ischial tuberosities, and greater trochanters. Pressure ulcers also commonly develop over the vertebrae, scapulae, elbows, knees, and heels in bedridden or immobile patients.

Preventing and managing pressure ulcers requires the efforts of the entire health care team. As a nurse, you're in the best position to coordinate these efforts. The treatment plan should include input from other members of the health care team. Treatments, consultations (such as for dietary planning and rehabilitation), equipment, supplies, and reimbursement may require a doctor's order. The team approach should emphasize consistency.

Expert nursing assessment is crucial in identifying at-risk patients who need preventive measures and detecting the specific factors placing them at risk. (See *Pressure ulcers: Who's at risk?* page 202.) You may use a validated risk assessment tool, such as the Braden Scale or the Norton Scale. Reassess your patient's risk for developing pressure ulcers periodically. Care goals for the high-risk patient include maintaining and improving tissue tolerance to pressure to prevent injury; guarding against the adverse effects of external mechanical forces, such as pressure, friction, and shear; and reducing the incidence of pressure ulcers through patient teaching.

Be sure to involve the patient and his family in treatment planning to elicit their cooperation. A pressure ulcer can cause a disturbance in the patient's self-esteem or body image and may even lead to significant distress in family members. A patient with a chronic pressure ulcer may be depressed about his debilitated

Pressure ulcers: Who's at risk?

Besides assessing every patient for signs of developing pressure ulcers, you should review the medical history for the following risk factors:
- advanced age
- chronic illness with bed rest
- dehydration
- diabetes mellitus
- diminished pain awareness
- immunosuppression
- incontinence
- malnutrition
- mental impairment (such as from coma, altered level of consciousness, sedation, confusion, or use of restraints)
- paralysis
- poor circulation
- previous corticosteroid therapy
- previous pressure ulcers
- significant obesity or thinness.

state, which in turn may affect his compliance with treatment.

The effectiveness and duration of therapy depend on the severity of the pressure ulcer. Ideally, prevention can help avoid the need for extensive therapy. When a pressure ulcer develops despite preventive efforts, treatment includes the use of mechanical devices, such as pressure-relieving cushions and mattresses, and frequent repositioning and exercise. Other measures include cleaning the wound meticulously using topical agents and applying dressings that are appropriate for the ulcer stage. (See *Staging and dressing a pressure ulcer,* pages 204 and 205, and *Topical agents for cleaning pressure ulcers,* page 206.)

The doctor may order debridement, hydrotherapy, and skin grafting to supplement other measures and to promote healing. The enterostomal nurse performs or coordinates these treatments according to hospital policy. The procedures detailed below address cleaning and dressing the pressure ulcer.

Indications

Pressure ulcer care relieves pressure on the skin, restores local circulation, and helps prevent or control related problems, such as infection. It aims to promote healing by providing a moist environment, protecting healthy skin, and avoiding putting pressure on the wound.

Contraindications and complications

Although the procedure has no contraindications, the pressure ulcer may lead to complications. Infection is the most common one, but others include breakdown of healthy skin around a wound and, in a deep wound, the formation of abscesses. Also, ischemia may be exacerbated by a wound that's packed too tightly.

Equipment

Nonallergenic tape or elastic netting • overbed table • sterile irrigation set with bulb syringe • two pairs of sterile gloves • 0.9% sodium chloride or other cleaning solution, as ordered • sterile 4″ × 4″ gauze pads • alcohol sponge • 18G to 20G needle and syringe • selected topical dressing (according to the ulcer stage) • linen-saver pads • impervious plastic trash bag • disposable wound-measuring device • sterile cotton-tipped applicators • optional: skin sealant, convoluted foam mattress, air-fluidized bed

Preparation

- Provide privacy.
- Explain the procedure to the patient and his family. Allow time for them to ask questions.
- Cut nonallergenic tape into strips for securing dressings.
- Assemble equipment at the patient's bedside.
- Loosen lids on cleaning solutions and medications for easy removal.
- Loosen existing dressing edges and tape before putting on gloves.
- Inspect packages of sterile supplies to make sure they have no openings, which could contaminate the supplies.
- Attach an impervious plastic trash bag to the overbed table to hold dressings and refuse.

Essential steps

• Before any dressing change, wash your hands and review the principles of universal precautions.

To clean the pressure ulcer

• Position the patient to increase his comfort and give you easy access to the pressure ulcer.
• Cover the bed linens with a linen-saver pad to prevent soiling.
• Open the sterile irrigation set. Carefully pour 0.9% sodium chloride solution into the irrigation container to avoid splashing. Put the bulb syringe into the opening provided in the irrigation container.
• Open the packages of sterile supplies and arrange them on the sterile field in order of use.
• Put on gloves. Remove the old dressing and expose the pressure ulcer. Discard the soiled dressing in the impervious plastic trash bag to avoid contaminating the sterile field and spreading infection.
• Inspect the wound. Note the color, amount, and odor of any drainage or necrotic debris. Measure the wound perimeter with the disposable wound-measuring device (a square, transparent card with concentric circles arranged in bull's-eye fashion and bordered with a straight-edge ruler).
• Using the bulb syringe, gently irrigate the pressure ulcer. If the wound contains necrotic debris, use a 30-ml syringe fitted with a 19G needle or a catheter instead of a bulb syringe.
• Remove and discard your soiled gloves and put on a fresh pair.
• Insert a sterile cotton-tipped applicator into the wound to assess wound tunneling. Gauge tunnel depth by determining how far the applicator can be inserted. (Use the disposable wound-measuring device. To avoid contamination, don't let the applicator touch the guide.) Tunneling usually signals wound extension and possible infection of underlying tissues.
• Using the sterile 4″ × 4″ gauze pads, blot the skin dry around the ulcer. Begin blotting at the center of the ulcer. Work with a spiral motion toward the edges to avoid contaminating the wound with microorganisms from the skin.
• Reassess the condition of both the skin and ulcer. Note the character of the cleaned wound bed and surrounding skin.
• Prepare to apply the appropriate topical dressing. Directions for typical hydrocolloid, transparent, and calcium alginate dressings follow. For other dressings or topical agents, follow your hospital's protocol or the supplier's instructions.

To apply a hydrocolloid dressing

• Choose a presized dressing or cut one to overlap the pressure ulcer by about 1″ (2.5 cm). Remove the dressing from its package, pull the release paper from the adherent side of the dressing, and apply the dressing to the wound. To minimize irritation, carefully smooth out wrinkles as you apply the dressing.
• If the dressing's edges need to be secured with tape, apply a skin sealant to the intact skin around the ulcer. After the area dries, tape the dressing to the skin. The sealant protects the skin and promotes tape adherence. Never use tension or pressure when applying the tape.
• Remove your gloves and discard them in the impervious plastic trash bag. Discard refuse according to your hospital's policy.
• Wash your hands.
• Change a hydrocolloid dressing every 1 to 7 days as needed; for example, if the dressing tears, the patient complains of pain, or leakage or foul odor occurs.

To apply a transparent dressing

• Clean and dry the wound as described above.
• Select a dressing to overlap the ulcer by 2″ (5 cm).
• Gently lay the dressing over the ulcer. To prevent shearing force, don't stretch the dressing. Press firmly on the edges of the dressing to promote adherence. Although the dressing is self-adhesive, you may have to tape the edges to prevent them from curling.
• If necessary, aspirate accumulated fluid with an 18G to 20G needle and syringe, using aseptic technique to preserve the dressing's integrity. After aspirating the fluid pocket, clean the aspiration site with an alcohol sponge and cover it with another strip of transparent dressing.

Staging and dressing a pressure ulcer

Assessing the stage of your patient's pressure ulcer can help ensure appropriate care. For instance, the type of dressing you'll use on a pressure ulcer depends on the ulcer stage. Use these descriptions and illustrations as a guide.

Stage I
In this stage, the skin lesion is erythematous, nonblanching, and intact—the heralding lesion of skin ulceration.
Note: Reactive hyperthermia normally occurs for a period lasting one-half to three-fourths as long as the pressure occluded blood flow to the area. Don't confuse this phenomenon with a stage I pressure ulcer.

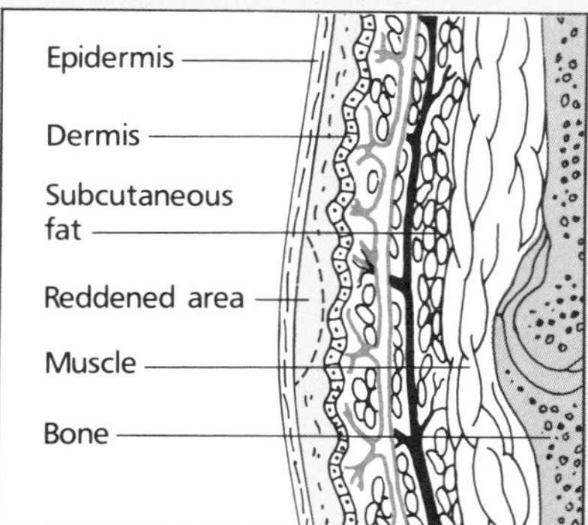

Dressing
A *film dressing* (such as Tegaderm, Bioclusive, Op-Site, or Uniflex) guards against shear and promotes eschar softening on deeper ulcers. It may be left in place up to 7 days if the occlusive seal remains intact. As a drawback, a film dressing doesn't allow wound assessment.

A *hydrocolloid dressing* (such as DuoDerm, Comfeel, or IntraSite Absorbent) also may be left in place up to 7 days if the occlusive seal remains intact.

Stage II
The ulcer is superficial and appears as an abrasion, blister, or shallow crater. Expect to assess partial-thickness skin loss involving the epidermis, dermis, or both.

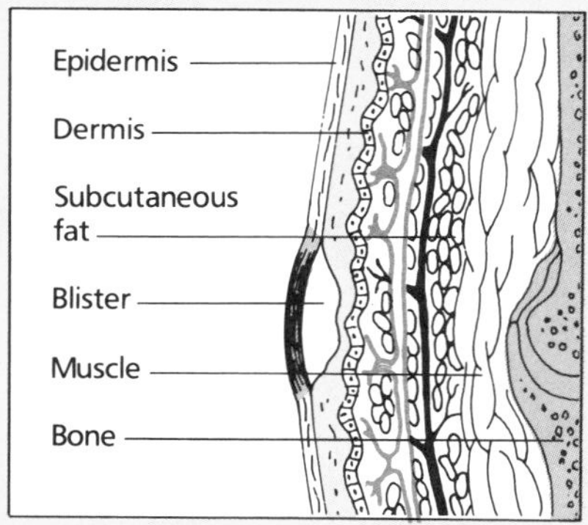

Dressing
A *composite dressing* (such as Viasorb or a film dressing over Telfa) provides an absorbent, nonadherent layer over the wound, with an occlusive cover. A *hydrogel dressing* (such as Vigilon, Geliperm, or J & J Gel Dressing) absorbs a draining ulcer. It usually requires a gauze dressing cover.

A *burn dressing* (such as Exu-dry) is absorbent and nonadherent and protects against shear. Nonocclusive, it may be used with a topical agent. A *hydrocolloid dressing* may also be used for a stage II ulcer.

• Change the dressing every 3 to 7 days, depending on whether the ulcer is infected and whether drainage is minimal or profuse.

To apply a calcium alginate dressing
• Irrigate the pressure ulcer with 0.9% sodium chloride solution. Blot the surrounding skin dry using the sterile 4″ × 4″ gauze pads.
• Apply calcium alginate to the ulcer surface. Cover the area with a second dressing, such as gauze pads, as ordered. Secure the dressing with tape or elastic netting.
• If the wound is draining heavily, change the dressing once or twice daily for the first 3 to 5 days. As drainage decreases, you can change the dressing less frequently—every 2 to 4 days, or as ordered.

Cautions
Some experts recommend using only physiologic solutions, such as 0.9% sodium chloride solution, to clean pressure ulcers because other solutions (such as povidone-iodine, hexachloro-

Stage III
The ulcer resembles a deep crater, with or without undermining of adjacent tissue. Expect full-thickness skin loss involving damage to or necrosis of subcutaneous tissue, which may extend to – but not through – underlying fascia.

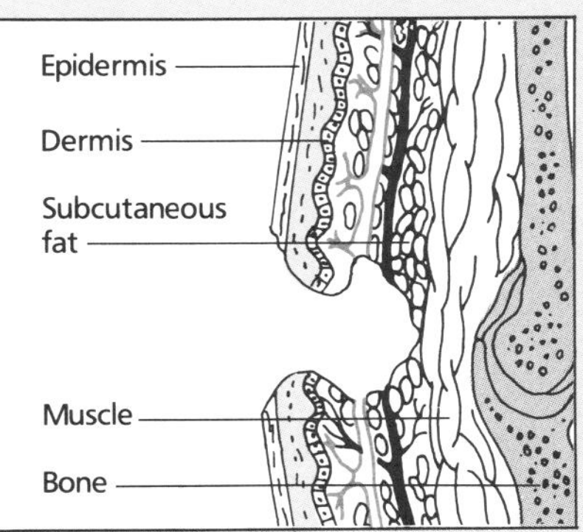

Dressing
A *hydrocolloid dressing* increases absorbency and wear time. However, it's not preferred because it may cause tissue damage if removed frequently (daily or more often). A *hydrogel dressing* may be used as a carrier for topical agents. A *burn dressing* is another option.

Stage IV
The ulcer involves full-thickness skin loss with extensive destruction, tissue necrosis, or damage to muscle, bone, or supporting structures (such as tendons or joint capsules). *Note:* Undermining and sinus tracts are also associated with stage IV pressure ulcers.

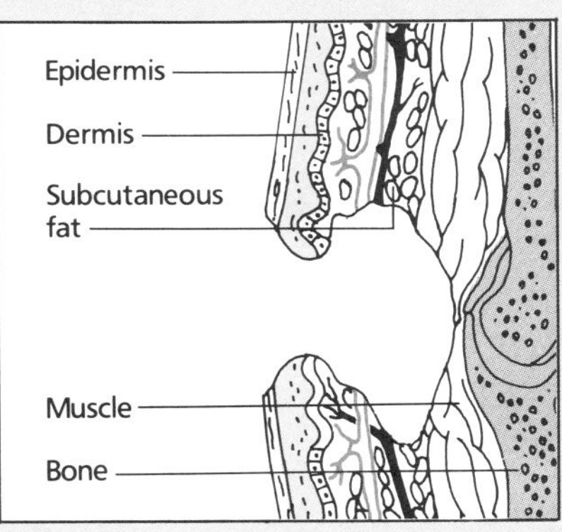

Dressing
A *gauze dressing* (such as a Kerlix dressing) is absorbent and nonocclusive. It usually must be changed every 8 to 12 hours. A *hydrogel dressing* is another option. A *hydrocolloid dressing* can be used. However, it may be contraindicated because of ulcer location, exposed bone, or the amount of drainage.

phene, sodium hypochlorite, and hydrogen peroxide) may injure cells and retard healing.

Don't use tincture of benzoin compound as a skin sealant because it triggers an allergic reaction in some patients.

Avoid using elbow and heel protectors that fasten with a single narrow strap. The strap may impair neurovascular function in the involved hand or foot.

Monitoring and aftercare

- Stay alert for signs of infection (which can lead to septicemia and osteomyelitis). These include leukocytosis; fever; increasing ulcer size; and odor, drainage, necrotic tissue, induration, warmth, and pain at the ulcer site.
- Turn and reposition the patient every 1 to 2 hours, unless contraindicated. For a patient who can't turn himself or who is turned on a schedule, use pressure-relieving and pressure-reducing devices, such as a 4" (10-cm) convoluted foam mattress or a low-air-loss or air-

Topical agents for cleaning pressure ulcers

TOPICAL AGENTS	NURSING CONSIDERATIONS
Antibiotics bacitracin (Neosporin Ointment, Polysporin Ointment)	• Use only for early-stage ulcers because these agents may not penetrate sufficiently to kill deeper bacterial colonies.
Antiseptics hydrogen peroxide, povidone-iodine (Betadine), sodium hypochlorite (Dakin's solution)	• Dilute standard 3% hydrogen peroxide solution to half-strength or quarter-strength. • Avoid using hydrogen peroxide after granulation tissue develops because its foaming action may cause blistering. Also avoid using it to clean deep or tunneled wounds because the wound may retain and absorb oxygen bubbles, creating air emboli. • Avoid using povidone-iodine on open wounds because it may damage granulation tissue, retard collagen synthesis, and irritate surrounding skin. • Apply diluted sodium hypochlorite, as directed, only for initial wound debridement. • Avoid multiple applications of sodium hypochlorite because it inhibits granulation tissue growth, delays epithelialization, and irritates surrounding skin.
Circulatory stimulants (Granulex, Proderm)	• Use these agents to promote blood flow. Both contain balsam of Peru and castor oil. However, Granulex also contains crystallized trypsin, an enzyme that promotes debridement.
Enzymes collagenase (Santyl), fibrinolysin and deoxyribonuclease (Elase), sutilains (Travase)	• Apply collagenase in thin layers after cleaning the wound with 0.9% sodium chloride solution. • Promote effectiveness by avoiding concurrent use of collagenase with agents that decrease enzymatic activity, including detergents, hexachlorophene, antiseptics with heavy-metal ions, iodine, or such acidic solutions as Burow's solution. • Use collagenase cautiously near the patient's eyes. If contact occurs, flush the eyes repeatedly with 0.9% sodium chloride solution or sterile water. • Use fibrinolysin only after surgical removal of dry eschar. • If using sutilains ointment and a topical antibacterial agent, apply sutilains ointment first. • Avoid applying sutilains to ulcers in major body cavities, to areas with exposed nerve tissue, or to fungating neoplastic lesions. Don't use sutilains in women of childbearing age or in patients with limited cardiopulmonary reserve. • Store sutilains at a cool temperature (35.6° to 50° F [2° to 10° C]). • Use sutilains cautiously near the patient's eyes. If contact occurs, flush the eyes repeatedly with 0.9% sodium chloride solution or sterile water.
Exudate absorbers dextranomer beads (Debrisan)	• Use dextranomer on secreting ulcers. Discontinue use when secretions stop. • Clean but don't dry the ulcer before applying dextranomer beads. Don't use in tunneling ulcers. • Remove gray-yellow beads (which indicate saturation) by irrigating with sterile water or 0.9% sodium chloride solution. • Use cautiously near the eyes. If contact occurs, flush the eyes repeatedly with 0.9% sodium chloride solution or sterile water.
Isotonic solutions 0.9% sodium chloride solution	• This agent moisturizes tissue without injuring cells.

fluidized bed. As appropriate, implement active or passive range-of-motion exercises to relieve pressure and promote circulation. To save time, combine these exercises with bathing, if appropriate.

• When turning the patient, lift him rather than slide him because sliding increases friction and shear. If necessary, use a turning sheet and get help from colleagues.
• Use pillows to position the patient and increase his comfort. Be sure to eliminate sheet

wrinkles that could increase pressure and cause discomfort.

• To prevent shearing pressure, avoid raising the head of the bed more than 30 degrees, except for brief periods.

• Post a turning schedule at the patient's bedside. Adapt position changes to his situation.

• Teach the patient and his family the importance of regular position changes. Encourage their participation in pressure ulcer prevention and treatment by having them perform a position change correctly after you demonstrate how.

• If your patient is confined to a chair or wheelchair, instruct him to shift his weight every 15 minutes to promote blood flow to compressed tissues. Show a paraplegic patient how to shift his weight by doing push-ups in the wheelchair. If he needs your help, sit next to him and help him shift his weight to one buttock for 60 seconds, then repeat the procedure on the other side. Provide pressure-relieving cushions as appropriate. However, avoid seating him on a rubber or plastic doughnut, which can increase localized pressure at vulnerable points.

• Adjust or pad appliances, casts, or splints as needed to ensure proper fit and avoid increased pressure and impaired circulation.

• If the patient has diarrhea or is incontinent, clean and dry soiled skin. Apply a protective moisture barrier to prevent skin maceration.

• Teach the patient to avoid heat lamps and harsh soaps because they dry the skin. Instruct him to apply lotion after bathing to help keep his skin moist. Also tell him to avoid vigorous massage because it can damage capillaries.

• As the patient's condition permits, recommend a diet containing adequate calories, protein, and vitamins. Dietary therapy may involve nutritional counseling, food supplements, enteral feeding, or total parenteral nutrition.

• If the patient will need to care for the ulcer after discharge, provide appropriate instruction. (See *Caring for a pressure ulcer.*)

• Document the date and time of initial and subsequent care procedures. Note the specific care provided. Describe preventive measures performed. Document pressure ulcer location and size (including length, width, and depth); color and appearance of the wound bed; amount, odor, color, and consistency of drainage; and condition of the surrounding skin. Also document patient teaching.

• Update the care plan as required. Note any change in the condition or size of the pressure ulcer and any elevation of skin temperature on the progress record. Document when the doctor was notified of any pertinent abnormal observations. Record the patient's temperature daily on the graphic sheet to allow easy assessment of body temperature patterns.

HOME CARE

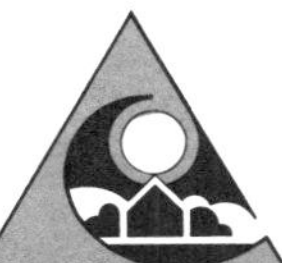

Caring for a pressure ulcer

After discharge, the patient with a pressure ulcer will need care similar to the professional care he received in the hospital. Follow these guidelines to ensure successful home care.

• Before discharge, have the patient or a family member demonstrate the proper technique for removing a dressing, cleaning the ulcer, and reapplying the dressing.

• When discussing which type of dressing to choose for home care, consider the cost as well as the patient's or caregiver's ability to apply the dressing properly. Teach the patient where to purchase dressing supplies, such as the local pharmacy or medical supply store.

• If the ulcer will be mechanically debrided at home, tell the patient he can use a hand-held shower head or forceful irrigation with a 20-ml syringe instead of whirlpool therapy.

• Teach the patient or caregiver about the signs and symptoms of infection. Urge him to follow a high-protein diet to promote wound healing.

• If appropriate, arrange for a home care nurse to follow the patient's progress.

• Stress that the patient and caregiver share responsibility in ensuring a successful treatment outcome and avoiding complications, such as ulcer infection and recurrence.

Vascular ulcer care

Vascular ulcers, which resemble pressure ulcers, occur when blood flow and cellular metabolism are disrupted. They result primarily from peripheral vascular insufficiency or underlying venous, arterial, or ischemic disease. Other causes include trauma, hematologic or metabolic disease, infection, neoplasms, drug reactions, insect bites, and certain rare diseases. This section addresses vascular ulcers related to venous and arterial disorders.

Venous disorders account for 70% to 90% of vascular ulcers. These ulcers result mainly from stasis caused by impaired valvular function. Arterial disorders, such as emboli, peripheral vascular disease (arteriosclerosis obliterans), and hypertension, account for most of the remaining 10% to 20% of vascular ulcers.

Vascular ulcers commonly lead to complications and financial burden. They've been a major cause of illness and disability for years. An aging population, cigarette smoking, and inactive life-styles—and the consequent increase in cardiovascular disease—have contributed to a their growing incidence. Other risk factors include diabetes mellitus, hypercoagulability, stasis, and immobilization. (See *Assessing your patient's risk for vascular ulcers.*)

Healing of a vascular ulcer requires adequate perfusion of the lower extremities. In patients with diabetes mellitus and incompressible arteries, blood pressure measured in the toes is a better predictor of ulcer healing than blood pressure measured in the ankle. A blood pressure of less than 30 mm Hg suggests poor healing.

When caring for a patient with a vascular ulcer, your responsibilities include promoting ulcer healing, providing emotional support, and teaching the patient how to prevent ulcers and thus avoid the need for prolonged therapy. (See *Managing vascular ulcers of the leg and foot.*)

Assessing your patient's risk for vascular ulcers

Compromised patients have an increased risk for both arterial and venous ulcers. If you're caring for an elderly or compromised patient, check his medical history for the following risk factors.

Arterial ulcers
- Arteriosclerosis obliterans
- Burns
- Collagen disease
- Diabetes mellitus
- Emboli
- Hypertension
- Neurogenic disorders
- Raynaud's disease
- Sickle cell anemia
- Trauma

Venous ulcers
- Cardiovascular disease
- Congenital or acquired valvular incompetence
- Dehydration
- Hypercoagulability
- Immobilization
- Impaired tissue metabolism
- Increased venous pressure
- Obesity
- Oral contraceptive use
- Orthopedic surgery
- Pregnancy
- Prolonged bed rest
- Prolonged standing
- Stasis
- Thrombosis
- Tissue edema
- Varicose veins

Indications

Indications for vascular ulcer care are the same as those for pressure ulcer care.

Contraindications and complications

Unna's boot, a common treatment for vascular ulcers, is contraindicated in patients with arterial ulcers, weeping eczema, or cellulitis.

Managing vascular ulcers of the leg and foot

Ulcer type	Assessment findings	Pain characteristics	Intervention
Arterial ulcer	• Two or three minor traumas • Skin atrophy • Thick, ribbed nails • Skin color variation: blanching on rising, deep red hue when limb is dependent, or pale or bluish color • Muscle atrophy • Subcutaneous fat tissue or no change in extremity size • Absence of hair on foot, ankle, and toes • Bruits heard over pulse points • Bilateral blood pressure variation • Normal or decreased skin turgor • Temperature variations (cool or cold extremity) • Delayed capillary refill on release of tactile pressure • Decreased or absent pulses of the femoral, popliteal, posterior tibialis, and dorsalis pedis arteries	• Intermittent claudication after walking 1 to 2 blocks, alleviated by rest • Pain relieved when limb is dependent (suggests severe arterial insufficiency) • Extremely painful ulcer • Paresthesia	• Patient teaching • Infection and trauma prevention • Hypertension control • Treatment of the underlying cause • Emotional support for the patient
Venous ulcer	• Previous ulcer history • Chronic, nonhealing superficial ulcer with jagged edges and granulation tissue • Varicose veins • Stasis on garter area of lower extremity • Normal capillary filling • Skin atrophy • Stasis dermatitis of ankle or lower leg • Hair present • Discoloration (brown staining) of ankle or lower leg • Cellulitis • Firm edema of ankle and lower leg • Old ulcer scars • Distention of superficial veins when legs are slightly dependent • Posterior tibialis and dorsalis pedis pulses present	• Moderately painful ulcer • Pain relieved by elevation • No intermittent claudication	• Patient teaching • Infection prevention • Elevation of extremity • Long-term wound care with Unna's boot or paste dressings • Topical antibiotics or steroids, as indicated • Compression bandages (elastic stockings and bandages) • Jobst extremity pump

Equipment
Overbed table • nonallergenic tape or elastic netting • sterile irrigation set with bulb syringe • two pairs of sterile gloves • 0.9% sodium chloride solution or other cleaning solution, as ordered • selected topical dressing (as for pressure ulcer dressings) • linen-saver pads • impervious plastic trash bag • disposable wound-measuring device • sterile cotton-tipped applicators • optional: skin sealant, low-air-loss or air-fluidized bed

Preparation
- Assemble equipment at the patient's bedside.
- Cut the nonallergenic tape into strips for securing dressings.
- Loosen existing dressing edges and tape.
- Put on gloves.
- Attach an impervious plastic trash bag to the overbed table to hold used dressings and refuse.
- Wash your hands.
- Review the principles of universal precautions.

How to wrap Unna's boot

If your patient has an uninfected, nonnecrotic leg or foot ulcer caused by venous insufficiency or stasis dermatitis, you may receive a doctor's order to wrap Unna's boot, a medicated gauze compression dressing, around the affected extremity.

First, clean the skin around the ulcer thoroughly. Then flex the patient's knee. Position the affected foot at a right angle to the leg, then wrap the dressing firmly, but not tightly, around the foot in overlapping turns. Continue overlapping the dressing up the leg. Smooth it with your free hand as you go, as shown here.

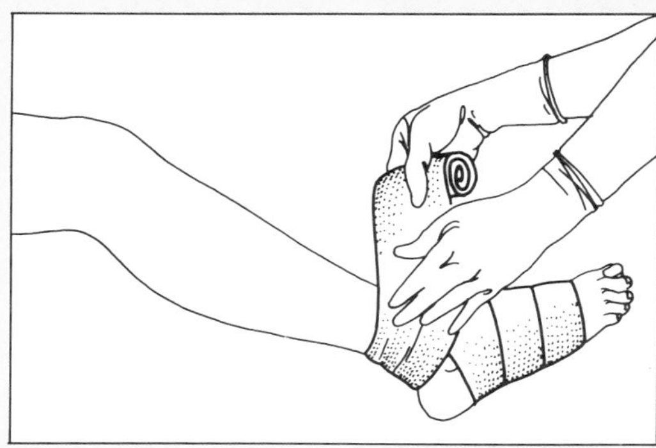

Stop wrapping about 1" or 2" (2.5 or 5 cm) below the knee. If necessary, you may make a 2" slit in the dressing just below the knee to relieve constriction that may develop as the dressing hardens. Repeat this procedure until the patient's leg has a three-layer boot.

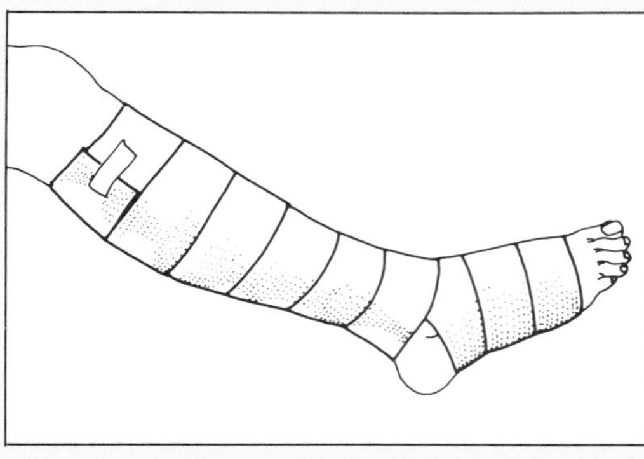

Essential steps

Follow the procedure described in "To clean the pressure ulcer," page 203.

If the doctor orders Unna's boot to treat your patient's ulcer, don't wrap nonexpandable tape completely around his leg because it may have a tourniquet effect, reducing blood supply. If swelling occurs between treatments, use small strips of duct tape. (See *How to wrap Unna's boot.*)

Cautions

Don't use benzoin compound as a skin sealant because it triggers an allergic reaction in some patients. Avoid using heel protectors that fasten with a single narrow strap because the strap may impair neurovascular function in the involved hand or foot.

Be aware that exercise and activity are contraindicated or restricted in patients with vascular ulcers because they increase metabolic tissue needs.

Monitoring and aftercare

• Monitor your patient's temperature daily, and record it on graphic progress notes.
• Stay alert for signs of infection (the most common complication of vascular ulcers). These include erythema, induration, foul-smelling drainage, and elevated skin and body temperature.
• Watch for other complications, such as cellulitis, gangrene, peripheral ischemia, and necrosis.
• Be aware that psychological and social factors can contribute to vascular ulcer formation. Assess your patient for uncertainty, anxiety, depression, anger (either direct or indirect), hopelessness, helplessness, poor self-esteem, and social withdrawal. Provide emotional support and, if necessary, refer the patient for psychological counseling.
• For a patient with a venous ulcer, perform meticulous foot and leg care daily. Observe for trophic changes. Help reduce dependent edema by elevating the legs.
• For a patient with an arterial ulcer, promote healing by elevating the head of the bed on 3" to 6" (8- to 15-cm) blocks to increase blood

flow to the extremities. Encourage him to actively participate in his care by following the prescribed diet, exercise, and drug therapy. Be aware that he may experience severe pain or further narrowing of the arteries supplying the extremity, and may fear becoming incapacitated or losing a limb (with recurrent occlusion). These fears may increase his anxiety and depression. Make sure the patient understands that treating the underlying problem may prevent ulcer recurrence. Help him develop appropriate coping strategies and relaxation techniques.

• If your patient has a venous ulcer secondary to thrombophlebitis, be aware that disruption in activities of daily living may cause anxiety and stress. The patient also may fear pulmonary embolism.

• Because venous insufficiency is a chronic illness, the patient with a venous ulcer may need long-term treatment (months to years) and may feel anxious and depressed. Encourage him to participate in his care to help speed recovery.

• Teach the patient to avoid cigarette smoking because nicotine promotes vasoconstriction and arterial spasms, reducing blood transport, while carbon monoxide decreases oxygen transport to tissues.

• If the patient has sensory deficits, teach him to avoid hot water bottles, heating pads, hot baths, and hot foot soaks because they increase tissue metabolism and may cause burns.

• Teach the patient measures to increase circulation, improve nutrition, prevent venous stasis, and avoid or minimize problems. Include the following points: Avoid obesity because excessive weight weakens the heart, diminishes blood flow, and increases venous congestion. Avoid standing or sitting in any position for a prolonged period. Get adequate rest. If appropriate, use crutches or a cast. Avoid trauma to the lower extremities. Avoid wearing constrictive clothing (such as garters, girdles, tight belts, and tight shoelaces) because these decrease blood flow. Follow a diet low in calories, fats, and cholesterol and high in protein, vitamin B complex, vitamin C, and iron. Refrain from crossing the legs at the knee because this constricts the popliteal vessels. Avoid stressful situations and chills because these can cause vasoconstriction. Try relaxation techniques or see a counselor. Know the name, purpose, dosage, administration schedule, and adverse effects of prescribed medications. Check with the doctor before taking any over-the-counter medications.

• Document the dates and times of initial and subsequent assessments and interventions. Record the location of the vascular ulcer; ulcer size (including length, width, and depth); color and appearance of the wound bed; amount, odor, color, and consistency of drainage; and condition of the surrounding skin.

Air therapy bed

Traditionally, air therapy beds have been used to prevent and treat pressure ulcers. They also provide therapeutic options for preventing and treating other complications of immobility, including pulmonary congestion and stasis of body fluids.

An air therapy bed consists of a standard hospital bed frame and a series of air-filled compartments. These compartments can be inflated to varying degrees to increase air pressure, providing different levels of support to different body parts. The level of support should be individualized to permit optimal pressure relief and reduce the risk of skin breakdown. (See *Using an air therapy bed,* page 212.)

An air therapy bed may combine air therapy with lateral rotation therapy (a continuous, gentle, side-to-side turning used to treat and prevent pulmonary complications) and continuous pulsation therapy (to stimulate blood flow). Other features of the bed include a quick deflation control to allow cardiopulmonary resuscitation (CPR), optional bed scales, and alarms to alert the nurse to a patient's exit from the bed.

Indications

• To prevent pressure ulcers in immobile patients at risk for skin breakdown

ADVANCED EQUIPMENT

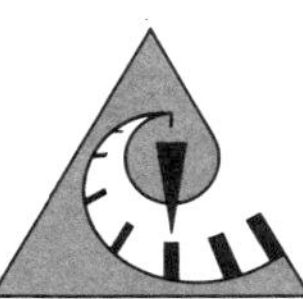

Using an air therapy bed

Patients with skin breakdown—and those who are at risk for it—may benefit from an air therapy bed without microspheres, an alternative to the air-fluidized bed. Its inflatable, air-filled compartments can provide different levels of support to different body parts.

Some air therapy beds have an optional pulsating or rotating motion that stimulates capillary blood flow, prevents venous stasis, increases peristalsis, and improves pulmonary hygiene. Because ordinary linen-saver pads block airflow, you'll need to use air-permeable pads, available from the manufacturer.

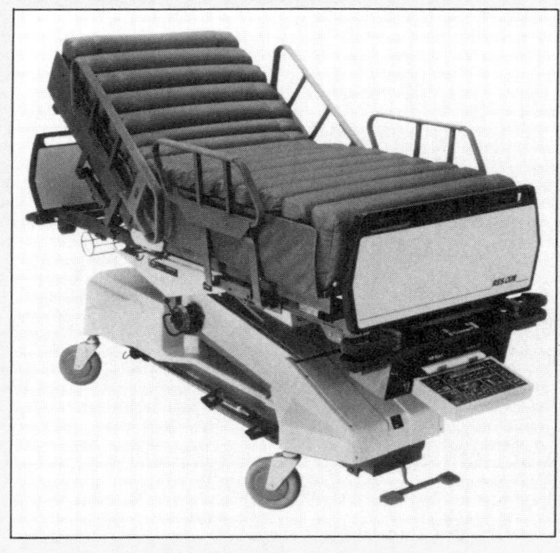

• To treat patients with stage I or II pressure ulcers
• To prevent other complications of immobility, such as pulmonary congestion

Contraindications and complications

Lateral rotation therapy is contraindicated in patients with unstable fractures or acute spinal cord injuries. Also, semiconscious patients may not tolerate the side-to-side motion of lateral rotation therapy.

Equipment

Air therapy bed, with or without lateral rotation and continuous pulsation options • flat sheet • air-permeable pads (if the patient is incontinent or has a copiously draining wound) • clamps to secure the sheet (optional)

Preparation

• Contact the manufacturer's representative or a trained hospital staff member to learn how to prepare the bed for use. Factors to consider when programming the bed's computerized controls for air therapy include the patient's height, weight, body composition, and skin condition. For lateral rotation therapy, assess the patient's pulmonary status and adjust the settings accordingly.
• Explain and demonstrate to the patient how to operate the bed. If lateral rotation or continuous pulsation will be used, describe how this will feel.

Essential steps

• Place a flat sheet over the mattress. Because the mattress is thick, you may have trouble tucking the sheet under it. If necessary, use special clamps to secure the sheet to the bed frame. (You may ask the manufacturer's representative for clamps or other materials to secure the sheet.)
• Turn on the bed to maximum inflation. With help from colleagues, transfer the patient to the bed using a lift sheet. Then remove the lift sheet.
• Using the control panel at the foot of the bed, set the air pressure to the settings that the patient requires (preset by the manufacturer's representative).

Cautions

Take care not to tear the air compartments. If a tear occurs, contact the manufacturer's representative to replace the torn section as soon as possible. Meanwhile, the air compartments surrounding the torn section will expand automatically to cover the space created by the deflated compartments.

For a patient who is incontinent or has a copiously draining wound, use only air-permeable pads (available from the manufacturer) because ordinary linen-saver pads will block the bed's airflow.

Monitoring and aftercare

- To position a bedpan, deflate the middle air compartments and roll the patient away from you. Position the patient on the bedpan. Reinflate the middle section to hold the bedpan in place. To remove the bedpan, again deflate the middle section of the bed, hold the bedpan steady, and roll the patient away from you. Remove the bedpan, reinflate the middle air compartments, and reposition the patient.
- When transferring or repositioning the patient, inflate the air compartments to maximum inflation. This setting will create a firm surface, easing patient repositioning or transfer.
- If the patient suffers cardiac arrest while on the air therapy bed, press the RAPID DEFLATE button on the control panel at the foot of the bed. Deflation will occur within 10 seconds, allowing CPR.
- Document the duration of therapy and the patient's response. Record the condition of the patient's skin, pressure ulcers, and any other wounds.

Colostomy and ileostomy care

A patient with an ascending or transverse colostomy or ileostomy must wear an external pouch to collect fecal discharge (unless the surgeon has created a continent internal or magnetic-ring fecal diversion). Besides collecting waste, the pouch helps to contain odor, and the appropriate skin barrier protects peristomal skin from emerging fecal matter.

A pouching system can be drainable or closed-bottomed, disposable or reusable, and one-piece or two-piece. The choice of a pouching system depends on the stoma type and anatomic location; effluent consistency; and the patient's visual acuity, manual dexterity, personal preference, life-style, finances, and ability to understand and perform stoma care. (See *Comparing ostomy pouching systems,* page 214.)

Most disposable pouching systems have an average wearing time of 5 days. The frequency of routine pouch changes depends on the type of stoma, the patient's abdominal shape, and the type and amount of fecal output. A protruding stoma is less likely to allow fecal matter to seep under the adhesive barrier. Leakage is more likely if the stoma is located in skinfold crevices or near scars, hernias, or bony prominences. Abundant watery discharge usually reduces wearing time.

The type of pouching system used affects wearing time because the material used in the skin barrier can vary in its ability to withstand erosion from fecal discharge. Skin protection is especially important for the patient with an ileostomy because his discharge contains active digestive enzymes that are extremely irritating to peristomal skin.

Indications

Colostomy and ileostomy care is needed to prevent skin irritation and leakage of fecal material.

Contraindications and complications

There are no contraindications.

Failing to fit the pouch properly over the stoma or using a belt improperly can injure the stoma. The patient may develop an allergic reaction to adhesives and other ostomy products.

Equipment

Pouching system • stoma measuring guide • stoma paste (if drainage is watery to pasty or if the stoma secretes excess mucus) • plastic bag • water • washcloth and towel • closure clamp • toilet or bedpan • water or pouch-cleaning solution • clean gloves • facial tissues • optional: ostomy belt, paper tape, mild non-moisturizing soap, shaving equipment, blunt-nose scissors, liquid skin sealant, pouch deodorant

Comparing ostomy pouching systems

Available in many shapes and sizes, ostomy pouches are designed for comfort, safety, and easy application. Some have closed ends, some are mini-pouches, and others have stomal caps to allow irrigation. Some patients may need drainable pouches, which can be either disposable or reusable. Pouches even come in pediatric sizes.

Disposable pouches

The patient who must empty his pouch often because of diarrhea or the ostomy location may prefer a one-piece, drainable, disposable pouch with a closure clamp attached to a skin barrier (see below, left). Patients who have established regular bowel elimination patterns may use a one-piece disposable closed-end pouch that combines the skin barrier and pouch (see below, right). The pouch is odor-proof and virtually undetectable under clothing.

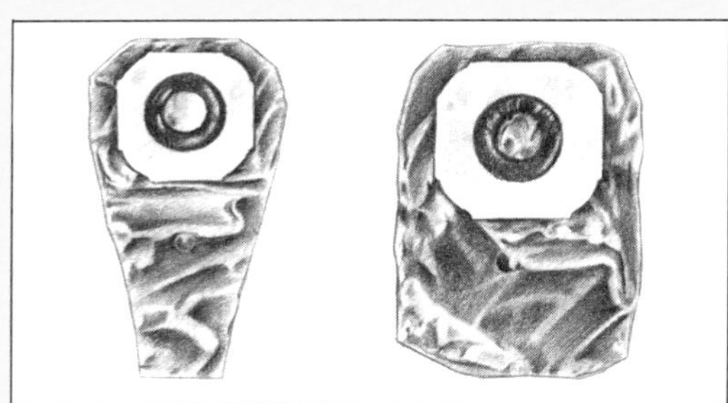

A two-piece, drainable, disposable pouch with a separate skin barrier permits frequent pouch changes and minimizes skin breakdown (see below).

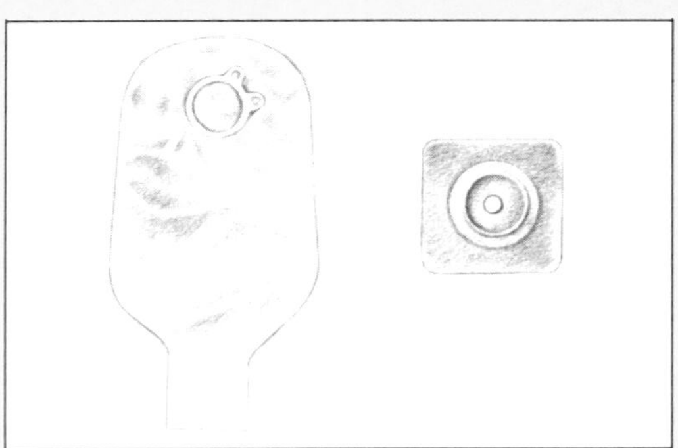

Made of transparent or opaque odor-proof plastic, this model comes with belt tabs and usually snaps to the skin barrier with a flange mechanism.

If the patient has a hard-to-manage stoma, he may prefer a convex disposable skin barrier in a one- or two-piece pouching system. In such a system, the area immediately next to the stoma curves outward, promoting stoma protrusion. This system is especially useful for managing a retracted or flush (nonprotruding and flat) stoma. The patient may add a belt for extra security.

Reusable pouches

Typically made of sturdy, opaque nonallergenic plastic, reusable pouches come with a separate custom-made faceplate and an O ring (see below).

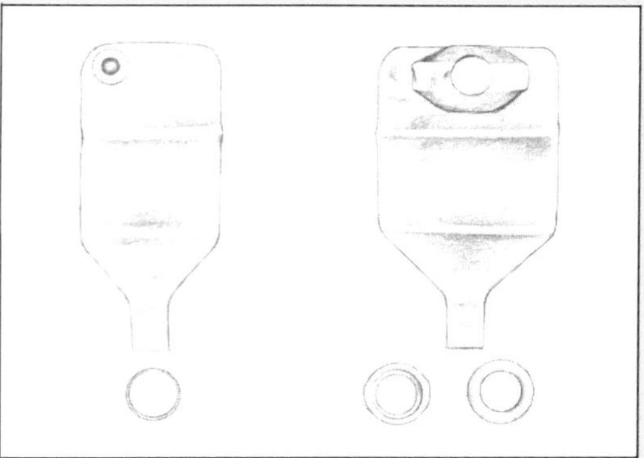

Some have a pressure valve for gas release. This device has a 1- to 2-month life span, depending on how frequently the patient empties it.

A reusable pouch may benefit a patient who needs a firm faceplate or who has limited finances. However, many reusable ostomy pouches aren't odor-proof.

Preparation

Provide the patient with privacy and emotional support.

Essential steps

To fit the pouch and skin barrier

- For a pouch with an attached skin barrier, measure the stoma with the stoma measuring guide. Select the opening size that either matches the stoma size or exceeds it by 1⁄16″. (You may use paste to protect peristomal skin.)
- For an adhesive-backed pouch with a separate skin barrier, measure the stoma with the measuring guide; then select the opening that matches the stoma. Trace the selected size opening onto the paper backing of the skin barrier's adhesive side. Cut out the opening. (If the pouch has precut openings, which can be handy for a round stoma, select an opening that's 1⁄8″ (0.3 cm) larger than the stoma. If the pouch lacks an opening, cut the hole 1⁄8″ wider than the measured tracing.) The cut-to-fit system works best for an irregularly shaped stoma. Note that the solid barrier wafer that will be attached to the adhesive-backed pouch should be sized to fit immediately next to the stoma base, but not touching the stoma.
- Avoid fitting the pouch too tightly because the stoma has no pain receptors. A constrictive opening could injure the stoma or skin tissue without the patient's feeling any discomfort as a warning. Also avoid cutting the opening too big because this could expose the skin to fecal matter and moisture.
- For 6 to 8 weeks after surgery, the stoma will shrink as edema subsides. Consequently, you must measure the stoma and alter the pattern as needed. Follow manufacturer's guidelines when selecting the correct size for a new or different product.

To apply or change the pouch

- Gather the necessary equipment.
- Wash your hands and provide privacy.
- Explain the procedure to the patient. As you perform each step, explain what you're doing and why because the patient eventually will have to perform the procedure himself. (See *Applying an ostomy wafer,* page 216.)
- Put on gloves.
- Gently remove and discard the old pouch. Wipe the stoma and peristomal skin gently with a facial tissue.
- Carefully wash the peristomal skin with soap and water, and dry it with a clean towel. Then inspect the peristomal skin and stoma. Shave surrounding hair or clip it with blunt-nose scissors, if necessary, to promote a better seal and avoid skin irritation from hair pulling against the adhesive.
- If applying a separate skin barrier, peel off the paper backing of the prepared skin barrier, center the barrier over the stoma, and press it gently to ensure adhesion.
- You may want to outline the stoma or the back of the skin barrier (depending on the product) with a thin ring of stoma paste to provide extra skin protection.
- Fill in any peristomal creases or crevices with stoma paste. This provides a smoother surface to adhere to the barrier and may extend the wearing time of the pouching system.
- Remove the paper backing from the adhesive side of the pouching system, and center the pouch opening over the stoma. Press gently to secure the pouch.
- If the pouching system has flanges, align the lip of the pouch flange with the bottom edge of the skin barrier flange. Gently press around the circumference of the pouch flange, starting at the bottom, until the pouch adheres securely to the barrier flange. (The pouch will click into its secured position). Holding the barrier against the skin, gently pull on the pouch to confirm the seal between flanges.
- Encourage the patient to stay quietly in position for about 5 minutes to improve adherence. Body warmth will promote adherence and soften a rigid skin barrier.
- Attach an ostomy belt to further secure the pouch, if desired. (Some pouches have belt loops or plastic adapters for belts.)
- Leave some air in the pouch to allow drainage to fall to the bottom.
- If the patient has a drainable pouch, apply the closure clamp.
- If desired, apply paper tape in a picture-frame fashion to the skin barrier edges for added security. Some skin barriers come with hypoaller-

HOME CARE

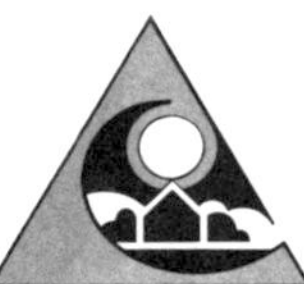

Applying an ostomy wafer

You might want to recommend to your patient that he wear an ostomy wafer to protect the skin around the colostomy site and make it easier for him to care for his colostomy. He may wear an ostomy wafer as long as it remains comfortable and secure. Instruct him to follow these guidelines when applying the wafer.

Applying the wafer

• Choose a flange size that's at least ½" (1 cm) larger in diameter than your stoma.

• Clean the area around the stoma with water and pat it dry thoroughly. Measure stoma size with the stoma measuring guide. Then trace the opening on the white paper backing of the Stomahesive wafer.

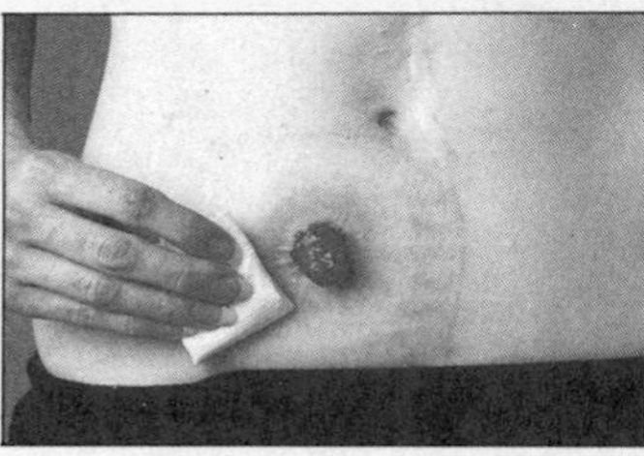

• With the white paper backing of the wafer still in place, cut a hole in the wafer in the same shape and size as the base of the stoma. For best results, cut from the reverse side of the wafer, using curved scissors with short blades.

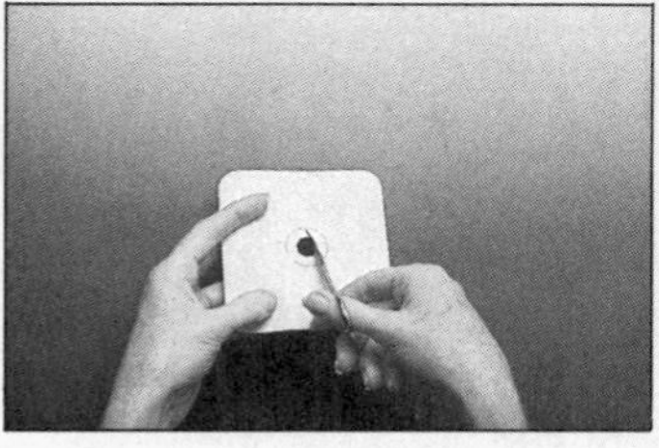

• Just before applying the wafer, peel off the white paper backing.

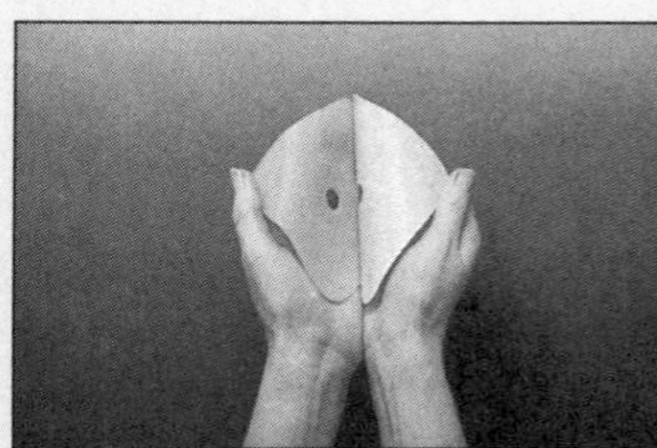

• Apply Stomahesive paste to the wafer, following the manufacturer's instructions, to further protect gaps between the wafer and the base of the stoma.

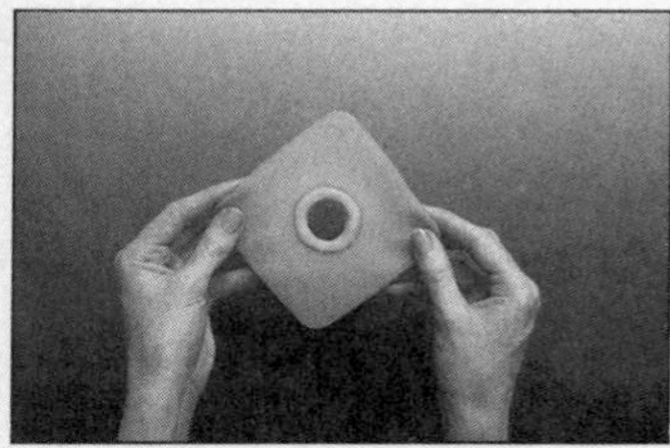

• Center the enlarged hole over the stoma. Then place it on your abdomen and apply light pressure.

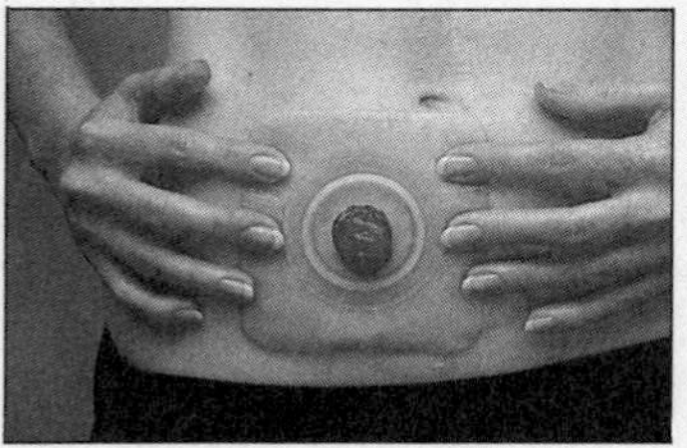

• Press the wafer down firmly, both inside and outside the flange. Pay special attention to the area close to the stoma. Make sure that the wafer adheres firmly to the skin within the area bordered by the flange. You may apply wide, water-resistant, hypoallergenic tape in a picture-frame fashion.

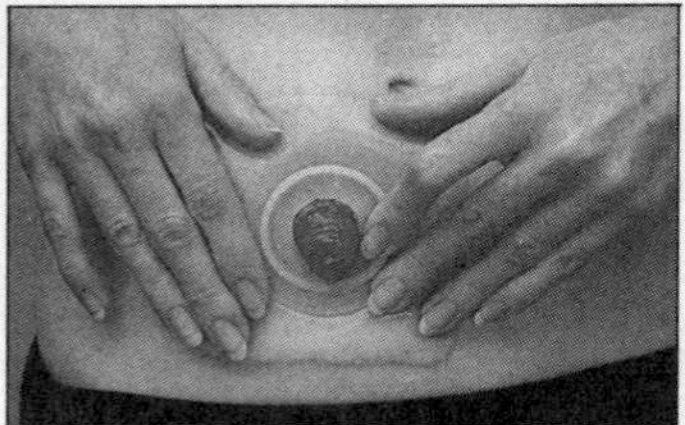

HOME CARE

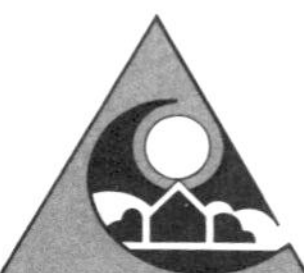

Applying an ostomy wafer *(continued)*

Attaching the Sur-Fit pouch

• Before attaching the pouch, make sure its inner surfaces are separated and the pouch contains some air. Position the outer lip of the pouch flange over the wafer flange at its bottom edge.

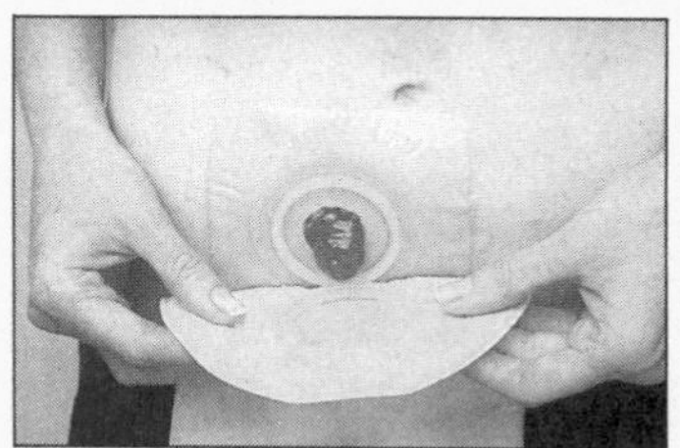

• Using your fingers, press the pouch flange firmly onto the wafer flange from bottom to top, using one continuous motion. You should feel the pouch snap into a secure position.

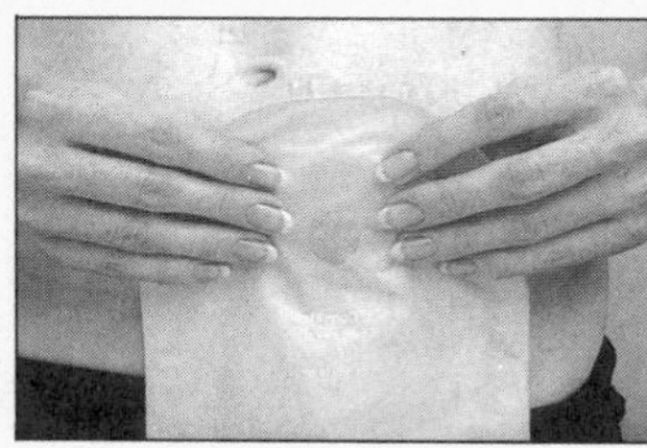

• To confirm that the pouch flange is firmly attached to the wafer flange, tug downward gently on the pouch.

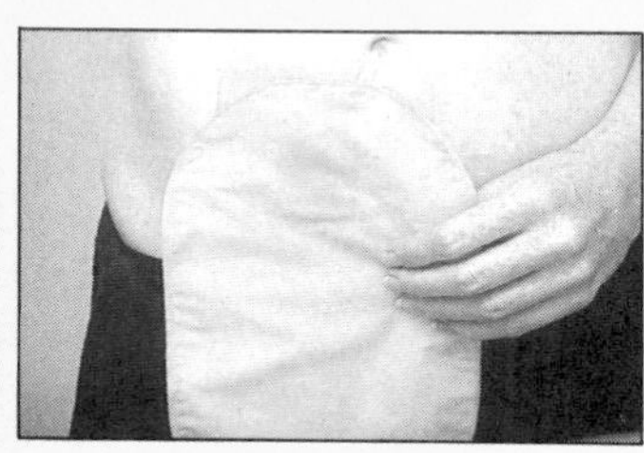

genic tape already adhering to the perimeter. With such barriers, remove the paper backing from the tape and smooth it to the abdomen, keeping it as wrinkle-free as possible.

To empty the pouch

• Tilt the bottom of the pouch upward and remove the closure clamp.
• Turn up a cuff on the lower end of the pouch, and allow it to drain into the toilet or bedpan. If you're draining the effluent directly into the toilet, reduce splashing by first placing some toilet tissue into the bowl.
• Wipe the bottom of the pouch with a towel moistened with water, and reapply the closure clamp. Clean both the inside and outside of the distal portion of the pouch (approximately 1" [2.5 cm]).
• If desired, rinse the bottom portion of the pouch with cool tap water. Don't aim water near the top of the pouch, however, because this may loosen the seal on the skin.
• Release flatus through the gas-release valve. If the pouch doesn't have a gas-release valve, release flatus by tilting the pouch bottom upward, releasing the clamp, and expelling flatus.

To release flatus from a flanged system, loosen the seal between the flanges.

Cautions

If a leak develops, change the pouching system immediately. Remove the pouching system if the patient reports burning or itching beneath it, if purulent drainage appears around the stoma, or if the patient complains of unexplained episodes of fecal odor (which may result from undetected contact of feces with the skin).

Be aware that a liquid skin sealant helps prevent epidermal stripping with tape removal. Most skin sealants must be completely dry before you can apply additional products. Be sure to follow the manufacturer's directions closely.

Use adhesive solvents and removers only after patch-testing the patient's skin because some products may irritate the skin or cause hypersensitivity reactions.

Because charcoal filters are ineffective when wet, use protective devices to keep the filters dry.

If the patient has severe allergies or sensitive skin or prefers not to use adhesive compo-

Colostomy irrigation

Colostomy irrigation serves several purposes. It lets a patient with a descending or sigmoid colostomy regulate his bowel function. It's also used to clean the large bowel before and after diagnostic tests, surgery, or other procedures and to relieve constipation on an infrequent, as-needed basis.

A history of a regular bowel pattern or of constipation suggests greater success than a history of diarrhea. Irrigation may not work if the patient has had radiation therapy to the abdomen or pelvis, has used certain medications long term, or has inflammatory bowel disease.

In a patient with a peristomal hernia, colostomy irrigation may predispose the bowel to perforation. In a patient with bowel prolapse (excessive protrusion at the stoma), it may trigger further prolapse. Irrigation is also contraindicated in patients with unstable fluid and electrolyte balance or any condition that contraindicates vagal stimulation.

Colostomy irrigation may begin as soon as the postoperative patient regains bowel function, but most experts recommend waiting until bowel movements are predictable.

Initially, you or the patient should irrigate the colostomy at the same time every day, recording the amount of output and any spillage between irrigations. Encourage the patient to assume as much responsibility as possible.

Procedure

- Gather the equipment you'll need: colostomy irrigation bag with cone tip, prescribed irrigating solution, irrigation sleeve, water-soluble lubricant, rubber glove, toilet paper and washcloths, bedpan or commode, new colostomy bag or pad, bed protector, and hook (for irrigation bag). (*Note:* You may irrigate with a soft red rubber catheter if the doctor orders this. If not, use a cone tip to keep the stoma dilated and to prevent bowel perforation by the tubing end.)
- Place the hook so that the bottom of the irrigation bag is at shoulder height when the patient is seated.
- Provide privacy. Explain the procedure to the patient in a calm, accepting manner. Position him as indicated by his condition. Then wash your hands.
- Have the patient lie on the protective pad or sit on the pad in bed. If you're doing the procedure in the bathroom, have him sit on the commode or in a chair next to it.
- Close the clamp on the tubing and fill the irrigation bag with 250 to 1,000 ml of the prescribed irrigating solution. Take the supplies to the bedside or bathroom.
- Position the bedpan so that gravity allows the sleeve to drain adequately. If irrigation will be performed in bed, place the bedpan on a bedside chair or at the patient's side. If you're irrigating in the bathroom, position the sleeve so that it drains into the commode.
- Lubricate the cone and expel air by letting the solution flow into the bedpan or commode. Test the warmth of the solution on your wrist. It should be warm, never hot or cold.
- Use 250 ml of solution for the initial irrigation; then increase the volume daily. If necessary and permitted by the doctor, you may use up to 1,000 ml.
- Place the sleeve around the stoma. If the patient has a one-piece system, put the belt on to keep the sleeve in place. With a two-piece system, the belt is optional.
- Dilate the stoma by lubricating the little finger of your gloved hand and gently inserting it into the stoma. Rotate your finger gently. Then lubricate and insert your index finger using the same gentle motion. Remove your finger.
- Gently insert the lubricated cone tip into the stoma, directing the water so that the flow follows the shape of the internal canal. Insert the cone tip far enough to make a seal, but don't insert it beyond its widest point. Make sure the solution flows slowly (one quart over 3 to 5 minutes).
- After inserting the entire volume of solution, turn off the clamp. Wait a few minutes; then slowly remove the cone from the stoma.
- Expect an initial return of fluid and stool within 15 minutes. Before removing the irrigation sleeve, wait another 30 minutes until you're sure all the stool has returned.
- Change the pouch. Or, if the colostomy is regulated, apply a colostomy pad.
- Clean all equipment thoroughly with a mild dishwashing detergent and warm water. Rinse thoroughly and drain dry. Then wash your hands thoroughly and assist the patient to a comfortable position.
- Document the amount and type of irrigating solution used, pouch contents before irrigation (the pouch may be empty or contain spillage), results of irrigation (stool color, amount, and consistency), appearance of the stoma and peristomal skin, the patient's response to the procedure, and his ability to participate.

Points to remember

- Dilate the stoma only when the doctor orders this.
- Never use force during irrigation.
- Cramping may occur if the solution flows too rapidly.
- If the patient doesn't want to sit for the entire procedure, you may clean, then clamp, the bottom of the sleeve. This will allow him to get up and perform other activities.
- Remove soiled laundry or trash from the patient's room immediately after the procedure.

nents, he may choose a nonadhesive pouching system. One such system (Cook VPI) consists of a reusable vinyl pouch with a silicone ring sized to fit around the stoma. An elastic belt secures the pouch.

Never make a pinhole in a pouch to release gas. This will destroy the odor-proof seal.

Monitoring and aftercare

- Empty the pouch when it's one-third to one-half full. Otherwise, weight from the discharge will pull the adhesive from the abdomen.
- Notify the doctor or enterostomal therapist of any skin irritation, breakdown, or rash, or of an unusual appearance of the stoma or peristomal area.
- Usually, the best time to change the pouching system is before breakfast, when the bowels are less active.
- Use commercial pouch deodorants, if desired. However, be aware that most pouches are odorless and that odor should be obvious only when the pouch leaks or is emptied. (Never use aspirin in the pouch to reduce odor because this could induce stomal bleeding.)
- After a patient with a descending or sigmoid colostomy regains bowel function, you may irrigate the colostomy, as ordered, to help restore a regular bowel elimination pattern. (See *Colostomy irrigation.*)
- Encourage the patient's increasing involvement in self-care.
- Suggest that the patient avoid or restrict intake of odor- and gas-forming foods (such as beans, cabbage, onions, yeast-containing foods, fish, garlic, and eggs). Inform him that flatus usually occurs 6 to 12 hours after ingestion of gas-forming foods.
- To help reduce gas-related noise, instruct the patient to apply manual pressure gently against the stoma and to layer clothing over the ostomy.
- If the patient has a reusable pouching system, recommend that he obtain two or more systems so that he can wear one while the other dries after it's cleaned with soap and water or a commercially prepared cleaning solution.
- Document the date and time of the pouch change and the color, amount, type, and consistency of drainage. Also record the reason for the pouch change (such as for routine changing or for leakage). Document the location of any leak to help identify and correct adherence problems. Describe the appearance of the stoma and peristomal skin.
- Document patient teaching, including teaching content. Record the patient's response to self-care and evaluate his learning. Note the involvement of family members in ostomy care and their emotional support in promoting the patient's rehabilitation. Document referrals (for example, to a social worker, a home health care nurse or nursing assistant, the United Ostomy Association, or the American Cancer Society).

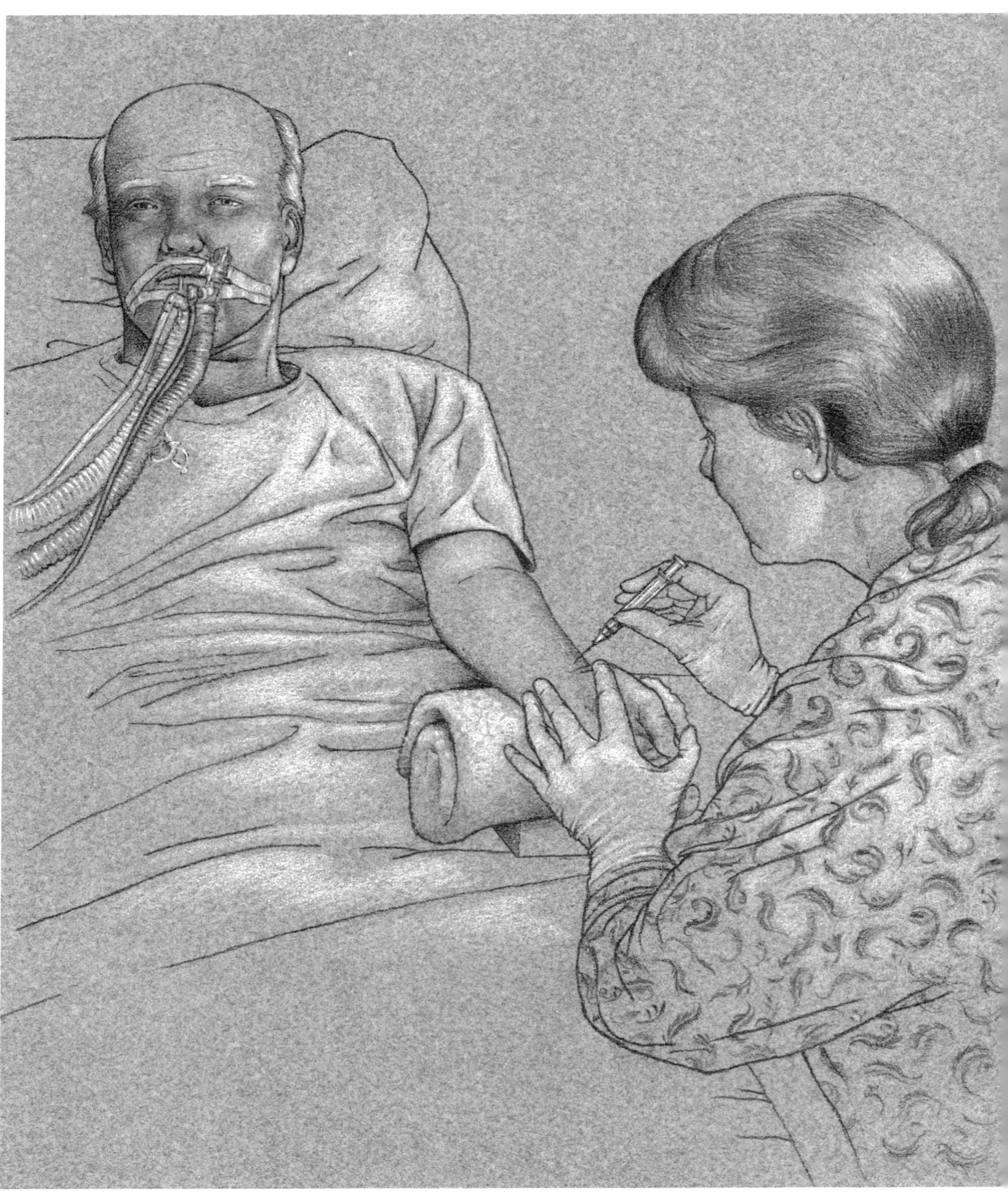

7

CHAPTER

Diagnostic procedures

Regardless of your clinical setting or practice area, managing diagnostic procedures is an important nursing responsibility. The scope of this responsibility goes beyond simply providing patient care during the procedure. In many cases, you must help implement the procedure—or even perform it independently. And for certain procedures, you may also interpret and analyze the results, which in turn helps you to improve and individualize patient care.

To manage a diagnostic procedure, you must integrate the nursing roles of clinician, caregiver, educator, and patient advocate. As a clinician and caregiver, you provide individualized care before, during, and after the procedure. As an educator, you explain the procedure to the patient and, in some cases, teach him how to perform it himself. As a patient advocate, you make sure that the patient understands the procedure adequately so he can give informed consent. As always, your specific duties depend on your hospital's and your state's nurse practice act.

This chapter describes diagnostic procedures in which you may play an important role. Most are performed at the patient's bedside. After describing each procedure and its purpose, the chapter details indications, contraindications and complications, equipment, preparation, essential steps, cautions, and monitoring and aftercare.

Arterial puncture for blood gas analysis

Arterial blood gas (ABG) analysis evaluates respiratory gas exchange and acid-base status by measuring blood pH and the partial pressures of oxygen (PaO_2) and carbon dioxide ($PaCO_2$) in arterial blood. The blood pH value reflects the blood's acid-base balance. The PaO_2 value shows how much oxygen the lungs are delivering to the blood, whereas the $PaCO_2$ value reflects the lungs' capacity to eliminate carbon dioxide. ABG samples can also be analyzed for bicarbonate content and for oxygen content and saturation.

Obtaining an ABG sample requires percutaneous puncture of the brachial, radial, or femoral artery or withdrawal of blood from an arterial line. A respiratory technician or a specially trained nurse can draw most ABG samples; a doctor usually collects blood from the femoral artery.

Indications

• To assess the adequacy of ventilation and oxygenation and the acid-base status of patients with chronic obstructive pulmonary disease, pulmonary edema, acute respiratory distress syndrome, myocardial infarction (MI), or pneumonia

• To evaluate and monitor acid-base balance and cardiopulmonary functioning during episodes of shock and after coronary artery bypass surgery, resuscitation from cardiac arrest, changes in respiratory therapy or status, or prolonged anesthesia

Contraindications and complications

If Allen's test on a patient's hand shows persistent signs of ischemia, arterial puncture for blood gas analysis should not be performed in that hand. Assess the opposite arm for possible use for arterial puncture. (See *How to perform Allen's test.*)

Complications can include ecchymosis, hematoma, infection, and pain at the puncture site.

If you use too much force when attempting to puncture the artery, the needle may touch the periosteum of the bone, causing pain; or you may advance the needle through the opposite wall of the artery. If this happens, slowly pull the needle back a short distance and check to see if you get a blood return. If blood still fails to enter the syringe, withdraw the needle completely and start with a fresh heparinized needle. Don't make more than two attempts to withdraw blood from the same site. Probing the artery may injure both it and the radial nerve. Also, hemolysis will alter test results.

If arterial spasm occurs, blood won't flow into the syringe and you won't be able to collect the sample. If this occurs, replace the needle with a smaller one and attempt the puncture again. A smaller-bore needle is less likely to cause arterial spasm.

Equipment

10-ml glass syringe or plastic luer-lock syringe specially made for drawing blood gases • 1-ml ampule of aqueous heparin (1:1,000) • 20G 1/4" needle • 22G 1" needle • povidone-iodine sponge or alcohol sponge • two 2" × 2" gauze pads • sterile gloves • rubber cap for syringe hub or rubber stopper for needle • ice-filled plastic bag • specimen label • laboratory request form • small adhesive bandage • 1% lidocaine solution (optional)

Note: Many hospitals use a commercial ABG kit that contains all the equipment listed above (except the adhesive bandage and ice). If your hospital doesn't use such a kit, obtain a sterile syringe specially made for drawing ABG samples and use a clean emesis basin filled with ice instead of the plastic bag to transport the sample to the laboratory.

SKILL TIP

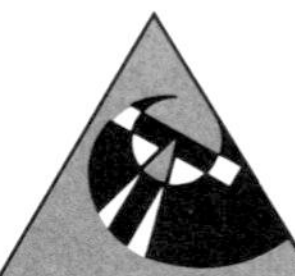

How to perform Allen's test

By performing Allen's test, which assesses blood supply to the hand, you can determine whether you can safely draw an arterial blood sample.

First, rest your patient's arm on the mattress or bedside stand, supporting his wrist with a rolled towel, palm side up. Have him clench his fist. Then, using your index and middle fingers, press on the radial and ulnar arteries. Hold this position for a few seconds.

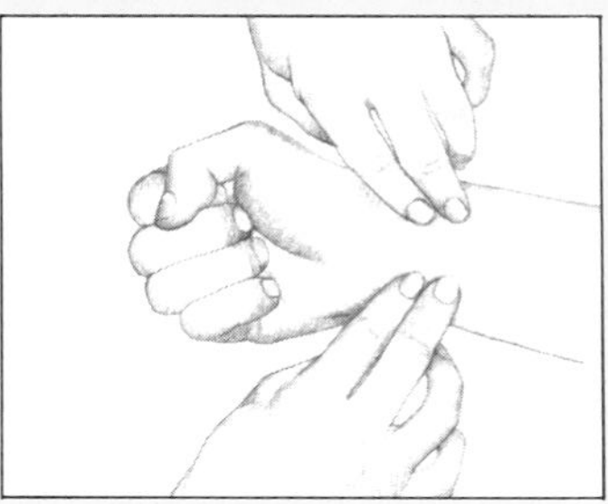

Without removing your fingers from the patient's arteries, ask him to unclench his fist and hold his hand in a relaxed position. The palm will be blanched because pressure from your fingers has impaired normal blood flow.

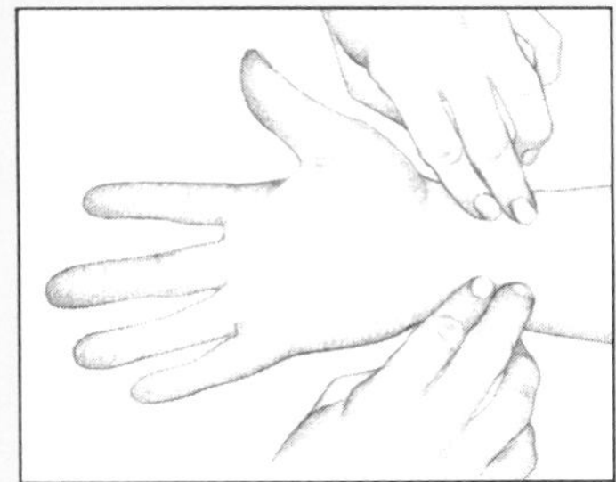

Release pressure on the ulnar artery. If the hand becomes flushed, which indicates blood filling the vessels, you can safely proceed with radial artery puncture. If the hand doesn't flush, perform the test on the other arm.

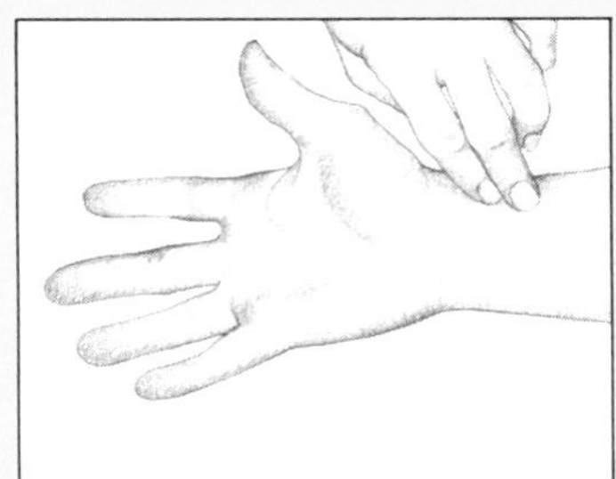

Preparation

• Prepare the collection equipment before entering the patient's room.
• Wash your hands thoroughly.
• Open the ABG kit and remove the specimen label and the plastic bag.
• On the label, write the patient's name and room number, the date and collection time, and the doctor's name.
• Fill the plastic bag with ice and set it aside.
• Heparinize the syringe by first attaching it to the 20G needle. Then open the heparin ampule. Draw all the heparin into the syringe to prevent the sample from clotting. Holding the syringe upright, slowly pull the plunger back to about the 7-ml mark. Rotate the barrel while pulling the plunger back to allow the heparin to coat the inside of the syringe. Then slowly force the heparin toward the hub of the syringe and expel all but about 0.1 ml of heparin.
• Heparinize the needle by first replacing the 20G needle with the 22G needle. Then, holding the syringe upright, tilt it slightly and eject the remaining heparin. (Excess heparin in the syringe alters blood pH and PaO_2 values.)
• Tell the patient you need to collect an arterial blood sample. Explain the procedure to help ease his anxiety and promote cooperation. Tell him that the needle stick will cause some discomfort but that he must remain still during the procedure.

Essential steps

• Wash your hands and put on gloves. Then place a rolled towel under the patient's wrist for support. Locate the artery and palpate it for a strong pulse.
• Perform Allen's test to assess the adequacy of blood supply to the patient's hand.
• If you use a povidone-iodine sponge to clean the puncture site, use a circular motion, start-

Arterial puncture technique

When you're obtaining an arterial blood gas sample, the angle of needle penetration depends on the artery to be sampled. For the radial artery (the most commonly used artery), the needle should enter bevel up at a 30- to 45-degree angle.

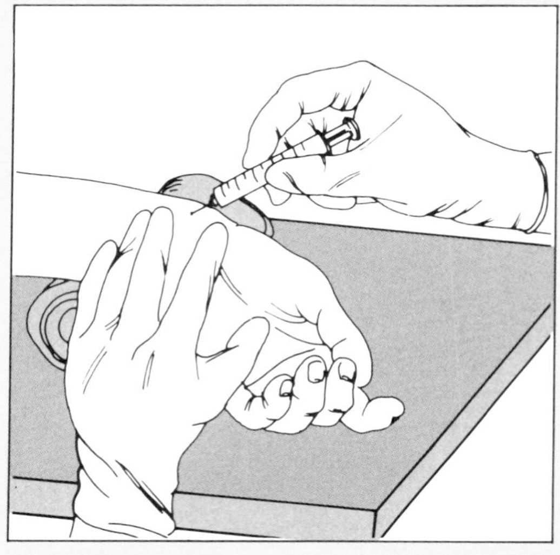

ing in the center of the site and spiraling outward to avoid introducing potentially infectious skin flora into the vessel during the procedure. Don't wipe off the povidone-iodine with alcohol because alcohol cancels the effect of povidone-iodine.

- If you use an alcohol sponge, apply it with friction for 30 seconds or until the final sponge comes away clean. Let the skin dry.
- Palpate the artery with the index and middle fingers of one hand while holding the syringe over the puncture site with the other hand. (See *Arterial puncture technique.*)
- Hold the needle bevel up at a 30- to 45-degree angle. (When puncturing the brachial artery, hold the needle at a 60-degree angle.)
- Puncture the skin and the arterial wall in one motion, following the path of the artery.
- Watch for blood backflow in the syringe. Don't pull back on the plunger because arterial blood should enter the syringe automatically. Fill the syringe to the 5-ml mark.
- After collecting the sample, press a gauze pad firmly over the puncture site until bleeding stops—at least 5 minutes. If the patient is receiving anticoagulant therapy or has a blood dyscrasia, apply pressure for 10 to 15 minutes; if necessary, ask a colleague to hold the gauze pad in place while you prepare the sample for transport to the laboratory. Don't ask the patient to hold the pad; if he fails to apply sufficient pressure, a large, painful hematoma could form, hindering future arterial punctures at that site.
- Check the syringe for air bubbles because these may alter PaO_2 values. If air bubbles appear, remove them by holding the syringe upright and slowly ejecting some of the blood onto a 2″ × 2″ gauze pad.
- Insert the needle into a rubber stopper, or remove the needle and place a rubber cap directly on the needle hub. This prevents the sample from leaking and keeps air out of the syringe.
- Put the labeled sample in the ice-filled plastic bag or emesis basin. Attach a properly completed laboratory request form and send the sample to the laboratory immediately.
- When the bleeding stops, apply a small adhesive bandage to the site.

Cautions

If your patient is receiving oxygen, make sure oxygen therapy has been underway for at least 15 minutes before drawing arterial blood. Unless ordered, don't turn off oxygen therapy before drawing the sample. However, be sure to indicate on the laboratory request form the amount and type of oxygen therapy the patient is receiving. If the patient isn't receiving oxygen, indicate that he's breathing room air.

If your patient has just received a breathing treatment or nebulizer treatment, wait about 20 minutes before drawing the sample.

If necessary, you may anesthetize the puncture site with 1% lidocaine solution. However, consider such use of lidocaine carefully because it delays the procedure, the patient may be allergic to the drug, or the resulting vasoconstriction may prevent a successful puncture.

Monitoring and aftercare

• Monitor the patient's vital signs and observe for signs of circulatory impairment, such as swelling, discoloration, pain, numbness, or tingling in the bandaged arm or leg. Also watch for bleeding at the puncture site.
• Document the results of Allen's test, the time the sample was drawn, the patient's temperature, the arterial puncture site, the length of time pressure was applied to the site to control bleeding and, if appropriate, the type and amount of oxygen therapy the patient was receiving.
• When filling out a laboratory request form for ABG analysis, be sure to include the following information to help the laboratory staff calibrate the equipment and evaluate results correctly: the patient's current temperature and respiratory rate, his most recent hemoglobin level, and the fraction of inspired oxygen and tidal volume if he's using a ventilator.

Lumbar puncture

To perform lumbar puncture, the doctor inserts a sterile needle into the subarachnoid space of the spinal canal, usually between the third and fourth lumbar vertebrae. A nurse assists during the procedure. Lumbar puncture requires sterile technique and careful patient positioning.

Indications

• To detect increased intracranial pressure (ICP) or to detect blood in cerebrospinal fluid (CSF), which indicates cerebral hemorrhage (See *CSF analysis findings,* page 226.)
• To obtain CSF specimens for laboratory analysis
• To inject contrast dyes or gases in radiologic studies of the brain and spinal cord
• To administer drugs or anesthetics
• To reduce ICP by removing CSF

Contraindications and complications

This procedure is contraindicated in patients with a lumbar deformity or an infection at the puncture site. It should be performed cautiously in patients with increased ICP because the rapid pressure reduction that follows CSF withdrawal may cause tonsillar herniation and medullary compression.

Headache is the most common complication of lumbar puncture. Tonsillar herniation and medullary compression (both rare) are the most serious complications. Other potential complications include a reaction to the anesthetic, meningitis, epidural or subdural abscess, bleeding into the spinal canal, CSF leakage through the dural defect that remains after needle withdrawal, local pain caused by nerve root irritation, edema or hematoma at the puncture site, transient voiding difficulty, and fever.

Equipment

Overbed table • one or two pairs of sterile gloves for the doctor • sterile gloves for the nurse • povidone-iodine solution • sterile gauze pads • alcohol sponges • sterile fenestrated drape • 3-ml syringe for local anesthetic • 25G 3/4" sterile needle for injecting anesthetic • local anesthetic (usually 1% lidocaine) • sterile 18G or 20G 3½" spinal needle with stylet (22G needle for a pediatric patient) • three-way stopcock • manometer • small adhesive bandage • three sterile collection tubes with stoppers • laboratory request forms • labels • light source, such as a gooseneck lamp

Note: Disposable lumbar puncture trays containing most of the needed sterile equipment are generally available.

Preparation

• Explain the procedure to the patient to ease his anxiety and promote cooperation. Tell him he may experience a headache after lumbar puncture, but reassure him that his cooperation during the procedure will minimize this problem. (*Note:* If the doctor suspects a central nervous system disorder, he usually withholds sedatives and analgesics before lumbar puncture because they may mask important symptoms.)
• Make sure that the patient has signed a consent form.
• Immediately before the procedure, provide privacy and instruct the patient to void.

CSF analysis findings

Test	Normal	Abnormal	Implications
Appearance	Clear, colorless	Cloudy	Infection (elevated white blood cell [WBC] count or many microorganisms) or elevated protein level
		Pink, red, or bloody	Subarachnoid, intracerebral, or intraventricular hemorrhage; subarachnoid obstruction; traumatic tap (usually noted only in initial specimen)
		Brown, orange, or yellow (xanthochromic)	Elevated protein, red blood cell (RBC) breakdown (blood present for at least 3 days)
Cell count	0 to 5 WBCs	Increase	Active disease: meningitis, acute infection, onset of chronic illness, tumor, abscess, infarction, demyelinating disease (such as multiple sclerosis)
	No RBCs	RBCs	Hemorrhage or traumatic tap
Chloride	118 to 130 mEq/liter	Decrease	Infected meninges (as in tuberculosis or meningitis)
Gamma globulin	3% to 12% of total protein	Increase	Demyelinating disease (such as multiple sclerosis), neurosyphilis, Guillain-Barré syndrome
Glucose	40 to 80 mg/dl (60% to 80% of blood glucose)	Increase	Systemic hyperglycemia
		Decrease	Systemic hypoglycemia, bacterial fungal infection, meningitis, mumps, postsubarachnoid hemorrhage
Gram stain	No organisms	Gram-positive or gram-negative organisms	Bacterial meningitis
Pressure	50 to 180 mm H_2O	Increase	Increased intracranial pressure due to hemorrhage, tumor, thrombosis, meningitis, or edema caused by trauma
		Decrease	Spinal subarachnoid obstruction above puncture site
Protein	15 to 45 mg/dl	Marked increase	Tumors, trauma, hemorrhage, diabetes mellitus, bacterial or fungal meningitis, polyneuritis, blood in cerebrospinal fluid (CSF), demyelinating disease (such as multiple sclerosis)
		Marked decrease	Rapid CSF production
Veneral Disease Research Laboratories (VDRL) and other serologic tests	Nonreactive	Positive	Neurosyphilis

• Wash your hands thoroughly.
• Provide adequate lighting at the puncture site.
• Adjust the height of the patient's bed so the doctor can perform the procedure comfortably.

Essential steps

• Open the equipment tray on an overbed table. When opening the wrapper, take care not to contaminate the sterile field.
• Have the patient lie on his side at the edge of the bed, with his chin tucked to his chest and his knees drawn up to his abdomen. Make sure his spine is curved and his back is at the edge of the bed. This position widens the spaces between the vertebrae, easing needle insertion. To help the patient maintain this position, place one of your hands behind his neck and the other hand behind his knees, then pull gently. Hold him firmly in this position throughout the procedure to prevent accidental needle displacement.
• After putting on sterile gloves, the doctor cleans the puncture site with sterile gauze pads soaked in povidone-iodine solution, wiping in a circular motion away from the injection site. He uses three different pads to prevent contamination of spinal tissues by the body's normal skin flora. Next, he drapes the area with the fenestrated drape to provide a sterile field. (If he uses povidone-iodine sponges instead of sterile gauze pads, he may remove his sterile gloves and put on another pair to avoid introducing povidone-iodine into the subarachnoid space with the lumbar puncture needle.)
• If the equipment tray doesn't include an ampule of anesthetic, clean the injection port of a multidose vial of anesthetic with an alcohol sponge. Then invert the vial 45 degrees so the doctor can insert a 25G needle and syringe and withdraw the anesthetic for injection.
• Before the doctor injects the anesthetic, tell the patient he'll experience a transient burning sensation and local pain. Ask him to report any other persistent pain or sensations because these may indicate nerve root irritation or puncture, necessitating needle repositioning.
• When the doctor inserts the sterile spinal needle into the subarachnoid space between the third and fourth lumbar vertebrae, instruct the patient to remain still and breathe normally.
• If lumbar puncture is being performed to administer a spinal anesthetic or contrast media for a radiologic study, the doctor injects the anesthetic or dye at this time.
• Once the needle is in place, the doctor attaches a manometer with a three-way stopcock to the needle hub to read CSF pressure. If ordered, help the patient extend his legs to provide a more accurate pressure reading.
• The doctor detaches the manometer and allows fluid to drain from the needle hub into the collection tubes. When he has collected approximately 2 to 3 ml in each tube, mark the tubes in sequence, stopper them securely, and label them properly.
• If the doctor suspects an obstruction in the spinal subarachnoid space, he may check for Queckenstedt's sign. To do this, he takes an initial CSF pressure reading. Then, as ordered, compress the patient's jugular vein for 10 seconds. This temporarily obstructs blood flow from the cranium, increasing ICP and—if no subarachnoid obstruction exists—causing CSF pressure to rise as well. The doctor then takes pressure readings every 10 seconds until the pressure stabilizes.
• After the doctor collects the specimens and removes the spinal needle, clean the puncture site with povidone-iodine solution and apply a small adhesive bandage.
• Send the CSF specimens to the laboratory immediately with properly completed laboratory request forms.

Cautions

During lumbar puncture, watch closely for signs of an adverse reaction: an increased pulse rate, pallor, or clammy skin. Alert the doctor immediately to any of these signs.

Monitoring and aftercare

• The doctor may order that the patient maintain the supine position for 8 to 12 hours after the procedure.
• Send CSF specimens to the laboratory immediately; they shouldn't be refrigerated for later transport.

• Document the time the procedure began and ended, the patient's response, administration of any drugs, number of specimen tubes collected, time of specimen transport to the laboratory, and the color, consistency, and any other characteristics of the collected specimens.

Paracentesis

In paracentesis, the doctor aspirates fluid from the peritoneal space through a needle, trocar, or catheter inserted in the abdominal wall. A bedside procedure, it is used for both diagnosis and therapy.

Indications

• To determine the cause of ascites
• To relieve pressure created by ascites
• To detect intra-abdominal bleeding after traumatic injury
• To obtain a peritoneal fluid specimen for laboratory analysis

Contraindications and complications

This procedure must be performed cautiously in pregnant patients and in those with bleeding tendencies or unstable vital signs.

Hypovolemic shock may result from the sudden shift of fluid from the circulatory system to the peritoneum to replace aspirated fluid. Other possible complications include perforation of abdominal organs by the needle or the trocar and catheter, hepatic coma from decreased systemic circulation and reduced tissue perfusion, wound infection, and peritonitis.

Equipment

Tape measure • sterile gloves • clean gloves • linen-saver pads • four Vacutainer laboratory tubes • two large sterile glass Vacutainer bottles (1,000 ml or larger) • dry sterile pressure dressings • laboratory request forms • povidone-iodine solution • local anesthetic (multidose vial of 1% or 2% lidocaine with epinephrine) • sterile 4″ × 4″ gauze pads • sterile paracentesis tray (containing needle, trocar, catheter, and three-way stopcock) • sterile drapes • felt-tip marking pen • 5-ml syringe with 22G or 25G needle • povidone-iodine ointment • optional: alcohol sponge, 50-ml syringe, scalpel, suture materials, I.V. salt-poor albumin

Preparation

• Explain the procedure to the patient to ease his anxiety and promote cooperation. Reassure him that he should feel no pain but mention that he may feel a stinging sensation from the local anesthetic injection and pressure from the needle or trocar and catheter insertion. Mention that he may sense pressure when the doctor aspirates abdominal fluid.
• Make sure that the patient has signed a consent form.
• Instruct the patient to void before the procedure. Or insert an indwelling urinary catheter, if ordered, to minimize the risk of accidental bladder injury from the needle or trocar and catheter insertion.
• Identify and record baseline values, including the patient's vital signs, weight, and abdominal girth. Use the tape measure to gauge abdominal girth at the umbilical level. Indicate the abdominal area measured with a felt-tip marking pen. Baseline data will be used to monitor the patient's status during and after the procedure.
• Help the patient sit up in bed so that fluid accumulates in the lower abdomen. Or help him sit on the side of the bed and use pillows to support his back. (See *Positioning your patient for paracentesis.*)
• Expose the patient's abdomen from diaphragm to pubis. Keep the rest of him covered so he won't get chilled.
• Make the patient as comfortable as possible. Place a linen-saver pad under him for protection from drainage.
• Remind the patient to stay as still as possible during the procedure to prevent injury from the needle or trocar and catheter.

Essential steps

• Wash your hands. Open the paracentesis tray, using aseptic technique to ensure a sterile field.
• Wear clean gloves to protect yourself from possible body fluid contamination. Assist the

doctor as he prepares the patient's abdomen with povidone-iodine solution, drapes the operative site with sterile drapes, and administers the local anesthetic.

- If the paracentesis tray doesn't contain a sterile ampule of anesthetic, wipe the top of a multidose vial of anesthetic solution with an alcohol sponge, and invert the vial at a 45-degree angle. This allows the doctor to insert the sterile 5-ml syringe with the 22G or 25G needle and withdraw the anesthetic without touching the nonsterile vial.
- Using the scalpel, the doctor may make a small incision before inserting the needle or trocar and catheter (usually 1″ to 2″ [2.5 to 5 cm] below the umbilicus). Listen for a popping sound, which means the needle or trocar has pierced the peritoneum.
- Assist the doctor with collecting specimens in the appropriate containers.
- If the doctor orders substantial drainage, connect the three-way stopcock and tubing to the cannula. Run the other end of the tubing to a large sterile Vacutainer collection bottle. Or aspirate the fluid with a three-way stopcock and 50-ml syringe.
- Gently turn the patient from side to side to enhance drainage, if necessary.
- As the fluid drains, monitor the patient's vital signs every 15 minutes. Observe him closely for vertigo, faintness, diaphoresis, pallor, heightened anxiety, tachycardia, dyspnea, and hypotension—especially if more than 1,500 ml of peritoneal fluid was aspirated at one time. This loss may induce a fluid shift and hypovolemic shock.
- When the procedure ends and the doctor removes the needle or trocar and catheter, he may suture the incision. Wearing sterile gloves, apply the dry sterile pressure dressing and povidone-iodine ointment to the site. Help the patient into a comfortable position.
- Label the Vacutainer specimen tubes and send them to the laboratory with the appropriate laboratory request forms. If the patient is receiving antibiotics, note this on the request form so that this information can be considered during fluid analysis.
- Remove and dispose of all equipment properly.

SKILL TIP

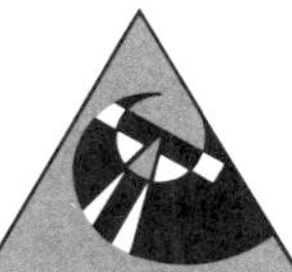

Positioning your patient for paracentesis

An ambulatory or bedridden patient must be properly positioned for paracentesis. Help the patient sit up in bed, or have him sit on the side of the bed with additional support for his back and arms. In this position, gravity helps fluid to accumulate in the lower abdominal cavity. Internal abdominal structures provide counterresistance and additional pressure to promote fluid flow.

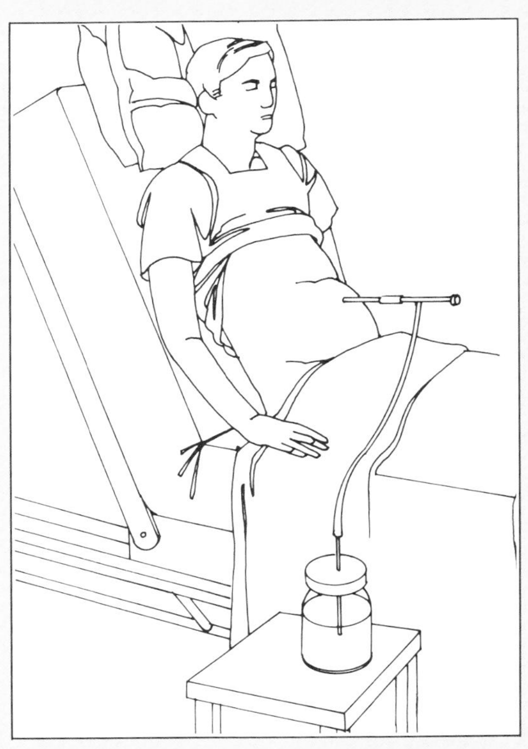

Cautions

Throughout this procedure, explain each step thoroughly to the patient and provide emotional support. Help him remain still to prevent accidental perforation of abdominal organs.

If the patient shows signs or symptoms of hypovolemic shock, reduce the vertical distance between the needle or the trocar and catheter and the drainage collection container to slow the drainage rate. If necessary, stop the drainage. Immediately report signs or symptoms of shock to the doctor, who may order you to administer I.V. salt-poor albumin to replace aspirated fluid and prevent hypovolemia.

To prevent fluid shifts and hypovolemia, limit aspirated fluid to between 1,500 and 2,000 ml. If peritoneal fluid doesn't flow easily, try repositioning the patient to promote drainage. Also verify suction in the Vacutainer collection bottle when you connect it to the drainage tubing, and be sure to use macrodrip tubing without a backflow device.

Monitoring and aftercare

• Monitor the patient's vital signs and check the dressing for drainage every 15 minutes for the first hour, every 30 minutes for the next 2 hours, every hour for the next 4 hours, then every 4 hours for the next 24 hours to detect delayed reactions to the procedure. Note drainage color, amount, and character.
• Observe for peritoneal fluid leakage. If this occurs, notify the doctor. Measure and record the patient's weight and abdominal girth daily. Compare daily values with baseline values to detect recurrent ascites.
• Document the date and time of the procedure, the puncture site location, and whether the wound was sutured. Record the amount, color, viscosity, and odor of aspirated fluid in your notes and in the fluid intake and output record. Document the patient's vital signs, weight, and abdominal girth measurements before and after the procedure. Also note his tolerance of the procedure and any signs or symptoms of complications. Record the number of specimens sent to the laboratory.

Peritoneal lavage

Following blunt trauma to the abdomen, peritoneal lavage is used to detect bleeding in the peritoneal cavity. It may proceed through several steps. First, the doctor inserts a catheter or trocar through the abdominal wall into the peritoneal cavity and aspirates peritoneal fluid with a syringe. (See *How peritoneal lavage works.*) If he can't see blood in the aspirated fluid, he infuses a balanced saline solution and siphons fluid from the cavity. Then he inspects the siphoned fluid for blood and sends fluid samples to the laboratory for microscopic examination. Normal peritoneal fluid appears clear to pale yellow. If peritoneal lavage results are abnormal, the patient may need a laparotomy and further treatment. (See *Abnormal findings in peritoneal lavage,* page 232.)

If the patient's condition is stable, a borderline positive result may suggest the need for additional tests, such as echocardiography and arteriography. If test results are questionable or inconclusive, the doctor may leave the catheter in place to repeat the procedure.

Indications

The procedure detects bleeding in the peritoneal cavity in patients with blunt abdominal trauma.

Contraindications and complications

Peritoneal lavage is contraindicated in patients who have had multiple abdominal operations (adhesions), those who are unstable and need immediate surgery, and those who can't be catheterized before the procedure. In pregnant patients, the procedure requires great caution and a different technique.

Complications include bleeding at the incision site or intra-abdominal bleeding from lacerated blood vessels. Visceral perforation may cause peritonitis, necessitating laparotomy for repair. In a patient with respiratory distress, infusing a balanced saline solution may cause additional stress and trigger respiratory arrest.

The bladder may be accidentally lacerated or punctured if it isn't emptied completely before peritoneal lavage. Use strict aseptic technique to prevent infection.

Equipment

Indwelling urinary catheter and drainage bag • nasogastric (NG) tube • gastric suction machine • shaving kit • I.V. pole • macrodrip I.V. tubing • I.V. solutions (1 liter of balanced saline solution, usually lactated Ringer's solution or 0.9% sodium chloride solution) • peritoneal dialysis tray • sterile gloves • antiseptic solution (such as povidone-iodine) • 3-ml syringe with 25G 1″ needle • bottle of 1% lidocaine with epinephrine • 5″ (12.7 cm) #14 intracatheter extension tubing and a small sterile hemostat (to clamp tubing) • scalpel • 30-ml syringe • 20G 1½″ needle • sterile towels • three containers for specimen collection, including one sterile tube for a culture and sensitivity specimen • labels • antiseptic ointment • 4″ × 4″ gauze pads • alcohol sponges • 1″ nonallergenic tape

Note: If you're using a commercially prepared peritoneal dialysis kit (containing a #15 peritoneal dialysis catheter, trocar, and extension tubing with roller clamp), make sure that the macrodrip tubing doesn't have a reverse flow (or backcheck) valve that prevents infused fluid from draining out of the peritoneal cavity.

Preparation

• Provide privacy and wash your hands.
• Clarify or reinforce the doctor's explanation of the procedure. Have the patient sign a consent form. Tell the patient to expect a sensation of abdominal fullness. Inform him that he may experience a chill if the lavage solution isn't warmed or doesn't reach his body temperature.
• Catheterize the patient with the indwelling urinary catheter; then connect the catheter to the drainage bag. This decreases bladder fullness, reducing the risk of accidental bladder puncture from the trocar or catheter used for lavage.
• Insert the NG tube; then attach it to the gastric suction machine (set for low intermittent suction) to drain stomach contents. Stomach decompression prevents vomiting and subsequent aspiration and minimizes the risk of bowel perforation during trocar or catheter insertion.
• Using the shaving kit, clip or shave hair from the area between the patient's umbilicus and pubis, as ordered.
• Set up the I.V. pole. Attach the macrodrip tubing to the lavage solution container. Clear air from the tubing to avoid introducing air into the peritoneal cavity during lavage.

How peritoneal lavage works

The doctor performs peritoneal lavage to detect bleeding in the peritoneal cavity. The top illustration shows the path the trocar or catheter takes through the abdominal wall. The bottom illustration shows how the doctor attaches a syringe to the catheter to aspirate fluid from the peritoneal cavity.

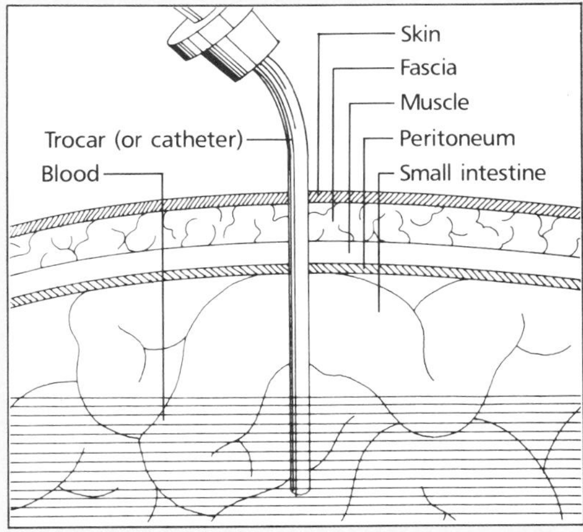

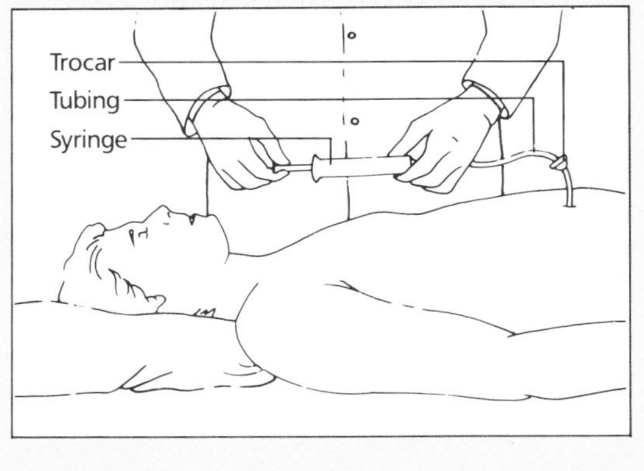

Essential steps

• Using aseptic technique, open the peritoneal dialysis tray.
• Wearing sterile gloves, the doctor wipes the patient's abdomen from the costal margin to the pubic area and from flank to flank with the antiseptic solution. Then he drapes the area

Abnormal findings in peritoneal lavage

If peritoneal lavage yields any of the following findings, your patient may need a laparotomy and further treatment:

- unclotted blood, bile, or intestinal contents
- red blood cell count over 100,000/mm³
- white blood cell count over 500/mm³
- bacteria, as identified by culture and sensitivity testing or Gram stain
- green, cloudy, turbid, or milky fluid
- bloody or pinkish-red fluid, dark enough to obscure reading newsprint through it. (If newsprint can be read through the fluid, test results are considered negative, although the doctor may order more tests.)

with sterile towels from the dialysis tray to create a sterile field.

• Using aseptic technique, hand the doctor the 3-ml syringe with the 25G 1″ needle. If the peritoneal dialysis tray doesn't contain a sterile ampule of anesthetic, wipe the top of a multidose vial of 1% lidocaine with epinephrine using an alcohol sponge and invert the vial at a 45-degree angle. This allows the doctor to insert the needle and withdraw the anesthetic without touching the nonsterile vial.

• The doctor injects the anesthetic directly below the umbilicus (or at an adjacent site if the patient has a surgical scar). Once the area is numb, he makes a small incision (about ¾″ [2 cm]) through the skin and subcutaneous tissues of the abdominal wall. He retracts the tissue, ligates severed blood vessels, and uses 4″ × 4″ gauze pads to absorb and keep incisional blood from entering the wound and causing a false-positive test result. Next, he directs the trocar through the incision into the pelvic midline until the instrument enters the peritoneum. Then he advances the peritoneal catheter (via the trocar) 6″ to 8″ (15 to 20 cm) into the pelvis. Using a syringe attached to the catheter, he aspirates fluid from the peritoneal cavity and looks for blood and other abnormal findings. With positive findings, the procedure ends, and you'll prepare the patient for laparotomy and further measures. If retrieved fluid looks normal, lavage will continue.

• Wearing sterile gloves, connect the catheter extension tubing to the I.V. tubing, if ordered. Instill 500 to 1,000 ml (10 ml/kg of body weight) of the warmed I.V. solution into the peritoneal cavity over 5 to 10 minutes, as ordered. Then clamp the tubing with the hemostat.

• Unless contraindicated by the patient's injuries (such as a spinal cord injury, a rib fracture, or an unstable pelvic fracture), gently tilt the patient from side to side to distribute the fluid throughout the peritoneal cavity. If the patient's condition contraindicates tilting, the doctor may gently palpate the sides of the abdomen to distribute the fluid.

• After 5 to 10 minutes, place the I.V. container below the level of the patient's body and open the clamp on the I.V. tubing. Lowering the container helps to drain excess fluid. Gently drain as much fluid as possible from the peritoneal cavity to the container. Take care not to disconnect the tubing from the catheter. The peritoneal cavity may take 20 to 30 minutes to drain completely.

• If you're using a glass I.V. container, be sure to vent it with a needle to promote flow. You don't need to vent a plastic bag container.

• To obtain a fluid specimen, use a 30-ml syringe and a 20G 1½″ needle to withdraw 25 to 30 ml of fluid from a port in the I.V. tubing. Clean the top of each specimen container with an alcohol sponge. Deposit fluid specimens in the containers.

Note: If you didn't obtain the culture and sensitivity specimen first, change the needle before drawing this fluid sample to avoid contaminating the specimen.

• Label the specimens and send them to the laboratory immediately for culture and sensitivity analysis, Gram stain, red and white blood cell count, amylase and bile determinations, and spun-down sediment evaluation. If blood is present in the peritoneal fluid, expect the doctor to perform a laparotomy. With a normal test result, expect him to close the incision.

• Wearing sterile gloves, apply antiseptic ointment to the site and dress the incision with a 4″ × 4″ gauze pad secured with 1″ nonallergenic tape.
• Discard disposable equipment. Return reusable equipment to the appropriate department for cleaning and sterilization.

Cautions

Be sure to maintain strict aseptic technique throughout this procedure to avoid introducing microorganisms into the peritoneum, which could cause peritonitis.

If the doctor orders abdominal X-rays, they will probably precede peritoneal lavage. X-rays taken after lavage may be unreliable because of air introduced into the peritoneal cavity.

Monitoring and aftercare

• Monitor the patient's vital signs frequently.
• Immediately report any signs or symptoms of shock, such as tachycardia, decreased blood pressure, diaphoresis, dyspnea, or vertigo.
• Check the incision site often for bleeding.
• Document the type and size of peritoneal dialysis catheter used, the type and amount of solution instilled and withdrawn from the peritoneal cavity, and the amount and color of fluid returned. Note whether the fluid flowed freely into and out of the abdomen. Record which specimens were obtained and sent to the laboratory. Also note any complications that occurred and the nursing action you took to manage them.

Bone marrow aspiration and biopsy

A specimen of bone marrow—the major site of blood cell formation—may be obtained by aspiration or needle biopsy. This procedure allows evaluation of overall blood composition by analyzing blood elements and precursor cells as well as abnormal or malignant cells. Aspiration removes cells through a needle inserted into the bone marrow cavity; a biopsy removes a small, solid core of marrow tissue through the needle. Usually, a doctor performs both procedures. However, some hospitals authorize specially trained chemotherapy nurses or nurse clinicians to perform them with the aid of an assistant.

Indications

For aspiration

• To diagnose various disorders and cancers, such as oat cell carcinoma, leukemia, and Hodgkin's disease and other lymphomas

For biopsy (usually performed simultaneously with aspiration)

• To stage the cancer
• To monitor the patient's response to treatment

Contraindications and complications

Bone marrow specimens should not be collected from irradiated areas because radiation may have altered or destroyed the marrow.

Bleeding and infection are potentially life-threatening complications of bone marrow aspiration or biopsy at any site. Complications of sternal needle puncture are uncommon but include puncture of the heart and major vessels, causing severe hemorrhage; puncture of the mediastinum, causing mediastinitis or pneumomediastinum; and puncture of the lung, causing pneumothorax.

Equipment

For aspiration

Prepackaged bone marrow set, which usually includes povidone-iodine sponges, two sterile drapes (one fenestrated, one plain), ten 4″ × 4″ gauze pads, ten 2″ × 2″ gauze pads, sterile pressure dressing, bone marrow needle, two 12-ml syringes, 22G 1″ or 2″ needle, 25G ½″ needle, scalpel, glass slides with coverslips, and labels • prescribed sedative • specimen containers • 70% isopropyl alcohol • 1% lidocaine (unopened bottle) • adhesive tape • sterile gloves

For biopsy
All of the equipment listed above • Vim-Silverman, Jamshidi, Illinois sternal, or Westerman-Jensen needle • Zenker's fixative or formaldehyde

Preparation
• Tell the patient that the doctor will collect a bone marrow specimen. Explain the procedure to ease his anxiety and promote cooperation. Make sure he or a family member understands the procedure and its implications and signs a consent form obtained by the doctor.
• Inform the patient that the procedure typically takes 5 to 10 minutes, that test results usually are available within 24 hours, and that more than one marrow specimen from the same site may be required.
• Check the patient's history for hypersensitivity to the prescribed local anesthetic. Tell him which bone (posterosuperior iliac crest, anterior iliac crest, or sternum) will be sampled. Inform him that he will receive a local anesthetic and will feel heavy pressure from insertion of the aspiration or biopsy needle as well as a brief pulling sensation when the marrow specimen is removed. If he has osteoporosis, mention that needle pressure may be minimal. If he has osteopetrosis, inform him that the doctor may use a drill. Explain that the doctor may make a small incision to avoid tearing the skin.
• Administer a sedative, as ordered.

Essential steps
• Position the patient according to the selected puncture site. For aspiration from the posterosuperior iliac crest (the preferred site), place the patient either in the lateral position with one leg flexed or in the prone position. If the anterior iliac crest will be used, place the patient in the supine or side-lying position.
• Using sterile technique, clean the puncture site with povidone-iodine sponges and allow to dry. Drape the area.
• To anesthetize the site, the doctor, using a 25G ½″ needle, infiltrates the area with 1% lidocaine, first injecting a small amount intradermally, then using a larger 22G 1″ to 2″ needle to anesthetize the tissue down to the bone.
• When the needle tip reaches the bone, the doctor anesthetizes the periosteum by injecting a small amount of lidocaine in a circular area about ¾″ (2 cm) in diameter. He withdraws the needle from the periosteum after each injection.
• After allowing about 1 minute for the lidocaine to take effect, the doctor may use a scalpel to make a small stab incision in the patient's skin to accommodate the bone marrow needle. This technique avoids pushing skin into the bone marrow and helps prevent unnecessary skin tearing to lessen the risk of infection.

Bone marrow aspiration
• The doctor inserts the bone marrow needle at the selected site and lodges it firmly in the bone cortex. If the patient feels sharp pain instead of pressure when the needle first touches bone, the needle was probably inserted outside the anesthetized area. In this case, expect the doctor to withdraw the needle slightly and move it to the anesthetized area.
• The doctor advances the needle by applying an even, downward force with the heel of the hand or the palm while twisting it back and forth slightly. A crackling sensation means the needle has entered the marrow cavity.
• Next, the doctor removes the inner cannula, attaches the syringe to the needle, aspirates the required specimen (usually about 1 ml), and withdraws the needle.
• Put on the sterile gloves. Then apply pressure to the aspiration site with a gauze pad for 5 minutes to control bleeding while an assistant prepares the marrow slides. Clean the area with alcohol to remove the povidone-iodine solution, dry the skin thoroughly with a 4″ × 4″ gauze pad, and apply a sterile pressure dressing.

Bone marrow biopsy
• The doctor inserts the biopsy needle into the periosteum and advances it steadily until the outer needle passes through the bone cortex into the marrow cavity.
• The doctor then directs the biopsy needle into the narrow cavity by alternately rotating the inner needle clockwise and counterclock-

wise. He removes a plug of tissue, withdraws the needle assembly, and expels the marrow specimen into a properly labeled specimen bottle containing Zenker's fixative or formaldehyde.

• Put on gloves and clean the area around the biopsy site with alcohol to remove the povidone-iodine solution. Firmly press a sterile 2" × 2" gauze pad against the incision to control bleeding; then apply a sterile pressure dressing.

Cautions

Faulty needle placement may yield too little aspirate. If the procedure fails to produce a specimen, the needle must be withdrawn from the bone (but not from the overlying soft tissue), the stylet replaced, and the needle inserted into a second site within the anesthetized field.

Monitoring and aftercare

• Observe the puncture site for a hematoma. If one forms, apply warm soaks.

• Administer an analgesic, as ordered, to relieve pain and tenderness at the puncture site.

• Document the time, date, location, the patient's tolerance of the procedure, and the specimen obtained.

Echocardiography

This widely used noninvasive test examines the size, shape, and motion of cardiac structures. It's useful in evaluating patients with chest pain, an enlarged cardiac silhouette on X-ray, electrocardiographic (ECG) changes unrelated to coronary artery disease, and abnormal heart sounds on auscultation.

The procedure usually is performed by cardiac technicians, who place a special transducer on an acoustic window on the patient's chest (an area lacking bones and lung tissue). The transducer directs ultra-high-frequency sound waves toward cardiac structures, which reflect these waves. After picking up the echoes, the transducer converts them to electrical impulses and relays them to an echocardiography machine for display on an oscilloscope screen and for recording on a strip chart or videotape. To time events in the cardiac cycle, ECG and phonocardiography may be performed simultaneously with echocardiography.

The most commonly used echocardiographic techniques are M-mode (motion-mode) and two-dimensional (cross-sectional). In M-mode echocardiography, a single, pencil-like ultrasound beam strikes the heart, producing a vertical view of cardiac structures. This method is especially useful for precisely recording the motion and dimensions of intracardiac structures.

In two-dimensional echocardiography, the ultrasound beam rapidly sweeps through an arc, producing a cross-sectional or fan-shaped view of cardiac structures. This technique is used to record lateral motion and reveal the correct spatial relationship between cardiac structures. Often, M-mode and two-dimensional echocardiography complement each other.

Normal results show a typical heart size and position and a typical motion pattern and structure of the four valves and chamber walls. Abnormal results help diagnose mitral stenosis, mitral valve prolapse, aortic insufficiency, aortic stenosis, subaortic stenosis, tricuspid valve disease, left atrial tumor, pericardial effusion, congenital heart disease, and an enlarged heart chamber. The doctor correlates results with the patient's clinical history, physical findings, and other test results.

Indications

• To diagnose and evaluate heart valve abnormalities

• To measure the size of the heart chambers

• To evaluate the heart chambers and valves in patients with congenital heart disorders

• To help diagnose hypertrophic and related cardiomyopathies

• To detect atrial tumors

• To evaluate cardiac function or heart wall motion after MI

• To detect pericardial effusion

Contraindications and complications

It may be difficult to perform echocardiography on patients whose chests have a thick layer of muscle or fat, or who have chronic obstructive pulmonary disease or chest wall abnormalities. The procedure doesn't involve any risk or discomfort.

Equipment

Conductive gel • transducer • echocardiography machine • oscilloscope screen

Preparation

• Explain or clarify the test purpose and procedure to the patient. Obtain a signed consent form. Tell him that a conductive gel will be applied to the skin under his left breast; then a transducer will be passed over the area, directing sound waves to the heart. Mention that the test is safe and painless, although he may feel pressure as the transducer passes over the skin.
• Inform the patient that he'll be asked to breathe in and out slowly, to hold his breath, or to inhale a gas with a slightly sweet odor (amyl nitrite) while a machine records changes in heart function. Describe the possible adverse effects of amyl nitrite (dizziness, flushing, and tachycardia), but assure the patient that these symptoms subside quickly.
• Tell the patient that he must remain still during the test because movement distorts test results. Mention that the procedure takes about 15 to 30 minutes to perform.

Essential steps

• Assist the patient to the supine position.
• The doctor or a technician applies conductive gel to the third or fourth intercostal space to the left of the sternum.
• The doctor or technician places the transducer directly over the site where the gel was applied, systematically angling it to direct ultrasonic waves at specific areas of the patient's heart.
• The doctor or technician observes the oscilloscope screen, which displays the returning echoes. Significant findings are recorded on a strip chart recorder (M-mode echocardiography) or a videotape recorder (two-dimensional echocardiography).
• For a different view of the heart, a transducer may be placed beneath the xiphoid process or directly above the sternum.
• For a left lateral view, you may position the patient on his left side.
• To record heart function under various conditions, the nurse or doctor may ask the patient to inhale and exhale slowly, to hold his breath, or to inhale amyl nitrite.

Cautions

Incorrect transducer placement and excessive movement interfere with test results.

Monitoring and aftercare

• Remove any remaining conductive gel from the patient's skin.
• Document the procedure and the patient's response to it.

Signal-averaged ECG

Signal-averaged ECG helps to identify patients at risk for sustained ventricular tachycardia. Because this cardiac arrhythmia can be a precursor of sudden death after an MI, the results of signal-averaged ECG can allow appropriate preventive measures.

Signal averaging detects low-amplitude signals or late electrical potentials, which reflect slow conduction or disorganized ventricular activity through abnormal or infarcted regions of the ventricles on a computer-based ECG. The signal-averaged ECG is developed by recording the noise-free surface ECG in three specialized leads for several hundred beats. Signal averaging enhances signals that would otherwise be missed because of increased amplitude and sensitivity to ventricular activity. For instance, on the standard 12-lead ECG, "noise" created by muscle tissue, electronic artifacts, and electrodes masks late potentials, which have a low amplitude.

Indications

This procedure identifies the risk for sustained ventricular tachycardia in patients with malignant ventricular tachycardia, a history of MI, unexplained syncope, nonischemic congestive cardiomyopathy, or nonsustained ventricular tachycardia.

Contraindications and complications

Because muscle movements may cause a false-positive result, patients who are restless or in respiratory distress are poor candidates for signal-averaged ECG. There usually are no complications associated with this procedure.

Equipment

Signal-averaged ECG machine • signal-averaged computer • record of the patient's surface ECG for 200 to 300 QRS complexes • three bipolar electrodes or leads • alcohol sponges • razor

Preparation

- Inform the patient that this procedure will take 10 to 30 minutes (considerably longer than obtaining a standard 12-lead ECG) and will help the doctor determine his risk for a certain type of arrhythmia. If appropriate, mention that it may be done along with other tests, such as echocardiography, Holter monitoring, and a stress test.
- Tell the patient he must lie as still as possible, should not speak, and should breathe normally during the procedure.
- If the patient has hair on his chest, shave the area, rub it with alcohol, and dry it before placing the electrodes.

Essential steps

- Place the patient in the supine position and instruct him to lie as still as possible.
- Place the leads in the X, Y, and Z orthogonal positions. (See *Placing electrodes for signal-averaged ECG.*)
- The ECG machine gathers input from these leads and amplifies, filters, and samples the signals. The computer collects and stores data for analysis. The crucial values are those showing QRS complex duration, duration of the portion of the QRS complex with an amplitude under 40 microvolts (μV), and the root mean square voltage of the last 40 milliseconds.

SKILL TIP

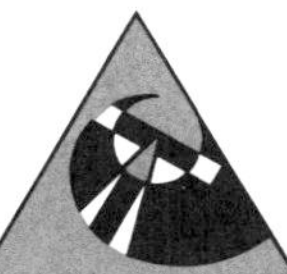

Placing electrodes for signal-averaged ECG

To prepare your patient for signal-averaged electrocardiography (ECG), place the electrodes in the X, Y, and Z orthogonal positions, as shown here. These positions bisect one another to provide a three-dimensional, composite view of ventricular activation.

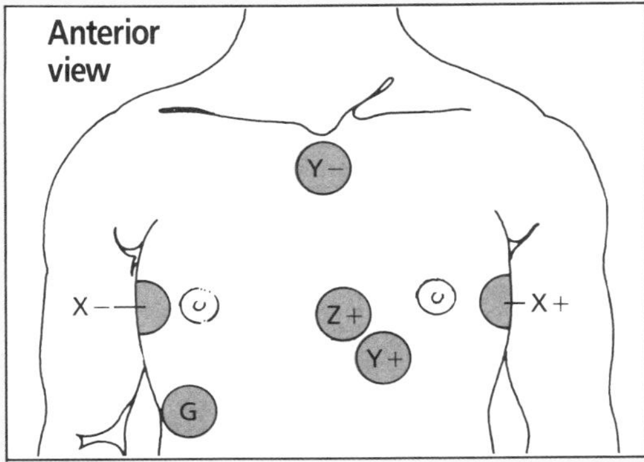

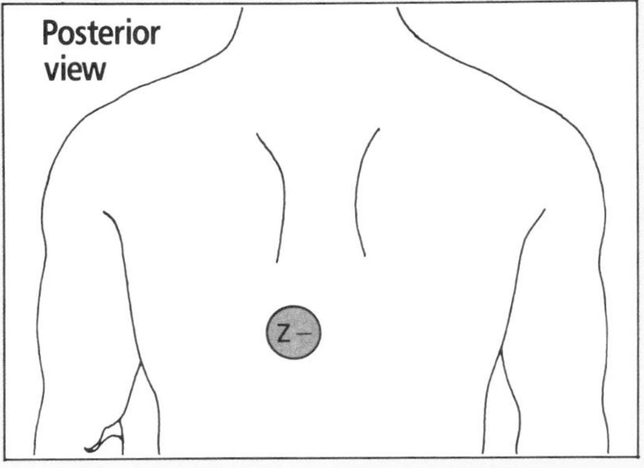

Key

X+	Fourth intercostal space, midaxillary line, left side
X−	Fourth intercostal space, midaxillary line, right side
Y+	Standard V_3 position (or proximal left leg)
Y−	Superior aspect of manubrium
Z+	Standard V_2 position
Z−	V_2 position, posterior
G	Ground; eighth rib on right side

Cautions

Proper electrode placement and skin preparation are essential to this procedure.

Results indicating low-amplitude signals include: a QRS complex duration greater than 110 milliseconds; a duration of more than 40 milliseconds for the amplitude portion under 40 μV; and a root mean square voltage of less than 25 μV during the last 40 milliseconds of the QRS complex. However, all three factors need not be present to consider the result positive or negative. The final interpretation hinges on individualized patient factors.

Monitoring and aftercare

• Results of signal-averaged ECG help the doctor determine whether the patient is a candidate for invasive procedures, such as electrophysiologic testing or angiography.
• Keep in mind that the significance of signal-averaged ECG results in patients with bundle-branch block is unknown. That's because myocardial activation doesn't follow the usual sequence in these patients.
• Document the time of the procedure, why the procedure was done, and how the patient tolerated it.

Esophageal ECG

Esophageal ECG is a semi-invasive procedure that records the activation of the heart's atria. It can be performed at the bedside or in a doctor's office. Because the left atrium is located near the esophagus, this procedure permits recording of atrial potentials.

Esophageal ECG causes only minor discomfort and requires little or no sedation. The procedure may be done in one of two ways – by having the patient swallow a bipolar pill electrode or by passing a bipolar catheter into the esophagus via the patient's nostril. The pill electrode consists of two electrodes spaced 13 mm apart. The electrodes are enclosed in a gelatin capsule that dissolves quickly after the patient swallows it with a glass of water.

The esophageal catheter, attached to thin, Teflon-coated stainless steel wires, can be placed faster than the time required to swallow and position the pill electrode. Also, the catheter is easier to use than the pill electrode in patients who have impaired consciousness or can't fully cooperate. (See *Pill electrode and electrode catheter for esophageal ECG.*)

This technique can also be used for transesophageal pacing of the atrium (with either the pill electrode or esophageal catheter). Such pacing may be done to initiate and terminate supraventricular tachycardias (SVTs) – usually to simulate stress and substitute exercise. Esophageal ECG always accompanies transesophageal pacing.

Indications

• To differentiate ventriculoatrial dissociation and narrow QRS-complex arrhythmias when a standard 12-lead ECG can't diagnose these disorders
• To distinguish between ventricular and supraventricular tachycardia in patients with tachycardia characterized by wide QRS complexes
• To diagnose ventriculoatrial dissociation (which confirms ventricular tachycardia)
• To diagnose the mechanism of arrhythmias characterized by narrow QRS complexes
• To distinguish atrioventricular-nodal-reentrant tachycardia from SVTs based on an accessory pathway with retrograde conduction

Contraindications and complications

If a pill electrode is required, this procedure is contraindicated in patients who can't swallow a gelatin capsule.

Equipment

Bipolar pill electrode or bipolar esophageal catheter • ECG machine or filtered esophageal ECG recorder • glass of drinking water (if a pill electrode will be used) • lidocaine jelly and benzocaine spray (if an esophageal catheter will be used)

Preparation

Explain the procedure to the patient. Inform him that this test will help diagnose his arrhythmia and ensure proper treatment. If a pill electrode will be used, teach him how to swallow it. Patient cooperation is vital.

Essential steps

With a pill electrode

• Give the patient a glass of water.
• The patient swallows the capsule with the water. The wire is then released, allowing the capsule to descend with normal esophageal peristalsis.

With an esophageal catheter

• The doctor anesthetizes the nostril with lidocaine jelly and the pharynx with benzocaine spray. Standard 5-mm electrodes are located at the distal end of the catheter and the electrodes.
• He connects the two proximal ends of the wires to the right and left arm leads of the ECG machine or filtered esophageal ECG recorder, which are displayed on an oscilloscope.
• The doctor withdraws the wire slowly until the atrial deflection in the esophageal ECG exceeds the ventricular deflection and is clearly visible. If the ventricular deflection is larger than the atrial deflection, he pulls the wire back to a higher level in the esophagus where it approaches the left atrium.
• The doctor compares the esophageal ECG to the surface ECG. If the ECG displays leads I, II, and III simultaneously, lead I will record a bipolar esophageal ECG and leads II and III will record unipolar ECGs with visible surface QRS complexes.

Cautions

For an accurate ECG, make sure that the patient remains still throughout the procedure.

Monitoring and aftercare

• Because the patient shouldn't require sedation or experience discomfort from esophageal ECG, monitoring and aftercare aren't necessary.
• Document when and why the procedure was done and how the patient tolerated it.

ADVANCED EQUIPMENT

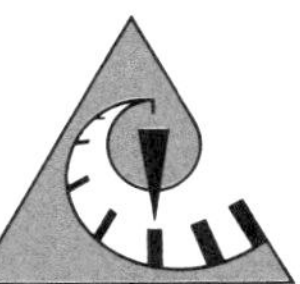

Pill electrode and electrode catheter for esophageal ECG

In esophageal electrocardiography (ECG), the patient swallows a bipolar pill electrode or the doctor inserts a bipolar esophageal electrode catheter into the patient's esophagus via a nostril. Inside a gelatin capsule, which dissolves quickly after the patient swallows it, are two electrodes that can record and pace the left atrium. The electrodes are attached to Teflon-coated wires, which are attached to an ECG machine to record bipolar atrial activation from the esophagus.

Pill electrode and wires

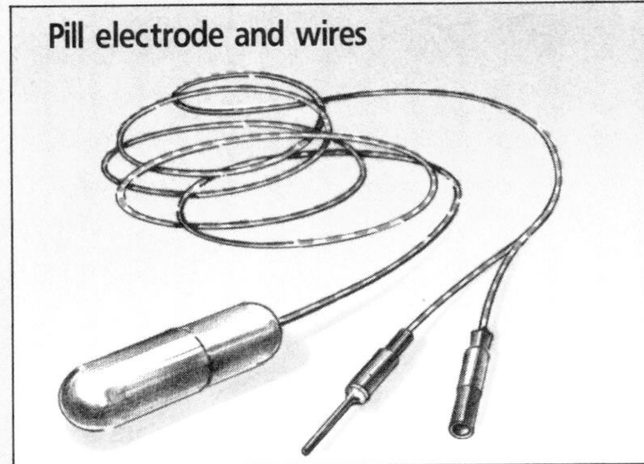

When a bipolar esophageal electrode catheter is used, the poles of the catheter can record and pace the left atrium from the esophagus.

Bipolar esophageal electrode catheter

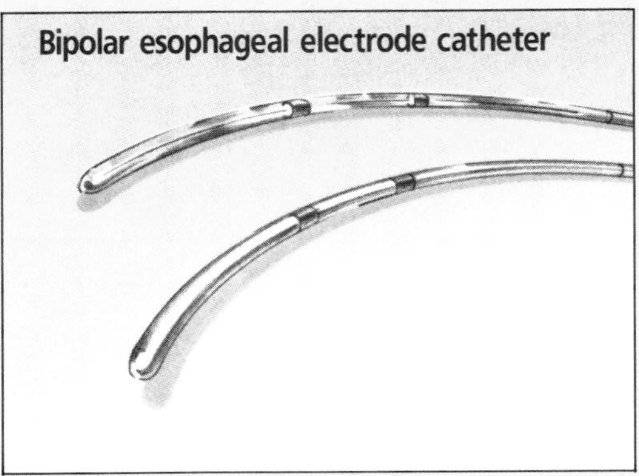

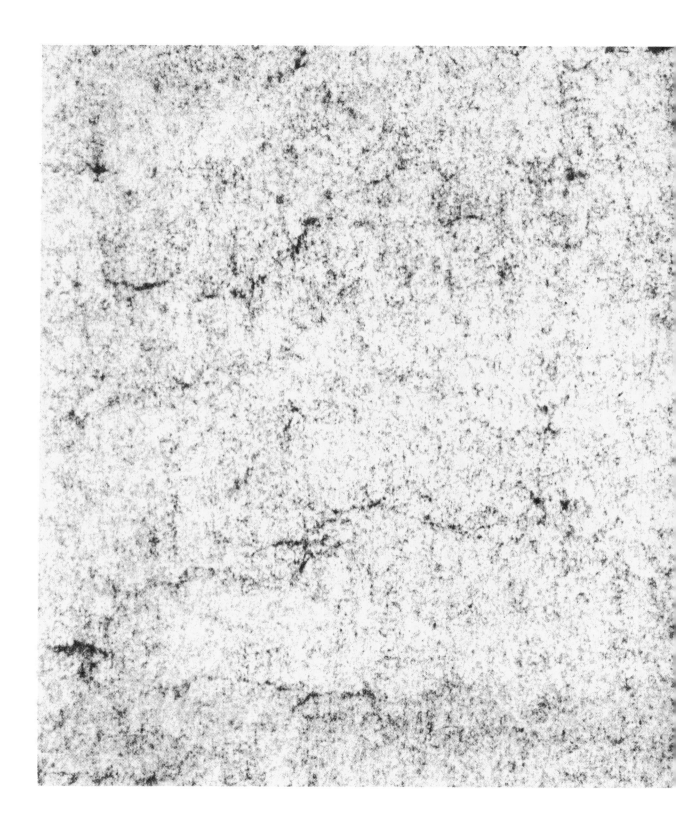

Suggested readings and acknowledgments

Abou-Awdi, N., et al. "New Support for the Failing Heart," *AJN* 91(1):38, January 1991.

Alspach, J.G., ed. *Core Curriculum for Critical Care Nursing.* Philadelphia: W.B. Saunders Co., 1991.

American Heart Association, Emergency Cardiac Care Committee and Subcommittees. "Guidelines for Cardiopulmonary Resuscitation and Emergency Cardiac Care, I: Introduction," *JAMA* 16(268):2172-83, October 1992.

Bayley, E. "Wound Healing in the Patient with Burns," *Nursing Clinics of North America* 25(1): 205-22, January 1990.

Brown, L. "Traumatic Amputation: Mechanisms of Injury, Treatment, and Rehabilitation," *AAOHN* 38(10):483-86, October 1990.

Camp, D., and Otten, N. "How to Insert and Remove Nasogastric Tubes Quickly and Easily," *Nursing90* 20(9):59-64, September 1990.

Cohen, A. "Body Image in the Person with a Stoma," *Journal of Enterostomal Therapy* 18(2):68-71, March-April 1991.

Colburn, L. "Preventing Pressure Ulcers: How to Recognize and Care for Patients at Risk," *Nursing90* 20(12):60-63, December 1990.

Cove, M., et al. "Cardiopulmonary Support in the Intensive Care Unit," *American Journal of Critical Care* 1:98-106, November 1991.

Craven, R., and Hirnle, C. *Fundamentals of Nursing: Human Health and Function.* Philadelphia: J.B. Lippincott Co., 1992.

Doughty, D., et al. "Your Patient: Which Therapy?" *Journal of Enterostomal Therapy* 17(4):154-59, July-August 1990.

Drago, S. "Banking on Your Own Blood," *AJN* 92(3):61-64, March 1992.

Duda, S., and Winn, E. "Home Care E.T. Nurses Improve Quality of Life," *Ostomy/Wound Management* 34:65-67, May-June 1991.

Gawron, C. "Colostomy Irrigations, Mechanism Guidelines and Considerations," *Ostomy/Wound Management* 28:56-61, May-June 1990.

Gift, A.G., et al. "Sensations During Chest Tube Removal," *Heart & Lung* 20(2):131-37, March 1991.

Grosso-Haacker, M. "Coping with an Ostomy," *Ostomy/Wound Management* 33:43-46, March-April 1991.

Guenter, P., et al. "Administering and Delivery of Enteral Nutrition" in *Clinical Nutrition: Enteral and Tube Feeding,* 2nd ed. Edited by Rombeau, J.L., and Caldwell, M.D. Philadelphia: W.B. Saunders Co., 1990.

Halfman-Franey, M., et al. "Using Stents in the Coronary Circulation: Nursing Perspectives," *Focus on Critical Care Nursing* 18(2):132-42, April 1991.

Ignatavicius, D., and Bayne, M. *Medical-Surgical Nursing: A Nursing Process Approach.* Philadelphia: W.B. Saunders Co., 1991.

Jaffe, A., ed. *Textbook of Advanced Cardiac Life Support,* 2nd ed. Dallas: American Heart Association, 1990.

Lewis, S., and Collier, I. *Medical-Surgical Nursing: Assessment and Management of Clinical Problems,* 3rd ed. St. Louis: Mosby-Year Book, Inc., 1992.

Maklebust, J. "Pressure Ulcer Update," *RN* 54(12):56-62, December 1991.

McErlean, E. "Ask the Experts," *Critical Care Nurse* 12(5):60-61, June 1992.

Murray, S., and Thompson, R. "We've Organized our Approach to Pressure Sores," *RN* 54(1):42-44, January 1991.

Nursing Procedures. Springhouse, Pa.: Springhouse Corp., 1992.

Pieper, B., et al. "Low and High Air-Loss Beds in Acute Care Hospitals," *Journal of Enterostomal Therapy* 17(3):131-36, May-June 1990.

Pierce, J.D., et al. "Effects of Two Chest Tube Clearance Protocols on Drainage in Patients after Myocardial Revascularization Surgery," *Heart & Lung* 20(2):125-30, March 1991.

Potter, P., and Perry, A. *Basic Nursing: Theory and Practice,* 2nd ed. St. Louis: Mosby-Year Book, Inc., 1991.

Reichman, R.T., et al. "Improved Patient Survival after Cardiac Arrest Using a Cardiopulmonary Support System," *Annals of Thoracic Surgery* 49(1):101-05, January 1990.

Rolstad, B. "Treatment Objectives in Chronic Wound Care," *Home Healthcare Nurse* 9(6):38-44, November-December 1991.

Rountree, W., et al. "The HEMOPUMP Cardiac Assist System: Nursing Care of the Patient," *Critical Care Nurse* 11(4):46-48, 50-52, 54-57, April 1991.

Standards of Care: Patient with Colostomy. Irvine, Calif.: International Association for Enterostomal Therapy, 1989.

Swearingen, P., and Keen, J., eds. *Manual of Critical Care,* 2nd ed. St. Louis: Mosby-Year Book, Inc., 1991.

Teplitz, L. "Update: Are Milking and Stripping Chest Tubes Necessary?" *Focus On Critical Care* 18(6):506-11, December 1991.

Trelstad, A., and Osmundson, D. "Water Piks: Wound Cleansing Alternative," *Plastic Surgical Nursing* 9(3):117-19, Fall 1989.

Weller, K. "In Search of Efficacy and Efficiency: An Alternative to Conventional Wound Cleansing Modalities," *Ostomy/Wound Management* 37:23-38, November-December 1991.

Acknowledgments

ConvaTec, a Bristol-Myers Squibb Company
Sur-Fit two-piece ostomy product application, p. 46

Doylestown (Pa.) Hospital

Advanced skilltest

Use these multiple-choice questions to test your knowledge of advanced procedures. The answers, along with rationales, appear on pages 245 to 246.

1. Which of the following arrhythmias calls for defibrillation?

a. Pulseless ventricular tachycardia
b. Atrial fibrillation
c. Electromechanical dissociation
d. Asystole

2. What should you teach a patient going home with a permanent pacemaker?

a. Signs and symptoms of pacemaker failure
b. Signs and symptoms of wound infection
c. Importance of regular follow-up care
d. All of the above

3. According to advanced cardiac life support (ACLS) guidelines, a patient with ventricular fibrillation needs immediate:

a. cardioversion.
b. cardiopulmonary resuscitation (CPR).
c. defibrillation.
d. epinephrine administration.

4. If you suspect a cardiac arrest victim has a neck injury, what should you do before CPR?

a. Perform a finger sweep.
b. Open the patient's airway with head-tilt, chin-lift maneuver.
c. Perform the abdominal thrust maneuver.
d. Open the airway with jaw-thrust maneuver.

5. After undergoing percutaneous balloon valvuloplasty for aortic stenosis, 72-year-old Rose White has returned to the coronary care unit. While monitoring her, you notice ventricular ectopy and a drop in blood pressure. As you assess her further, you note a sudden weakness in her left side and observe that she can't speak. You suspect:

a. MI.
b. calcium embolization.
c. ventricular tamponade.
d. hemorrhage.

6. Cardiopulmonary support (CPS) can help a patient suffering from any of the following conditions *except:*

a. cardiogenic shock.
b. septic shock.
c. trauma.
d. a drug overdose.

7. Before deflating a pneumatic antishock garment (PASG), make sure that the patient:

a. has an adequate fluid volume.
b. has been intubated.
c. has a systolic blood pressure of at least 130 mm Hg.
d. has an arterial pH of at least 7.4.

8. Which of the following conditions calls for the use of extracorporeal membrane oxygenation (ECMO)?

a. Profound neurologic impairment
b. Bacterial or viral pneumonia
c. Incurable neoplasm
d. Uncontrollable bleeding disorder

9. You should use an esophageal tube instead of an endotracheal tube on a patient with a suspected spinal cord injury because:

a. it seals off the trachea from the GI tract, decreasing the risk of aspiration.
b. it causes less tissue trauma.
c. insertion doesn't require hyperextending the patient's neck.
d. it poses less risk of nasal necrosis from pressure.

10. Before being weaned from a ventilator, a patient should:

a. have a maximum inspiratory pressure of less than -20 cm H_2O.

b. be able to maintain spontaneous resting minute ventilation.

c. have no infections, acid-base or electrolyte imbalances, arrhythmias, renal failure, anemia, fever, or excessive fatigue.

d. have a vital capacity of less than 10 cc/kg of body weight.

11. All of the following require cerebrospinal fluid (CSF) drainage *except:*

a. disorientation, memory loss, and aphasia.

b. intracranial pressure monitoring through a ventriculostomy.

c. direct administration of drugs into the spinal column.

d. aspiration of CSF.

12. Which type of skeletal tongs requires drilling holes in the exposed skull?

a. Gardner-Wells

b. Vinke

c. Halo-vest

d. Crutchfield

13. What steps can you take to check the placement of a nasogastric tube?

a. Try to aspirate stomach contents from the tube with a syringe. Then place a stethoscope over the epigastric region and listen for a whooshing sound while injecting 5 cc of air into the tube.

b. Aspirate stomach contents from the tube with a syringe and place the end of the tube into a cup of water. If air bubbles appear, the tube is in the lungs.

c. Have the stomach X-rayed.

d. Watch the patient for signs of respiratory distress.

14. You'd provide all of the following care for a patient with an esophageal tube *except:*

a. irrigating the gastric aspiration port with 0.9% sodium chloride solution.

b. injecting air into the esophageal aspiration port to maintain patency.

c. applying low suction to the gastric and esophageal aspiration ports.

d. keeping the head of the bed flat for 2 hours after tube placement.

15. When administering a tube feeding, you'd do all of the following *except:*

a. place the patient in semi-Fowler's or high Fowler's position for the feeding.

b. check the placement of the feeding tube.

c. administer the feeding within 15 minutes.

d. assess the patient's bowel sounds before beginning the feeding.

16. To prevent skin irritation around the exit site of a gastrostomy tube, you would:

a. place a dressing under the button or peg tube.

b. rotate the external button or bumper daily.

c. apply skin protectant before applying tape.

d. use Stomahesive around the site.

17. What treatment improves circulation in a patient with an arterial ulcer that won't heal?

a. Exercise

b. Vasodilators

c. Sympathectomy

d. Vascular surgery

18. Vascular insufficiency can worsen:

a. muscle tremors.

b. warm feet.

c. subcutaneous fatty tissue atrophy.

d. leg and foot ulcers.

19. To assess the adequacy of the blood supply to a patient's hand before performing a radial puncture, you'd:

a. perform Allen's test.

b. use a pulse oximeter.

c. take the patient's health history.

d. determine the patient's pulse pressure.

20. Bone marrow aspiration allows the diagnosis of all of the following *except:*

a. oat cell carcinoma.

b. adenocarcinoma of the lung.

c. leukemia.

d. Hodgkin's disease.

21. Signal-averaged electrocardiography allows the detection of which of the following potentially life-threatening arrhythmias?

a. Atrial fibrillation

b. Ventricular fibrillation

c. Ventricular tachycardia

d. Electromechanical dissociation

Answers and rationales

1. a. Only pulseless ventricular tachycardia requires immediate defibrillation. Atrial fibrillation calls for drug treatment and elective cardioversion (for a rapid rate). A patient with electromechanical dissociation requires drugs and CPR. A patient with asystole needs CPR, endotracheal intubation, drug treatment and, possibly, pacemaker insertion.

2. d. A patient with a permanent pacemaker needs to know all the signs and symptoms he must watch for as well as understand the importance of regular follow-up care.

3. c. Although CPR can help a patient survive until a defibrillator becomes available, ACLS guidelines recommend defibrillation as the first step for treating ventricular fibrillation. A patient shouldn't receive epinephrine until after defibrillation has begun. Cardioversion – a procedure that generates a burst of electricity to coincide with the heart's R wave – won't work because a fibrillating heart doesn't generate an R wave.

4. d. Although you'd usually use the head-tilt, chin-lift maneuver to open a patient's airway, the jaw-thrust maneuver poses the least risk of further neck injury. A finger sweep can further obstruct the patient's airway. You'd use the abdominal thrust only to dislodge a foreign object blocking a patient's throat or bronchus.

5. b. Although it rarely happens, debris from the calcified valve could result in an embolism that would cause Ms. White's signs. An MI would cause chest pain and electrocardiogram (ECG) changes, but not weakness or an inability to speak. Ventricular tamponade results in pale skin, decreased or absent pulses, hypotension, and a paradoxical pulse. Hemorrhage decreases blood pressure and increases heart rate but doesn't cause unilateral weakness.

6. c. Because a trauma patient receives systemic anticoagulants, CPS could result in massive hemorrhage.

7. a. If the patient doesn't have an adequate fluid volume, removing the PASG could cause further hemodynamic instability. A patient who's breathing adequately doesn't need intubation. You can start deflating the PASG when the patient's systolic blood pressure reaches 100 mm Hg. The patient's arterial pH doesn't usually affect the use of a PASG.

8. b. ECMO can help in the treatment of adults with bacterial or viral pneumonia. But because the benefits must outweigh the risks of this dangerous procedure, ECMO is contraindicated for patients with profound neurologic impairment, incurable neoplasm, or uncontrollable bleeding disorders.

9. c. Because insertion of an esophageal tube doesn't require hyperextension of the patient's neck, it decreases the risk of further spinal cord injury. An esophageal tube doesn't seal off the trachea from the GI tract and can actually cause tissue damage and nasal necrosis.

10. c. The patient should meet all of these criteria before weaning. He should also have a maximum inspiratory pressure above -20 cm H_2O, be able to double his spontaneous resting minute ventilation, and have a vital capacity above 10 cc/kg of body weight.

11. a. These are only symptoms. The others are procedures that require direct access to the spinal column.

12. d. Only Crutchfield tongs need holes drilled into the exposed skull. Gardner-Wells and Vinke tongs use spring-loaded pins. Halo-vest tongs provide traction by immobilizing the head and neck after traumatic spinal cord injury.

13. a. These two steps allow you to double-check tube placement. Placing the end of the tube in a glass of water might cause the patient to aspirate some water. The doctor would order an X-ray to check placement only if aspiration and auscultation can't confirm placement. You may not observe any signs of respiratory distress in a comatose or an anesthetized patient.

14. d. You'd usually elevate the head of the bed 45 degrees. Even when using traction to keep the tube in place, you'd elevate the head of the bed 25 degrees to produce countertraction, and 35 to 45 degrees if you're using a football helmet for traction.

15. c. A tube feeding should take place over at least 30 minutes to prevent abdominal distention and dumping syndrome.

16. b. Rotating the external bumper or button daily helps prevent skin maceration. Placing a dressing under the bumper or button could lead to skin breakdown. You'd apply skin protectant around the exit site only if the doctor orders a dressing over the site. If the patient receives proper exit site care, he shouldn't need Stomahesive.

17. d. Exercise, vasodilators, and sympathectomy would not be effective. Only vascular surgery—either endarterectomy or arterial bypass—improves circulation.

18. d. The decreased blood flow caused by vascular insufficiency hinders the ability of leukocytes and erythrocytes to reach damaged tissue, interfering with healing. Muscle tremors occur in response to nerve stimulation; warm feet indicate sufficient circulation; and subcutaneous fatty tissue atrophy can occur following prolonged inactivity.

19. a. Allen's test indicates an adequate blood supply if the patient's hand blanches when you compress his radial and ulnar arteries, then quickly flushes when you release pressure. A pulse oximeter measures oxygen saturation. A health history doesn't include the physical assessment necessary to determine the adequacy of the blood supply. Pulse pressure is the difference between the systolic and diastolic pressures.

20. b. Unlike the other three neoplasms, adenocarcinoma of the lung doesn't result in detectable changes in bone marrow.

21. c. Signal-averaged electrocardiography allows the detection of ventricular tachycardia. This type of ECG picks up low-level, high-frequency signals found late in the QRS complex and is ineffective for detecting atrial fibrillation, ventricular fibrillation, and electromechanical dissociation.

Index

i refers to an illustration; t refers to a table

i refers to an illustration; t refers to a table